Cognitive and Behavioral Interventions in the Schools

Rosemary Flanagan • Korrie Allen • Eva Levine
Editors

Cognitive and Behavioral Interventions in the Schools

Integrating Theory and Research into Practice

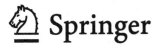 Springer

Editors
Rosemary Flanagan
Touro College
New York, NY, USA

Korrie Allen
Innovative Psychological Solutions
Fairfax, VA, USA

Eva Levine
Touro College
New York, NY, USA

ISBN 978-1-4939-1971-0 (hardcover)   ISBN 978-1-4939-1972-7 (eBook)
ISBN 978-1-4939-3489-8 (softcover)
DOI 10.1007/978-1-4939-1972-7
Springer New York Heidelberg Dordrecht London

Library of Congress Control Number: 2014954345

Printed on acid-free paper

Springer is part of Springer Science+Business Media (www.springer.com)

To my parents, Angela and Patrick Flanagan,
you are missed everyday.

Rosemary Flanagan

To my wonderful children
Olivia and Charlie.

Korrie Allen

To my father, Norman, who guides me
through my memories of his wisdom,
kindness and friendship.

Eva Levine

Preface

Cognitive and Behavioral Interventions in the Schools is the product of our collective years of training and experience in clinical and school psychology. Although we are similarly trained, we have followed varied career paths as psychologists, serving in settings that include academia, the school system, independent practice, and pediatric mental health facilities. In our work with cognitive and behavioral approaches, we have successfully applied these methods with high functioning children needing specific assistance in one or two specific areas of difficulty, children with mild but more chronic difficulties, and children with severe and persistent mental health problems that significantly compromise functioning. We have designed this book to assist clinical and school psychologists working with a similarly diverse client base.

The training competencies of school psychologists are quite varied with regard to cognitive and behavioral treatment approaches. There are a number of reasons for this variability. Most importantly, as school psychologists can be trained at either a specialist (certificate) or doctoral level, there are significant differences in the amount of clinical-training school psychologists receive and the range of practice areas for which they obtain supervised experience. While those trained at the specialist level will typically have some training in cognitive and behavioral interventions, the certificate programs tend to place more emphasis on the areas of psychoeducational assessment (including social-emotional assessment), school consultation, academic interventions, childhood disorders, learning theory, counseling, research design, and psychometrics. Those trained at the doctoral level have more room in the curriculum for training in cognitive and behavioral interventions, and also have the benefit of a second internship, which often takes place in a more "clinically" focused setting with children exhibiting more complex and severe mental health presentations.

With regard to actual practice, the work of school psychologists ranges from a primarily "test and place" role, emphasizing the matching of children's learning and socio-emotional needs to services in the special education system, to more of a "response to intervention role," which gives more space for the implementation of individually tailored clinical protocols. Psychologists with a high level of testing/placement responsibilities will often have less time available to conduct clinically based individual or group interventions. Importantly, as hospital clinic settings are increasingly being downsized, and more children with disabilities are being served locally, public schools have seen an increase in the numbers of youth with unaddressed and significant mental health and behavioral needs. Thus, the role and function of school psychologists continues to evolve, as we face ongoing changes in the health care delivery system and funding streams. As a notable case in point, school psychologists are among the providers named in the Affordable Care Act! We believe that school psychologists are in a unique position to provide much needed mental health support in this new environment. School psychologists are unique in the breadth and depth of their training, and they are well positioned to provide a wide array of services. Unfortunately, their diverse skill sets and knowledge bases are often underutilized, if not unutilized.

Indeed, school psychologists can theoretically be faced (and often are) with just about any problem facing children and families. Schools are one of the most diverse practice settings, and the school psychologist is often the first mental health professional to come in contact with a child and family in need of assistance. Being able to navigate such a broad range of presentations requires considerable knowledge and skill. This book is a resource that can provide school psychologists with specific practice guidelines and the research support for designing interventions within a cognitive and behavioral framework. Information is provided about techniques and strategies that may serve as a "tool kit" or resource to provide psychoeducation and assistance to children, parents, teachers, and other school professionals who interact with children facing mental health difficulties.

While a number of competing texts have focused on presentations of important empirically validated treatment packages, we have chosen to emphasize the component techniques and strategies that are incorporated into these packages, with the expectation that school psychologists may need to draw on these strategies in more idiosyncratic ways to meet the specific needs of their students and treatment settings. We acknowledge that it may often not be within the practice or job-description role for the school psychologist to directly deliver clinical services to children with identified mental health needs; however, in that scenario the school psychologist is often central in developing an appropriate treatment plan and in identifying adequate referral sources to provide children with the support they need. The knowledge this book provides will also be of guidance for school psychologists needing to make such referrals to community-based settings.

We are particularly excited to also have included in this text a segment on the use of technology in applying cognitive and behavioral interventions to school settings. While psychologists should not dismiss historically proven treatment modalities and treatment aids, there are a number of interesting developments in the interface between technology and mental health practice that school psychologists should start to become familiar with; it is our experience that students are also particularly interested in interventions that utilize these techniques.

Working in school systems has many differences from the settings in which many clinical trials are designed and implemented. Thus, providing school psychologists with an understanding of the underlying principles of treatment and the key issues for treatment fidelity can position them to make adjustments to interventions in a way that fits the school environment while minimizing threats to treatment integrity. Further, as the need for research on transportability of interventions and their sustainability is imperative, school psychologists with a greater knowledge of cognitive and behavioral interventions would be natural partners with the researchers wishing to conduct clinical trials in schools.

Finally, while clinical psychologists are well trained to deliver services in typical mental health outpatient settings, they are often less well trained in the logistics and challenges of working in school settings. This volume also specifically addresses aspects of navigating and entering school systems to provide clinical interventions. This is intended to assist psychologists first venturing into the school setting, as well as those working as independent practitioners who are treating youngsters whose problems are manifest in the school setting. We hope readers will find this book engaging and useful.

New York, NY, USA   Rosemary Flanagan
Fairfax, VA, USA   Korrie Allen
New York, NY, USA   Eva Levine

Contents

Contributors

Korrie Allen Innovative Psychological Solutions, Fairfax, VA, USA

Marie-Christine André Clinical Psychology Department, Suffolk University, Boston, MA, USA

Jose Arauz Clinical Psychology Department, Suffolk University, Boston, MA, USA

Prerna Arora Division of Child and Adolescent Psychiatry, University of Maryland School of Medicine, Baltimore, MD, USA

Allison D. Barnard Department of Educational & Counseling Psychology, Counseling, and College Student Personnel, University of Louisville, Louisville, KY, USA

Rebecca Rialon Berry Department of Psychiatry and Behavioral Sciences, Stanford School of Medicine, Stanford, CA, USA

Jared A. Bishop Department of Educational Psychology, Ball State University, Muncie, IN, USA

Jill Haak Bohnenkamp Center for School Mental Health, University of Maryland School of Medicine, Baltimore, MD, USA

Brian C. Chu Department of Clinical Psychology, Graduate School of Applied and Professional Psychology, Rutgers University, Piscataway, NJ, USA

Graduate School of Applied and Professional Psychology, Rutgers, The State University of New Jersey, Piscataway, NJ, USA

Lisa W. Coyne Clinical Psychology Department, Suffolk University, Harvard Medical School/McLean Hospital, Boston, MA, USA

Kathleen I. Diaz Department of Psychology, University of Miami, Coral Gables, FL, USA

Caroline J. Ehrlich Department of Psychology, University of Miami, Coral Gables, FL, USA

Eva Feindler Clinical Psychology Program, C.W. Post, Long Island University, Brookville, NY, USA

Rosemary Flanagan Touro College, Graduate School of Psychology, New York, NY, USA

Dominick A. Fortugno School of Health Sciences, Touro College, New York, NY, USA

Anna K. Gogos Department of Psychology, University of Miami, Coral Gables, FL, USA

Jenny Herren Judge Baker Children's Center & Harvard University, Boston, MA, USA

Rachel Hodas Psychological, Organizational, and Leadership Studies in Education, Temple University, Philadelphia, PA, USA

Lauren Hoffman Department of Clinical Psychology, Graduate School of Applied and Professional Psychology, Rutgers University, Piscataway, NJ, USA

Alyssa Johns Department of Clinical Psychology, Graduate School of Applied and Professional Psychology, Rutgers University, Piscataway, NJ, USA

Judith Kaufman School of Psychology, Fairleigh Dickinson University, Teaneck, NJ, USA

Betty S. Lai Division of Epidemiology and Biostatistics, School of Public Health, Georgia State University, Atlanta, GA, USA

Matthew Liebman Clinical Psychology Program, C.W. Post, Long Island University, Brookville, NY, USA

Department of Child Psychology/Psychiatry, Montefiore Medical Center, Bronx, NY, USA

Kristy A. Ludwig Department of Psychiatry and Behavioral Sciences, University of Washington School of Medicine, Seattle, WA, USA

Aaron R. Lyon Department of Psychiatry and Behavioral Sciences, University of Washington School of Medicine, Seattle, WA, USA

Robert W. Motta Department of Psychology, Hofstra University, Hempstead, NY, USA

Matthew P. Mychailyszyn Department of Psychology, Towson University, Towson, MD, USA

Division of Psychology and Neuropsychology, Mt. Washington Pediatric Hospital, Baltimore, MD, USA

Erik Newman University of California, San Diego, CA, USA

Integrative Psychotherapy Services of San Diego, CA, USA

Camilo Ortiz Clinical Psychology Program, C.W. Post, Long Island University, Brookville, NY, USA

Patrick Pössel Department of Educational and Counseling Psychology, Counseling, and College Student Personnel, University of Louisville, Louisville, KY, USA

Linda Reddy Department of Applied Psychology, Graduate School of Applied and Professional Psychology, Rutgers University, Piscataway, NJ, USA

Carlos E. Rivera Villegas Clinical Psychology Department, Suffolk University, Boston, MA, USA

Erin Rotheram-Fuller Division of Educational Leadership and Innovation, Arizona State University, Tempe, AZ, USA

Julie L. Ryan School of Psychology, Fairleigh Dickinson University, Teaneck, NJ, USA

Janay B. Sander Department of Educational Psychology, Ball State University, Muncie, IN, USA

Mitchell L. Schare Department of Psychology, Hofstra University, Hempstead, NY, USA

Rebecca B. Skolnick Department of Psychology, Hofstra University, Hempstead, NY, USA

Alex Stratis Clinical Psychology Program, C.W. Post, Long Island University, Brookville, NY, USA

Yvette N. Tazeau Independent Practice, San Jose, CA, USA

Mark Terjesen Department of Psychology, St. John's University, Jamaica, NY, USA

Arielle Verdesco Department of Applied Psychology, Graduate School of Applied and Professional Psychology, Rutgers University, Piscataway, NJ, USA

Kristin P. Wyatt Department of Psychology, Hofstra University, Hempstead, NY, USA

Part I
Intervention Planning

Chapter 1
Introduction: The Future Is Now—Challenges in the New Age of Psychological Practice

Judith Kaufman

"Do not confine your children to your own learning for they were born in another time."

Hebrew proverb

"The real difficulty in changing any enterprise lies not in developing new ideas, but escaping old ones."

John Maynard Keynes

The Changing Landscape of School Psychology: Contributing Factors

Schools are microcosms of society at large, and as such, school personnel deal with the impact of social challenges and problems as they are reflected in the children they serve. Economic concerns, unemployment and underemployment, family and school violence, immigration, and acculturation have both direct and indirect impacts on learning and academic achievement. More and more children and adolescents are in need of mental health support, but are underserved (NAMI, 2013). While the current practice trend is directed at implementing a Public Health model of intervention in schools (Nastasi, 2004) (e.g., school-wide prevention programs, Response to Intervention (RTI) (Adelman & Taylor, 2010)), there are a large number of students who require individual and group intervention strategies.

J. Kaufman, Ph.D., A.B.P.P. (✉)
School of Psychology, Fairleigh Dickinson University, Teaneck, NJ, USA
e-mail: judith@fdu.edu

© Springer Science+Business Media New York 2015
R. Flanagan et al. (eds.), *Cognitive and Behavioral Interventions in the Schools*, DOI 10.1007/978-1-4939-1972-7_1

Contemporary Risk Factors

There are more than 73 million children under the age of 18 living in the United States. This is expected to increase to 80 million by the year 2020 (Federal Interagency Forum on Child and Family Statistics, 2007). There is a steady increase in the public school population, with over 49 million children now attending public schools (the private school sector has remained constant, accounting for 11 % of school-aged population). There has been a significant increase in the minority population in the public schools, which is currently at approximately 42 % and growing. These increases reflect greater demographic shifts in the general population, with the largest growth in the Hispanic population. A related increase in the free and reduced lunch program nationwide further indicates increased levels of poverty in our public school youth, with an estimated 12.5 million children living in poverty in the United States today. Importantly, higher poverty rates exist among minority groups (Annie E. Casey Foundation, 2007). The consequences of poverty and minority group membership together predict greater risk for school failure, lack of completion of high school, and mental and physical health issues (Borman & Rachuba, 2001; Larson, Russ, Crall, & Halfon, 2008).

Recent national reports of the educational progress in the public schools indicate that a growing number of children have not met national proficiency levels (Hemphill & Vanneman, 2011; Lee, Grigg, & Donahue, 2007). The achievement gap is particularly evident in comparing Hispanic students to White students. While scores in mathematics have generally increased, the performance gap has remained the same when measured in fourth and eighth grades. Similar trends in reading were found as well (Hemphill & Vanneman, 2011). Academic performance is typically assessed through standardized achievement tests often referred to as *high-stakes testing* (Kruger, Wandle, & Struzziero, 2007). High-stakes testing can be viewed as a critical stressor for school administrators, their teachers, and pupils. There may be sanctions imposed on underachieving schools including school restructuring and removal of staff (Nichols, Glass, & Berliner, 2006). There has been some research suggesting that high-stakes testing might be a considerable source of stress for students (Cornell, Krosnick, & Chang, 2006). Students who do not meet the test standards may be particularly vulnerable leading to feelings of depression and anxiety and potentially have a negative impact on mental health (Cornell et al., 2006). For those individuals where there is an existing achievement gap, the consequences may be even greater. Grant et al. (2004) report that multiple stressful life events predict psychological problems in adolescents.

Approximately 12 % of children between the ages of 3 and 21 receive special education services under IDEA (http://disabilitycompendium.org/compendium-statistics/special-education. No date). About 80 % of these students spend more than 40 % of their time in regular classroom settings. Of the youth exiting IDEA services, 20 % dropped out of school compared to the 7 % in regular education. Providing effective and evidence-based interventions to students with special needs is an additional challenge for mental health providers within the school setting.

Negative school climate has been demonstrated to be a potential risk factor and can potentially contribute to the increase in bullying and victimization (Wilson, 2004). National data suggest that one in four children are either face-to-face or cyber bullied on a regular basis (http://www.bullyingstatistics.org/content/school-bullying-statis. No date). The long-term mental health consequences of being bullied have been well documented (Rigby, 2007). The confluence of changing demographics and poor academic and behavioral outcomes along with increased environmental stressors provide a strong argument for the need for quality psychological services in the schools, both within the regular education and special education frameworks.

Children and Mental Illness: Schools and Mental Health

Over four million children and adolescents, or 12–20 %, suffer from serious mental disorders (SED) that cause significant impairment at home, at school, and with peers (NAMI, 2011). The lifetime prevalence of mental disorders is 46 %, with no significant difference between males and females. The estimated cost of providing services is approximately $247 billion per year, although only 40 % of children and youth suffering with mental illness receive mental health services (NAMI, 2011).

About half of all lifetime cases of mental disorders begin by age 14. Approximately 50 % of students age 14 and older living with serious mental illness drop out of high school, the highest rate of any disability group (US Department of Education, 2006). While already alarming, these numbers and the magnitude of the problems keep increasing without a parallel increase in available services (Center for Disease Control and Prevention, 2013; US Department of Health and Human Services, 1999).

Gender differences exist when examining prevalence rates of mental disorders (Eaton et al., 2012). ADHD is the most prevalent diagnosis in children between the ages of 3 and 17, with males impacted at a higher prevalence rate than females (see Reddy et al. 2015). With the exception of autistic spectrum disorder (ASD), the number of children with mental health diagnoses increases with age (NAMI, 2013). Females present with internalizing disorders, while males exhibit more externalizing disorders (Eaton et al., 2012). By the age of 15, two times more girls than boys demonstrate symptoms of depression, generalized anxiety disorders, and eating disorders (NAMI, 2013). Boys demonstrate a greater percentage of antisocial behavior, aggression, and substance abuse (Eaton et al., 2012).

School is a natural environment for mental health service delivery. The majority of youth receiving such services do so within the school setting (Rones & Hoagwood, 2000). It has been noted that 96 % of families who were offered school-based mental health services followed through, while only 13 % referred to community-based clinics availed themselves of services (Mennuti & Christner, 2010). School-based health centers which encompass mental and behavioral health care are often operated in partnership with the community and have proven to be successful in addressing both the physical and mental health needs of children and youth (HRSA.gov retrieved, 1/27/14). School-based mental health services have received empirical support in demonstrating not only an increase in emotional well-being but also directly impacting on increased academic achievement (Research and Training Center for Children's Mental Health, retrieved 1/29/14). There is an increasing emphasis on a tiered model of school-based mental health services, with the primary entry point being universal or systemic prevention/intervention (Nastasi, 2004), followed by targeted interventions addressing particularly at-risk populations. However, although prevention efforts have proven to be successful, there are significant numbers of children who require more intensive interventions (Mennuti & Christner, 2010). Such interventions are typically provided on an individual or small group basis and involve symptom reduction, enhancement of coping skills, building resiliency, and risk reduction (Compas et al., 2005; Smallwood, Christner, & Brill, 2007). Although it is essential to consider the broader role of the school psychologist in systems-level interventions, expanding the intensive intervention skill set is likewise imperative, as research supports the relationship between improved mental health and children's academic competencies in the school context (Adelman & Taylor, 2010).

Impact of the Affordable Care Act (ACA)

The Affordable Care Act of 2010 (ACA) provides a major focal point for the change in the delivery of health services, particularly for children and youth. Children, in particular, will benefit as a result of ACA, as almost double the number (from about 7 million to 11 million) will be eligible to receive both physical and mental health care because of expanded coverage (Kaiser Family Foundation, 2010). Provisions of ACA encompass the funding for school-based health clinics (SBHC), expanding services, and the identification of new treatment sites. The ACA appropriated $50 million in competitive grant funds for each fiscal year from 2010 to 2013 to develop SBHCs (Section 4101a, The Patient Protection Act of 2010). SBHCs are typically located in schools or on school grounds and cooperate with the school and community to meet the unique needs of the community population. Currently, there are about 2,000 SBHCs in 46 states and the District of Columbia serving about two million children and youth (Strozer, Juszczak, & Ammerman, 2010).

If the potential of the ACA is realized, there are opportunities to significantly change mental health service delivery models. As an outgrowth of and in conjunction with ACA, Healthy People (2020) has as one of its primary goals to improve mental health through prevention and by ensuring access to appropriate quality mental health services (healthypeople.gov, retrieved 10/2013). A broader range of services and new approaches to treating complex problems can be offered to underserved populations (School Psychology in Illinois, 2013). With the expansion of mental health services to a broader population, mental health professionals will be compelled to expand their skill sets incorporating prevention and integrated primary care (Rozensky, 2012).

In order for school psychology to take advantage of ACA provisions, a reframing of role, and function is essential. A shift from primarily providing assessment and placement services to delivering intervention services is required (Mennuti & Christner, 2010). Included in this change of role would be the exploration of specific questions—for example, what are the competencies that would be required to offer integrated care in a school setting? What evidence-based services need to be available? How do we develop collaborative interdisciplinary working relationships?

The Ethics of Change: Professional Considerations

The practice of school psychology has undergone significant changes as a result of evolving social trends, federal legislation, and societal challenges. There has been increased attention to issues of social responsibility and the protection of the rights of children (McNamara, 2011). The prevailing influence of technology, security of records, and personal information, as well as storage and access to information, provide additional challenges in the protection of patient confidentiality.

New challenges raise new ethical considerations. School psychologists express concerns as to what appropriate services are to be provided in a school setting and what competencies are necessary to provide such services (Dailor, 2007). A critical ethical principle is that of "responsible caring," requiring professionals "to attain and maintain competence in the delivery of professional services, and to guard against practices that may result in harmful or damaging consequences" (McNamara, 2011, pg 768). Among the conditions of responsible caring are that school psychologists must continually assess and maintain competency in their areas of professional practice, monitor their own practices and decisions, and assist in the identification and execution of evidence-based practices. Further, the school psychologist must consider the integrity or fidelity by which these practices are executed. An additional ethical consideration is how to protect confidentiality within the school system (Dailor, 2007). The National Association of School Psychologists in the *Blueprint for Training and Practice* (Ysseldyke et al., 2006) and the Ethical Principles and Code of Conduct of the American Psychological Association (2010) specify that psychologists must work within the bounds of their professional competence. With the critical need for evidence-based mental health services, it is essential that school psychologists have the necessary training to be effective therapists.

The "half-life" of specialty training is a concept used to indicate the amount of time that the acquired information can be considered current and relevant. Thus, the half-life of a doctorate degree in psychology is considered to be 10–12 years. The estimated half-life of knowledge in school psychology is 9 years and, with the proliferation of research and information, is moving to 8 years. In clinical child psychology, the half-life is 8 years with movement toward 6.75 years (Rozensky, 2012). Rozensky, a 2013 APA award winner for Distinguished Career Contributions to Education and Training in Psychology, states that "education and training in, and the practice of, professional psychology must adopt and adapt to changes in accountability and quality expectations in the evolving health care system brought about by the implementation of the Patient Protection and Affordable Care Act"

(Rozensky, 2013 pg 703). "The ultimate contract is between society and the profession...a mature, autonomous self- regulating profession" (Belar, 2012 pg 548). While there is great importance in understanding the foundations of knowledge, it is critical to remain informed of contemporary issues and changing cultural and clinical concerns.

With the impetus of ACA, the potential for role expansion for school psychologists is evident. While school psychologists are ideally positioned to provide mental health services, are they prepared to meet the challenge of providing counseling and mental health services? (http://csmh.umaryland.edu/Resources/Briefs/HealthCareReformBrief.html). School Psychologists have always been seen as the mental health providers in the schools. However, there is great variation in the emphasis in training programs across the United States as well as local differences in job priorities and demands. Therefore, there are many practitioners in the field requiring further training and knowledge.

Research Supported Treatment

In response to the concerns about the efficacy of mental health treatment and the results of such treatment, the American Psychological Association created the Task Force on the Promotion and Dissemination of Psychological Procedures (1993). The Task Force developed a model with three levels to evaluate empirically supported treatments (EST):

1. *Well-established* treatments that require two or more studies using between group research designs done by different investigators which demonstrated the superiority of the treatment to a placebo or different treatment or its equivalence to another empirically supported treatment. The treatment must be manualized to permit replication of treatment.
2. *Probably* efficacious treatment that require at least two studies with superior outcomes compared to untreated control groups or two studies by the same investigators yielding superior results or series of single case studies with withdrawal designs and multiple replications.
3. *Experimental* treatment that is newly developed and awaiting study.
4. All other treatments that lack empirical verification without research support (APA Presidential Task Force on Evidence-based Practice, 2006).

Evidence-based treatment (EBT), a categorization similar to EST, upholding similar criteria, however, is less specific in the standards and does not necessarily require manualized treatment in order to be considered to be "well established" and permits a wider range of treatments to be acceptable (Kazdin, 2008; Steele et al., 2008). Recent research has indicated that not every patient benefits from every treatment component in an indicated protocol. Thus, a modular treatment approach has been introduced (Comer & Barlow, 2014). Protocols are structured as freestanding modules, rather than a linear approach as seen in manualized treatment. Clinicians can select modules and design a sequencing that is most appropriate to the specific concern or patient, while preserving the authenticity of an evidence-based approach (Comer & Barlow, 2014).

While data-based decision making is critical (Ysseldyke et al., 2006), along with the need for developing an evidence base to support a form of treatment, there are questions which remain unanswered when solely applying a data driven approach. Of primary concern is *how* (emphasis added) the treatment works or what factors other than the treatment itself are important sources of the treatment effectiveness. These factors include the client/therapist relationship, the cultural relevance of the treatment, and the setting where the treatment occurs. In a close examination of the evidence-based studies, the population diversity is often not reflected. Further, much evidence is gathered in "clean" settings as contrasted to implementation in a school context and with adult rather than child populations, where treatments are often downward extensions of interventions without regard to the developmental implications. It is important to remember that clinical practice with children and adolescents may bear little resemblance to treatments evaluated in efficacy research (Messer, 2004).

The evaluation of what works by examining the process of successful treatments in contrast to the specific content is referred to as the "common factors" approach (Messer, 2004; Norcross, Pfund, & Prochaska, 2013). There is a trend in the literature to more closely examine the process and mechanisms of change across evidence-based treatments and not necessarily on the specific treatment (Krueger & Glass, 2013). The issue of efficacy of treatment vs. effectiveness of a particular treatment has been a primary issue for discussion and debate (Kazdin, 2008). Integrative approaches are becoming more common among clinicians treating children and adolescents, with more than 50 % of therapists reporting the use of a mixture of techniques (Fonagy, Target, Cottrell, Phillips, & Kurz, 2002; Stricker, 2010). The integrative approach focuses on taking techniques from a variety of models and applying them to treatment while examining the relationship between practice and theory (Stricker, 2010). However, there is little empirical research on the application of integrative therapy for children.

Irrespective of the model of treatment provided, and in consideration of both NASP (2010) and APA (2010) guidelines particularly with the diversity of the populations, we need to respect the dignity and rights of all persons. This includes fostering autonomy and self-determination, protection of privacy and confidentiality, and assuring fairness and justice. *Informed* consent and assent for the minor receiving treatment are essential and include sharing of the reasons for treatment, goals, the frequency and duration, the format and methods, anticipated benefits, potential risks, and alternatives to the methods proposed. For self-referred minors, one or several meetings to assess the need for services and the extent the minor may be in danger may be engaged in within the school system without parental consent. Subscribing to the professional codes of ethics first and foremost protects the individual and secondarily the practitioner.

New Roles, New Functions

The confluence of the aforementioned factors is evolving to redefine the role and function of psychology in the schools. No longer is a "test and place" model adequate for the practice of school psychology. Today's role and function is more varied and may include consideration of universal prevention strategies and the integration of a public health model; the impact of data-based decision making and multi-tiered problem solving encompassing Response to Intervention (RTI) has shifted assessment and intervention paradigms (Eckert, 2011). These shifts suggest that with a greater emphasis on prevention and early intervention, those identified as requiring intervention at an individual level may present with the more challenging issues and potentially require more in-depth and extensive services. School psychologists need to consider the knowledge necessary to support expanding roles in a multicultural and global society. Examining the impact of technology on communication and practice is essential. For example, the ethics of cyber-counseling and the role of social media and electronic communication are just being examined and potentially could have significant impact on training and practice (DeAngelis, 2012).

Schools are unique practice settings, reflecting a diversity of gender, race, ethnicity, religion, and ability level and may, in fact, be the most diverse environment (Flanagan & Miller, 2010). There are opportunities to work systemically, introducing prevention programs as well on an individual level. School psychologists have the advantage of observing and intervening with children in their ecological environment. Treatment can be provided on a consistent basis without depending on family members bringing children to the proscribed services. However, ethical challenges often concern the provision of appropriate treatment within the legal and legislative constraints of the educational system (see Mychailyszyn, 2015). How then do we prepare for the future which is now?

This Volume

Despite the fact that intervention is an important domain of training within the National Association of School Psychologist Standards, historically school psychologists have not been extensively involved in school-based interventions (Ball, Pierson, & McIntosh, 2011). In contrast, demographics and contemporary issues suggest an important role that school psychologists can play in the direct provision of therapy services. School psychologists are well positioned to deliver quality interventions. Their understanding of the educational process, the relationship between mental health and academic health, and knowledge of the sociocultural school environment provide a critical basis to determine the most effective interventions (see Flanagan, 2015).

To address the challenges of providing effective intervention services to diverse populations, psychologists working in schools need to evaluate their knowledge base and repertoire of intervention strategies. To meet professional and ethical responsibility, it is essential to build upon already existing skills and to develop more in-depth and sophisticated skill sets, particularly within the cognitive behavioral framework. Cognitive behavioral therapy (CBT) has consistently achieved research support, particularly with children and adolescents. CBT has proven to be flexible with fidelity, allowing the practitioner to tailor interventions to the individual, problem, or setting (Kendall, 2006). The emphasis on problem-solving approaches, cognitive information processing, coping skills, and interpersonal relationships while remaining performance-based fits naturally in a school environment (Kendall, 2006). The focus on "learning" provides ample opportunity for the transfer of skills to the classroom and to the home. Techniques are applicable for both individual and group interventions.

This volume is divided into five sections that provide a systematic approach to treatment planning, examining the trajectory from clinical assessment to intervention strategies for specific clinical disorders. Difficulties in implementation of these strategies in school settings are addressed and comprehensively discussed (see Mychailyszyn, Chap. 14). Maintaining integrity and fidelity to treatment may be difficult given the daily scheduling and the time for treatment balanced with academic demands. Engaging parental participation may present an additional challenge.

The treatment approaches presented in this book are helpful for all mental health professionals working with children, particularly for psychologists working in the schools who are often on the frontlines of intervention planning. Each chapter presents a comprehensive review of the disorder and the evidence-based CBT interventions supported by case examples highlighting important aspects of assessment and intervention planning. The variety of chapters in this volume provides a wide range of information on contemporary evidence-based treatment and offers the knowledge to expand treatment options. The chapters answer important questions such as the following: what state-of-the-art, evidence-based treatment interventions are available that could be tailored to a school setting? How do we treat internalizing and externalizing disorders with the most efficacious approaches? What techniques and strategies can be imported to assist the psychologists in the school setting? How do we overcome obstacles and barriers in school-based treatment? We are ethically bound to provide the best evidence-based treatment to a particular patient given the sociocultural context, with respect for diversity and special needs. The focus of this book provides us with knowledge to meet our commitment to the populations we serve.

The mental health profession is changing. ACA provides opportunities to provide a wider range of services to underserved populations. There is a greater emphasis on implementing evidence-based treatment and evaluating the outcomes of that treatment. Cyber treatment and enhanced technology present both practice and ethical concerns. Children with severe disabilities and chronic illnesses formerly excluded from public education are now included in the mainstream and more often in inclusionary environment. This volume responds to the need to meet contemporary practice challenges, to continue to develop professional competencies, and to be responsive to the ethical commitment for responsible caring. CBT interventions have demonstrated efficacy in facilitating change with school-age populations; this volume is an important step in making these interventions accessible to professional working in the school setting.

References

Adelman, H. S., & Taylor, L. (2010). *Mental health in the schools*. California: Corwin.

Annie E. Casey Foundation. (2007). *2007 KIDS COUNT data book: State profile of child well-being*. Baltimore, MD: Annie E. Casey Foundation.

APA. (2010). *Ethical principles of psychologists and code of conduct*. Washington: APA.

APA Presidential Task Force on Evidence-Based Practice. (2006). Evidence-based practice in psychology. *American Psychologist, 61*, 271–285.

Ball, C., Pierson, E., & McIntosh, D. (2011). The expanding role of school psychology. In M. A. Bray & T. J. Kehle (Eds.), *The Oxford handbook of school psychology* (pp. 47–60). New York, NY: Oxford Handbooks.

Belar, C. D. (2012). Reflections on the future: Psychology as a health profession. *Professional Psychology: Research and Practice, 43*, 545–550.

Borman, G. D., & Rachuba, L. T. (2001). *Academic success among poor and minority students. Report number 52*. Maryland: CRESPAR.

Center for Disease Control and Prevention. (2013). Mental health surveillance among children in the United States 2005-2011. *Morbidity and Mortality Weekly Report 62*(suppl), 1–35.

Comer, J. S., & Barlow, D. H. (2014). The occasional case against broad dissemination and implementation. *American Psychologist, 69*(1), 1–18.

Compas, B. E., Champion, J. E., & Reeslund, K. (2005). Coping with stress: Implications for preventive interventions with adolescents. *The Prevention Researcher, 12*, 17–20. http://www.mh.umaryland.edu/Resources/Briefs/HealthCareReformBrief.html.

Cornell, D. G., Krosnick, J. A., & Chang, L. (2006). Student reactions to being wrongly informed of Eailvagahegh Stakes: The case of the Minnesota Basic Standards Test. *Educational Policy, 20*(5), 718–751.

Dailor, A. N. (2007). *A national study of ethical transgressions and dilemmas reported by school psychology practitioners*. Unpublished Master's thesis, Central Michigan University.

DeAngeis, T. (2012). Practicing distance therapy, legally and ethically. *Monitor in Psychology, 43*(3), 52. Retrieved from https://www.apa.org/monitor/2012/03virtual.aspx.

Eaton, N. R., Keyes, K. M., Krueger, R. F., Balsis, S., Skodol, A. E., Markon, K. E., et al. (2012). An invariant dimensional liability model of gender differences in mental disorder prevalence: Evidence from a national sample. *Journal of Abnormal Psychology, 121*(1), 282–288.

Eckert, T. L. (2011). Conclusion: Evolution of school psychology. In M. A. Bray & T. J. Kehle (Eds.), *The Oxford handbook of school psychology* (pp. 860–876). New York: Oxford.

Federal Interagency Forum on Child and Family Statistics. (2007). *Americas children: key national indicators of well-being. 2007*. Washington, DC: US Government Printing Office.

Flanagan, R., & Miller, J. A. (2010). *Specialty competencies in school psychology*. New York: Oxford University Press.

Flanagan, R. (2015). Professional issues in cognitive and behavioral practice for school psychologists. In R. Flanagan, K. Allen, & E. Levine (Eds.), *Cognitive and behavioral interventions in the schools: Integrating theory and research into practice* (pp. 303–317). New York, NY: Springer.

Fonagy, P., Target, M., Cottrell, D., Phillips, J., & Kurtz, Z. (2002). *What works for whom a critical review of treatments for children and adolescents*. New York: Guilford.

Grant, K. E., Compas, B. E., Thum, A. E., McMahon, S. D., & Gipson, P. Y. (2004). Stvesson's and child and adolescent psychopathology: Measurement issues and prospective effects. *Journal of Clinical Child and Adolescent Psychology, 33*, 412–425.

Hemphill, F. C., & Vanneman, A. (2011). *NCES 2011–485 achievement gaps: How hispanic and white students in public schools perform in mathematics and reading on the NAEP: Highlights*. Washington, DC: US Department of Education Publications.

Kaiser Family Foundation. (2010). *Summary of new health reform law*. Menlo Park: Henry J. Kaiser Family Foundation.

Kazdin, A. E. (2008). Evidence-based treatment and practice. *American Psychologist, 63*(3), 146–159.

Kendall, P. C. (Ed.). (2006). *Child and adolescent therapy: Cognitive-behavioral procedures.* New York: Guilford Press.

Krueger, S. J., & Glass, C. R. (2013). Integrative psychotherapy for children and adolescents: a practice-oriented literature review. *Journal of Psychotherapy Integration, 23*(4), 331–344.

Kruger, L. J., Wandle, C., & Struzziero, J. (2007). Coping with stress of high stakes testing. *Journal of Applied School Psychology, 23*(2), 109–128.

Larson, K., Russ, S. A., Crall, J. J., & Halfon, N. (2008). Influence of multiple social risks on children's health. *Pediatrics, 121*(2), 337–344.

Lee, J., Grigg, W., & Donahue, P. (2007). *The nations report card reading 2007 (NCES 2007-496).* Washington, DC: National Center for Education Statistics, Institute of Education Sciences, U.S. Department of Education.

McNamara, K. (2011). Ethical considerations in the practice of school psychology. In M. A. Bray & T. J. Kehle (Eds.), *The Oxford handbook of school psychology* (pp. 762–773). New York: Oxford.

Mennuti, R. B., & Christner, R. W. (2010). School-based mental health: Training school psychologists for comprehensive service delivery. In: Garcia-Vazquez, E., Crespi, T. D., & Riccio, C. A. (Eds.), Handbook of education, training and supervision of school psychologists in school and community (Vol. I, pp. 235–257). New York: Routledge.

Messer, S. B. (2004). Beyond empirically supported treatments. *Professional Psychology Research and Practice, 35*(6), 580–588.

Mychailyszyn, M. (2015). Transporting cognitive behavior interventions to the school setting. In R. Flanagan, K. Allen, & E. Levine (Eds.), *Cognitive and behavioral interventions in the schools: Integrating theory and research into practice* (pp. 283–301). New York, NY: Springer.

Nastasi, B. K. (2004). Meeting the challenges of the future: Integrating public health and public education for mental health promotion. *Journal of Educational and Psychological Consultation, 15*, 295–312.

National Alliance on Mental Illness (NAMI). (2013). *Mental illness facts and numbers.* Arlington: NAMI. Retrieved from www.nami.org.

National Association of School Psychologists. (2010). *Principles for professional ethics. Guidelines for the provision of school psychological services. Professional conduct manual.* Bethesda, MD: National Association of School Psychologists. Retrieved from http://www.nasponlline.org.

Nichols, S. L., Glass, G. V., & Berliner, D. C. (2006). High-stakes testing and student achievement: Does accountability pressure increase student learning? *Education Policy Analysis Archives, 14*(1), 1–172.

Norcross, J. C., Pfund, R. A., & Prochaska, J. O. (2013). Psychotherapy in 2022: A Delphi poll on its future. *Professional Psychology: Research and Practice, 44*(5), 363–370.

Reddy, L., Newman, E., & Verdesco, A. (2015). Attention deficit hyperactivity disorder: Use of evidence-based assessments and interventions. In R. Flanagan, K. Allen, & E. Levine (Eds.), *Cognitive and behavioral interventions in the schools: Integrating theory and research into practice* (pp. 137–159). New York, NY: Springer.

Research and Training Center for Children's Mental Health, University of South Florida. http://rtckids.fmhi.usf.edu/sbmh/default.cfm

Rigby, K. (2007). *Bullying in schools: And what to do about it.* Camberwell, VIC: ACER Press.

Rones, M., & Hoagwood, K. (2000). School-based mental health services: A research review. *Clinical Child and Family Psychology Review, 3*(4), 223–241.

Rozensky, R. H. (2012). Health care reform: Preparing the psychological workforce. *Journal of Clinical Psychology in Medical Settings, 19*, 5–11.

Rozensky, R. H. (2013). Quality education in professional psychology flowers, blooming, Flexner, and the future. *American Psychologist, 68*(8), 703–716.

School Psychology in Illinois. (2013). What school psychologists need to know about the affordable health(care) act (ACA). *Illinois School Psychology Association, 34*(3), 18–19.

Smallwood, D. L., Christner, R. W., & Brill, L. (2007). Applying cognitive behavioral therapy groups in school settings. In R. L. Christner, J. L. Steward, & A. Freeman (Eds.), *Handbook of*

Cognitive Behavior Group Therapy Specific settings and presenting problems (pp. 89–105). New York: Routledge.

Steele, R. G., Roberts, M. C., & Elkin, T. D. (2008). Evidence-based therapies for children and adolescents: Problems and prospects. In R. G. Steele, T. D. Elkin, & M. C. Roberts (Eds.), *Evidence-base therapies for children and adolescents bridging science and practice* (pp. 3–8). New York: Springer.

Stricker, G. (2010). *Psychotherapy integration*. Washington, DC: American Psychological Association.

Strozer, J., Juszczak, L., & Ammerman, A. (2010). *2007-2008 National school-based health care census*. Washington, DC: National Assembly on School-Based Health Care.

The Patient Protection and Affordable Care Act of 2010, Section 4101(a), 111th Congress, H.R. 3590.

U.S. Department of Education. (2006). *Twenty-eighth annual report to Congress on the implementation of the Individuals with Disabilities Education Act, 2006* (Vol. 2). Washington, DC: U.S. Department of Education.

U.S. Department of Health and Human Services. (1999). *Mental health: A report of the surgeon general*. Rockville: U.S. Department of Health and Human Services, Substance Abuse and Mental Health Services Administration, Center for Mental Health Services, National Institutes of Health, National Institute of Mental Health.

U.S. Department of Health and Human Services Office of Disease Prevention and Health Promotion. (n.d.). *Healthy people 2020*. Washington. Retrieved December 23, 2013, from www.cdc.gov/nchs.heathy_people/hp

Wilson, D. (2004). The interface of school climate and school connectedness and relationships with aggression and victimization. *Journal of School Health, V74*(7), 293–299.

Ysseldyke, J., Burns, M., Dawson, M., Kelley, B., Morrison, D., Ortiz, S., et al. (2006). *School psychology: A blueprint for training and practice III*. Bethesda, MD: National Association of School Psychologists.

Chapter 2
Behavioral Assessment in School Settings

Eva Feindler and Matthew Liebman

Introduction to Behavioral Assessment

Assessment is an indispensable component in the treatment of child behavior disorders and can be a complex and lengthy process. Assessment results are often the basis for diagnosis and classification as well as for the selection of targets for intervention. Further, data from various assessment methods can assist in the design and evaluation of intervention efforts. The assessment process also helps to draw inferences about causal variables and assist in the functional analysis of problem behavior patterns. Behavioral assessment encompasses methods and concepts derived from behavioral construct systems and is most frequently identified with an emphasis on quantification of observable and minimally inferential constructs. The methods of assessment differ from traditional assessment methods in their structure, focus, specificity, level of interest, and underlying assumptions. A recent comprehensive volume, *Diagnostic and Behavioral Assessment in Children and Adolescents* by McLeod, Jensen-Doss, and Ollendick (2013), attests to the developments in the field and can be consulted for greater theoretical and methodological information.

This chapter is an overview of behavioral assessment methods that might be useful in the development and evaluation of interventions for children in the school setting. As such, the authors will review a number of methods, namely, interviewing, screening measures, other paper–pencil inventories, behavioral observation, analogue

E. Feindler, Ph.D. (✉)
Clinical Psychology Program, C.W. Post, Long Island University, Brookville, NY, USA
e-mail: elfphd@aol.com

M. Liebman, M.A., M.S.
Clinical Psychology Program, C.W. Post, Long Island University, Brookville, NY, USA

Department of Child Psychology/Psychiatry, Montefiore Medical Center, Bronx, NY, USA
e-mail: mattgliebman@gmail.com

© Springer Science+Business Media New York 2015
R. Flanagan et al. (eds.), *Cognitive and Behavioral Interventions in the Schools*, DOI 10.1007/978-1-4939-1972-7_2

methods, archival records, and self-monitoring. The chapter will then further address developmental issues as well as issues related to reliability and validity in general. Further, suggestions are made for adaptation of methods for individualized use. One of the hallmarks of behavioral assessment is the idiographic nature of most methods: each can be tailored to specific situation, specific behaviors, and specific children.

Some additional principles of behavioral assessment that make it a unique approach are worth mentioning here as well. First, behavioral assessment is considered an ongoing process wherein data is collected at multiple points from intake and referral throughout the duration of treatment. Gathering of baseline data prior to the implementation of any intervention is recommended and can serve as a way to evaluate changes across time. If continuous data, i.e., daily or weekly, are not possible to obtain, repeated assessment is still encouraged. Secondly, we encourage data collection across settings. Rarely is a behavior pattern the same across and throughout different environments and with different people, and it is important to be thorough in this regard. Inconsistencies across settings help determine the mechanisms that elicit and maintain behavior problems. Thirdly, we suggest that any comprehensive assessment includes multiple informants (child, parents, teacher, and others) and multiple methods in order to obtain the most comprehensive picture of a child's functioning. It is often that informants do not agree (parents often rate their child differently than the child rates him/herself) and that there are inconsistencies across methods (self-report data are often quite different than behaviors directly observed in the natural environment). Recent research has indicated that youth are more accurate informants of their internalizing symptoms and caregiver more accurately reports external behaviors (Penney & Skilling, 2012) and correlations between cross-informants remain only moderate (Althoff, Rettew, Ayer, & Hudziak, 2010). However, these inconsistencies are what are the most interesting and compelling aspects of the behavioral assessment process.

Functional Analysis

It is reasonable to consider the development of a *functional analysis* , the conceptually based integration of data from all pre-intervention assessments, to be the only foundation for an individualized intervention plan. The *FA* (functional analysis) is an explanation of a student's target behaviors based on the synthesis of: (a) interacting behavioral, cognitive, and psychological causal factors; (b) associated behavioral assets and deficiencies; (c) situational sources of variance; (d) the context in which behavior occurs; and (e) any other mediating variables. The *FA* will help the practitioner determine whether to intervene, how best to select intervention strategies, and how to evaluate treatment impacts. Functional assessment provides accountability for treatment outcomes and increases the validity of clinical judgments. Practitioners should design a comprehensive assessment plan, based upon multiple informants, using multiple methods of assessment and with data collection continuing across time to test clinical hypotheses about "*why*" problem behavior occurs. Rather than relying on inferential or "best guess" answers to the question of "*why?*," FA helps to uncover all of the variables presently maintaining the target behaviors and can lead directly toward intervention strategies most likely to be effective.

Interviewing

There are several types of clinical and diagnostic interviews that can be conducted with children and their family members. General clinical interviews are designed to obtain overall demographic and family information and information about social–emotional development, academic functioning, and the referral concerns. Often, each person interviewed has a different perspective on the problem behaviors and situations, and the interviewer should expect inconsistencies and even be intrigued by them. In a clinical setting, a general intake might be followed by a diagnostic interview of which there are three types: unstructured, semi-structured, and structured interviews. The unstructured approach allows for a more conversational approach to information gathering and helps develop an initial therapeutic alliance and obtain information on possible diagnoses; however, these interviews do not have much diagnostic accuracy.

Semi-structured interviews have a specific set of questions to be included, but the exact sequence is not predetermined. This allows for greater flexibility and for opportunity to gather other relevant information. A skilled interviewer will be able to cover all of the required sections of the *Mental Status Exam* , for example, but in a way that puts the student/family member at ease. Sometimes, these semi-structured interviews ask a series of questions about specific child/adolescent diagnostic categories such as ADHD or conduct disorder, and this information is then used to substantiate a diagnostic formulation. Other forms of semi-structured interviews require training to administer. These include: *ISCA*–Interview Schedule for Children and Adolescents, *K-SADS*–Schedule for Affective Disorders and Schizophrenia for School-Age Children, and *DICA-R*–Diagnostic Interview for Children and Adolescents–Revised. Phillips and Gross (2010) provide an excellent description and overview of diagnostic interviewing for children and adolescents under the auspices of structured interviewing (i.e., *DISC-IV, CAPA, ChIPS*), though these types of interviews are actually rarely used in clinical practice (Brunchmuller, Margraf, Suppier, & Schneider, 2011) and most likely are not part of the assessment protocol in school contexts.

Behavioral Interviewing

In contrast to many forms of interviewing in clinical psychology, the primary objective of *behavioral interviewing* is to obtain accurate information that will be helpful in formulating a functional analysis of the presenting problem (Haynes & O'Brien, 2000).

Although unstructured, the focus is on describing and understanding the relationships among specific antecedent triggers, problematic behaviors, and reinforcing and maintaining consequences. The treatment provider should plan for a behavioral interview with the student, the parents, and perhaps the referral source to begin the assessment process. Kratochowill (1985) suggests that behavioral interviews follow the following four-step problem-solving format:

1. *Problem identification*: a specific problem is identified and explored and procedures are selected to measure target behaviors across time.
2. *Problem analysis*: conducted by assessing the student's resources and the contexts in which the problematic behaviors are likely to occur and by gathering some historical information about problematic situations.
3. *Assessment planning*: the treatment provider helps establish an assessment plan to be implemented. This plan might include a number of behavioral assessment methods (questionnaires, self-monitoring, role-play assessments) and ongoing procedures to collect data relevant to assessment and intervention. Methods are selected such that data can be gathered across time and contexts in order to evaluate treatment outcomes.

Thus, the behavioral interview is focused not only on obtaining information within the interview session, but also on making plans to gather information on behavior outside the interview, in the environment in which the behavior naturally occurs and from the perspectives of others (i.e., teachers and parents). Certainly there are different approaches to interviewing children versus their parents/teachers as often, the child is not in agreement that there are any difficulties. There are developmental considerations for the child interview as often children are unable, due to a limited verbal repertoire, or unwilling to report on their own behaviors and/or internal states. Adults are usually the powerful agents in a child's life and therefore may provide information from their own perspective. Further, the actual interview situation allows the interview to "observe" the student and family members interacting and relating to the interview context itself.

One simple format for guidelines for the behavioral interview is the "ABC" format. The interview should elicit specific descriptions of *Antecedents* or triggers of the problematic behaviors. A specific *Problem List* should be developed and centered on problem *Behaviors* defined in observable and measurable ways. Hypothetical constructs (i.e., "he is an angry child"; "she is so neurotic") are translated into overt behavioral responses ("he has pushed others while standing in line"; "she continuously asks the teacher whether her work is correct") so that baseline measurement can be obtained. If the target behaviors do include covert phenomena such as subjective emotional states ("worry," "shame," etc.) or distorted thoughts and interpretations of situations ("nothing ever works out for me"; "nobody cares about me"), then self-monitoring methods can be developed. Lastly, immediate and long-term *Consequences* thought to be shaping and maintaining the target behaviors are identified and earmarked for inclusion in intervention strategies.

Interviewing Parents

The parent interview is a key component in assessment and treatment planning and should occur soon after the referral of the student for services. In addition to obtaining key information about the background and current picture of the presenting problems, parents can provide critical information about situational antecedents and maintaining conditions that occur outside of the school context. The parent interview also allows for an early assessment of parenting, current behavior management strategies in use, and receptivity to school interventions.

An excellent example of behavioral interviewing is found in the work of Barkley (1990) who developed extensive interview protocols for the behavioral assessment of ADHD. One portion of the interview generates information on the nature of specific parent–child interactions that are related to the defiant and oppositional child behaviors often associated with ADHD. The interviewer reviews a series of situations that are frequent sources of difficulty between children and parents and solicits detailed information about particularly problematic situations. For example, parents may report that their child has temper tantrums, during which the child cries, whines, screams, hits, and kicks. A behavioral interview will be used as a first step in determining precisely what these behaviors look like when they occur, in which situations the behaviors occur (e.g., while the parent is on the telephone, in public places, at bedtime), and in which situations they do not occur (e.g., when the child is playing alone, playing with other children, at mealtimes). Additional information is then sought regarding the sequence of events, including the behaviors of the parents and the child that unfold during a tantrum. This type of situationally focused interview provides a detailed picture about how the parent perceives the antecedents and consequences that surround the child's problem behaviors. Often, the interviewer will ask for a "recent example" of the target behavior problem and a detailed "*Critical Incident Analysis*", which includes the details leading up to the problem (i.e., everything that went on in the house that Tuesday when Jimmy refused to go to school), everything the child and other family members did in response, and what the eventual outcomes were for that particular day. These sequential details will help to flesh out the functional analysis. It is suggested that initial behavioral interviews be held with the referral source for the student. Most likely this will be teachers and parents who have expressed concerns. Specific information and initial functional hypotheses can be generated which should be confirmed by interviewing the student. Although the information obtained from multiple sources often seems inconsistent, discrepancies themselves are always of interest. *The behavioral interview* should result in (1) initial hypotheses about the occurrence and maintenance of the target behaviors and (2) a plan for a multi-method, multi-informant assessment process. Included in this plan will be ideas about repeated assessment to help determine treatment outcomes and further treatment planning.

Screening Measures

When a student has been identified for intervention services, it is difficult to know how best to assess and subsequently address their needs. It becomes imperative to gather data in the most accurate, concise, and noninvasive way possible to design and evaluate any potential treatment program. Choosing an initial screening measure that is most developmentally and diagnostically appropriate for both the student and the situation at hand can be complicated. The intent of this section is to outline some easily accessible measures that school psychologists can use to quickly and accurately obtain a diagnostically informative snapshot of an identified student.

It is often the case that despite having been identified as in need, a student's pending diagnostic considerations may elude even the keenest observer. In these instances, it is worth using a broader-based tool to narrow the focus. The *Behavioral Assessment Scale for Children, 2nd Ed* (BASC-2) is a widely used and valid self-report assessment to measure behavior. As a multifaceted tool, the BASC boasts the ability to integrate the Self-Report of Personality (SRP) which is filled out by the student (or via an interview by a trained clinician), the Teacher Rating Scales (TRS) which can be completed by any educator who would have more than surface-level insight regarding the individual's behavior, and the Parent Rating Scales (PRS) which should be completed by either or both parents. Assessors should be mindful that the BASC has male and female norms for the parent rating form, which is indicative that fathers typically rate their children less stringently (tend to minimize issues more) than mothers.

The ability to compare and contrast the different reports across several potential diagnostic categories, including propensity toward anxiety, depression, and a range of externalizing and internalizing behaviors, makes the *BASC* a strong tool for use in better narrowing the focus for diagnostic consideration. Even more compelling is its reliable and valid predictability regarding symptom picture across a wide age range. The BASC can be used from ages 2:0 through 21:11 for both the TRS and the PRS. Equally notable is the net for the SRP—ages 6:0 through college (Lane et al., 2009). It should be noted that the *BASC* can be used to *guide* treatment planning in schools and should not really be used as or considered to be a complete personality assessment. It is a reasonable alternative to the Achenbach System of Empirically Based Assessment (AESBA) with solid psychometric properties and should be used in this vein. The *BASC* also has the capacity to rate adaptive and maladaptive characteristics of an individual, much like the AESBA—a notable strength of the tool overall.

Feasibility remains an issue in assessment planning. Fortunately, within the school setting, this is likely less of an issue with the *BASC*. In other clinical settings, it often borders on impossible to enlist the participation of both the parent(s) *and* the teacher in addition to completing the inventory with the student. Within the schools, this tool is likely able to give all parties involved a voice. In this regard, there are some positives to note. Though the comparative nature of different perspectives on individual behavior yields more compelling diagnostic information, the SRP can still be used as an individual tool to gain insight regarding a student's view of himself.

The question of truthfulness in response, or even potential malingering, may arise. The *BASC* comes equipped with validity of response scales that are used to determine whether the data are valid for interpretation. . If there is a question as to whether or not a student in need of services may even be able or willing to complete this questionnaire in the first place, a clinician can use the SRP as an interview tool and ask the student questions via structured interview. However, it is important to note that this is likely to only hold true in extreme circumstances (i.e., a child simply does not want to do it themselves). One of the primary purposes in the development of this powerful tool was for use in Special Education Evaluations. In this capacity, it is inherently sensitive to those who may not be able to adhere to its prescribed completion. Regardless of the methodology, this measure appears to yield strong data useful in guiding direction for both clinicians and diagnosticians. It should be noted that the BASC is not a diagnostic tool; however, it yields symptom pictures that can suggest diagnostic categories consistent with DSM-IV-TR classifications. It should be used to guide and inform, not to firmly categorize. Maintaining mindfulness in this capacity is a useful tool for clinicians to carry with them through the use of most behavioral monitoring and screening.

School psychologists and other professionals may also decide that rather than diagnostically focusing the screening of an identified individual, a more categorical assessment of behaviors that are both adaptive and maladaptive is indicated. The *Strengths and Difficulties Questionnaire* (*SDQ*; Goodman & Goodman, 2009) is a brief measure that can be used with multiple informants. The SDQ quantifies externalized behaviors by asking about 25 different attributes—some positive, others negative. It can be completed in an average of 5 min, making it quite appealing for use with children exhibiting oppositional behaviors or attentional deficits. This measure can be used with individuals ages 4–16 and can be given as an interview if the student is unable to complete the form on his or her own. It has also been used as a predictor of the presence of potential psychiatric disorders. More information on clinical utility and questionnaire practicality can be found on the publisher's website: http://www.sdqinfo.org/a0.html.

Another tool that can be given to parents and teachers is the *Disruptive Behavior Rating Scale* (Barkley, 2012). These 41- and 26-item paper and pencil inventories, respectively, are scored using a 0–3 Likert scale indicating whether certain behaviors interfere with functioning in school and/or in the home within the last 6–12 months. Similar to other measures, these rating tools are appropriate for youngsters aged 6–18 years.. These inventories are not particularly diagnosis specific, but rather, they can be used to supplement screening measures that solely focus on the identified student. Gathering information on behavior across settings is an integral piece of the puzzle, yielding crucial data regarding the support and perspectives of significant others across settings (Barkley & Murphy, 2006).

Common referral problems exhibited by adolescents are anxiety and depression. Viable and widely used screening and assessment tools have been the various Beck inventories. The *Beck Anxiety Inventory* (BAI; Beck & Steer, 1990) is a brief paper and pencil screening tool designed to help differentiate among emotional, behavioral, and physiological symptoms in individuals struggling with both anxiety and depression.

It is a self-report measure that can be used as both a tool for the clinician to inform diagnosis and act as a potential intervention in and of itself. This particular clinical tool brings awareness of generalized symptoms of anxiety to an individual's attention. In this way, it can provide just enough education for the willing participant to know that some new behaviors or experiences are worth noticing. Interestingly, Leyfer et al. (2006) purport that it assesses and screens for panic symptomatology. Individuals with symptoms similar to panic disorder have been found to endorse significantly higher scores on the *BAI* than those with other anxiety disorders (Beck & Steer, 1990), though the measure itself can still be used to both screen for and assess symptoms of globalized anxiety before and after intervention. While it cannot provide enough information to definitively diagnose an anxiety disorder, the BAI is a useful start to assess any child's behavior reflective of anxiety.

Its sister screener, the *Beck Depression Inventory II*, is also a paper and pencil measure for rating self-reported symptoms of depression through a 21-question scale based on symptom frequency and severity rated from 0 to 3. This measure detects the dichotomous or extremely positive or extremely negative thinking in some individuals with severe depression. So while a tool like the BDI-II can be useful for those who are honestly self-reporting, it also has a built in security net for that will reflect a true depression by means of either under- or overreporting symptoms (Beck, Steer, & Brown, 1996).

The *Beck Youth Inventory (BYI-II)* may be warranted in cases where impressions are not as clear as to which diagnosis the individual may exhibit. Essentially, the BYI-II has been validated as a screener for emotional and social impairment in five areas: depression, anxiety, anger, disruptive behavior, and self-concept. Each domain is assessed through its own separate inventory of 21 questions each, 105 questions total (i.e., BDI and BAI are both 21 items long). While the screening process itself will likely take longer for a student to complete, a full BYI-II will yield a symptom profile across each of these domains. The profile can then be compared to profiles similar to individuals who had been diagnosed with different sets of symptoms (i.e., depression, oppositional defiant disorder, attention-deficit/hyperactivity disorder). It is important to note that the use of this assessment tool has shown benefits as a screening measure, an outcome measure, and equally as importantly as a method for monitoring ongoing progress in treatment. Providing a level of buy-in exists and there is adherence to self-monitoring needed to complete an assessment at this length (five domains of functioning, average of 21 questions per area), the BYI-II can be a powerful, useful tool.

The intricacies of each useful screening tool that our profession may choose to employ are beyond the scope of this chapter. Often there may be concerns about a student's ability to effectively problem-solve and use planning skills in social and/ or academic situations. When a more specific analysis of behavior is warranted, there exists an array of choices for professionals. The *Behavior Rating Inventory of Executive Functioning (BRIEF)* is a targeted and simple self-report paper and pencil survey of behaviors accompanying disorders of executive function, such as ADHD. While not a diagnostic tool, the BRIEF can be used to quantify difficulty with focus and attention. Parents and teachers can be surveyed as well. Much like the BASC-2 in this way, the BRIEF can be used as part of a larger battery or as its own screening measure, which yields data that helps the student.

In general, what should be gleaned here is that there are a number of broad-based tools in addition to more narrowly focused tools that can be used at different points throughout the screening and treatment processes alike and for different purposes. Let us consider, for example, a child who is beginning to display infrequent yet severe angry outbursts in the classroom. This behavior could potentially be a marked qualifier of several diagnoses (i.e., attention-deficit/hyperactivity disorder, oppositional defiant disorder, Asperger's disorder, major depressive disorder). Clinicians may consider a *BYI-II* for use at the initial intervention stage to gain a more clear understanding of the breadth of symptom picture. It may turn out that this individual has been experiencing symptoms concordant with a depressive diagnosis. Without proper screening, it is likely that this behavior would have been classified as externalizing rather than a product of a truly internalizing disorder such as depression. Throughout what may now be a more efficient and focused treatment protocol, the clinician could ask the student to fill out a *BDI-II* weekly or perhaps even every other week as a means of evaluating intervention effectiveness. The more effective the screening, the more sure a clinician can be that he or she is providing the best care for the individual. An interesting consideration here is the hesitancy that many professionals feel when asking students to engage in frequent assessments, as there may be a sense of guilt, as if their time is being wasted and could otherwise be spent in a more effective way. Frequent monitoring can be a genuinely effective tool for informing care in an environment where time is often of the essence because it provides a basis for making adjustments to treatment in progress.

In sum, there is an increased awareness in the field for data collection for use in not only justifying treatment strategies, but also for providing concrete data to evaluate outcomes and to inform future practice. Without a proper screening assessment to gather baseline information regarding symptom presentation and maintenance, data in this capacity may be skewed, inaccurate, or simply not sufficient to provide diagnostic qualifiers. With this in mind, any of the aforementioned inventories can be used as such, as long as they are executed and maintained appropriately to each situation.

Parent Measures

Sometimes, it is not the child that requires intervention. It may be determined that although a child's behavior has warranted intervention, the parent or parents are likely at the root of an externalized presentation. Truthfully, there are many times when parents are and in fact may *need* to be referred for treatment. Parents struggling with depression, for example, tend to not seek services. They instead typically bring their children for various treatments without acknowledging their own need, thus not acknowledging the impact their potential pathology may have on the functioning of their child. One construct worth considering is the perceived level of parental competence and confidence. The *Parenting Sense of Competence Scale* (*PSOC*) (Johnston & Mash, 1989) is a 16-item paper and pencil survey designed to assess individual perception of parenting skill. This measure can yield a quick and accurate snapshot of sense of confidence and satisfaction with parenting. Scoring simply consists of tallying Likert-style responses which then correspond to one of the three acuity ranges: low, moderate, or high. The PSOC is particularly useful for assessing parental resources to make effective or positive decisions regarding their child's behavior, as well as to give the clinician enough information to guide intervention strategies for use with the child. A copy can be found and reproduced here:

http://www.afterdeployment.org/sites/default/files/pdfs/assessment-tools/parenting-confidence-assessment.pdf.

If it is suspected that there is a high level of parental and/or familial stress contributing to the identified child's behavior, the school psychologist may consider administering the *Parenting Stress Index, Fourth Edition* (*PSI-4*) (Abidin, 1995). The PSI is a screening measure available in both pencil and paper format and electronically. It can aid in identifying and evaluating the level of stress in a family system by focusing on parent characteristics and child characteristics, while highlighting situational and demographic aspects of life stressors. This 120-item inventory is designed for parents of children from 0 to 12 years of age and can be completed in approximately 20 min. A validity scale (Defensive Responding) is available designed to indicate whether the parent completing this tool is responding in a defensive manner regarding them or their child. Should a clinician suspect that a high level of parental stress is likely influencing both their own and the child's pathology, this tool may be used to better guide treatment in a way that can provide support for the child by validating that circumstances out of one's control (i.e., parental behavior, financial/living situation).

Clinicians might also consider aspects of family functioning that may be intertwined with a student's presenting problems. Pritchett and colleagues (Pritchett et al., 2011) provide a comprehensive overview of measures that target parent–child relationships, parental practices and discipline, parental beliefs, marital functioning, and general family dynamics and that might be considered in the assessment process. The *Parenting Scale* (see Salari, Terreros, & Sarkadi, 2012) is one of the most widely used measurements of parental discipline. This 30-item self-report inventory consists of three subscales: laxness, overreactivity, and verbosity. Laxness identifies a parent's permissive and inconsistent parenting style. Its counterpart, overreactivity, highlights aspects of parenting that are harsh or punitive. Hostile parenting, which is more extreme, examines the extent to which a parent might resort to hitting, cursing, or insulting their child. This scale can be useful in identifying gaps or lapses in style that parents may inadvertently or intentionally be resorting to in their parent–child relationship. A free copy of this scale can be found here:

http://www.pti-sf.org/yahoo_site_admin/assets/docs/PS_English.242164902.pdf.

Behavioral Observation: Direct Behavior Ratings

One of the hallmark strategies of behavioral assessment has been direct observation of behavior problems and their correlates in their natural environment. This allows for precision assessing discrete behaviors in one or more of the natural settings as they occur. This method requires that behaviors of interest are operationally defined in terms that can be observed, so that the frequency and duration of the behaviors, as well as the mechanics of where and when the behavior occurs, can be documented. The collection of data can be completed by an external and objective observer or a participant observer, someone already in the natural environment (e.g., a teacher), and should be conducted across many observations in order to gain a reliable estimate of target behaviors.

Often a place to begin would be with an *ABC recording*: a more descriptive narrative recording of antecedents, behaviors, and consequences occurring for the target student in the natural environment. Figure 2.1 is an example of this type of ABC narrative.

This recording can be rich in detail and allow a focus on multiple behavioral sequences prior to treatment planning. Although this method requires little actual observer training, it may be time consuming and not amenable to observations of multiple students. *Anecdotal recording* is a briefer narrative account describing a single incident of a student's behavior that is of interest to the observer, i.e., physical fight with a peer. Often written after the incident, the anecdotal record describes (a) what happened, (b) how it happened, (c) when and where it happened, and (d) what was said and done in response. This narrative is certainly less time consuming and helps focus on behaviors of interest and no special training is needed. It is suggested that a standard incident form be used and collected throughout the school year.

Once an observer has completed this preliminary observation, initial functional hypotheses can be developed relative to target behaviors and the antecedent and consequent events thought to be related to the maintenance of these behaviors across time. *Home-based or school-based observations* are designed to more naturalistically capture particular child behaviors of interest within the context of routine daily activities. Usually, a trained observer watches and codes any number of a student's behaviors during predetermined structured observation sessions. This will help to establish baseline frequencies of target behaviors and correlates and will help to develop treatment strategies. The main two methods of direct observation used by school personnel are *Time Sampling* and *Event Sampling*. Both first require complete behavioral definitions of each behavior to be observed in the natural environment. These definitions must be objective, clear, and reliable across observers. In *Time Sampling* the observer records the frequency of the behavior's occurrence over specific time intervals, i.e., during 15 min of snack time. This is an easy way to measure the occurrence of high-frequency, easily observable behaviors for one or more children. However, context-specific information (i.e., antecedents and consequences) is not obtained. In *Event Sampling*, the observer waits for and records a specific preselected behavior and the subsequent events and associated behaviors

Narrative ABC Record

Directions: Complete a narrative account of the situation using the boxes on the attached sheet. For each behavior observed, record what happen immediately before (Antecedents) and after (Consequences) each behavior. Note that sometimes a consequence leads directly to another behavior.

Student: Jack

Setting: Classroom - Snack + Independent Seatwork

Date/Time: Monday   October 16, 2006

ANTECEDENTS	BEHAVIORS	CONSEQUENCES
Students instructed to read silently & eat snack	Yells across the room to classmate	teacher redirects
	Rips paper out of notebook	no response
	goes to teacher's desk	no response
	gets a piece of tape from the dispenser	no response
	hops, shakes, wiggles	teacher redirects
	gets a piece of tape from the dispenser	teacher redirects
	walks back to desk	no response
	tapes a piece of paper to front of his desk	attention from peer
	returns for more tape	teacher redirects
	talks to some kids	attention from peers
	finishes taping paper to desk	attention from peer
	runs to classmate to say something	attention from peer
	runs back to his desk	no response
	talking and humming to himself	attention from peer
	swaying and dancing at his desk	attention from peers

Fig. 2.1 Narrative ABC record

(i.e., temper tantrum). This can be used to study low-frequency behaviors as well as setting events, which may have direct implications for treatment planning. The Event Sampling method will help to further the functional assessment of specific target behaviors each time they occur in a far more detailed fashion than Time Sampling. However, the burdens of both of these direct observation methods for either the participant teacher or an outside observer are many and may not be easily implemented in a school setting. Most behavioral intervention research studies have relied upon direct observation of behaviors in the natural environment to examine fluctuations in responding during various treatment conditions repeatedly across time. This is referred to as idiographic *time-series measurement* rather than snapshot measurement at any single point in time and is the hallmark of the behavioral assessment approach. This will provide continuous feedback across time to aid in treatment decisions.

The emphasis on the response to intervention (RTI) model highlights the necessity for a greater need for easy and frequent monitoring methods, perhaps daily, so that intervention efforts can be designed, implemented, and evaluated more efficiently. Often, in the school setting, there are limited resources for such methods of data collection across multiple observation times. *DBR (Daily Behavior Rating)* refers to a class of behavioral observation methodologies that can be used to document the effects of a behavioral and/or academic intervention. The recent advancement of DBR research is the analysis of the assessment potential of these methods. DBR, like systematic direct observation, may also fulfill educational accountability standards because the data provide valid and reliable information about the effects of behavioral interventions (Schlientz, Riley-Tillman, Walcott, Briesch, & Chafouleas, 2009). DBR methods require that behaviors to be observed are specified and operationally defined as with SDO methods. Ratings or Likert-type scores are then entered at the end of some predetermined observation period (e.g., 5 min, 1 h, half day, or daily) in specific settings. The data can be easily charted and summarized to share with parents, counselors, school psychologists, or administrators.

Riley-Tillman, Kalberer, and Chafouleas (2005) provide a comprehensive overview of one such DBR, the *DBRC: Daily Behavior Report Cards used to rate* both academic (such as on task, hand raising, work completion) and social (such as disruptive or aggressive) behaviors. The parameters they note about the DBRC are similar to the recommendations for conducting direct observations:

1. The behavior of interest is operationally defined.
2. The observations should be conducted under standardized procedures to ensure consistency in data collection.
3. The DBRC should be used in a specific time and place with a predetermined frequency.
4. The data can be scored and summarized in a consistent manner across raters, settings, and even across students.

Also included in their review is a conceptual flowchart model which will help determine the appropriateness of using the DBRC to monitor student behaviors that are not severe or frequent enough to warrant immediate intervention. Behaviors are clearly defined and each is given a Likert-type scale rating. For example, if hand raising was a target behavior, the assessor would rate either a "1" (0 times), "2" (1–2 times), "3" (3–4 times), "4" (5–6 times), or 5 (7+ times). The range would be based upon baseline observations and the goals of the intervention. The assessor, usually the teacher, would complete this either at a specific time point each day or at multiple predetermined data points across the day. As such, multiple behaviors can be assessed via a single DBRC. A case example that illustrates the method is available from Riley-Tilman et al. (2005). An available resource in the development of student specific monitoring tools is found at Intervention Central: the Report Card Generator (http://www.jimwrightonline.com/php/tbrc/tbrc.php).

DBRs have several advantages when compared to other methods of direct behavioral observation. First, a natural participant, the teacher, is used as the observer which may result in less reactivity from those observed than the use of an outside observer which is often required when using other direct observation methods. Second, *DBRs* are quite socially acceptable among teachers: over 60 % of the teachers contacted via a national database reported using DBRs periodically (Chafouleas, Riley-Tillman, & Sassu, 2006).

Analogue Assessment

Since it is often impossible or impractical to observe students' behavior in the natural environment, analogue assessment methods have been developed to help understand the functional relationships associated with target behaviors and to obtain baseline levels of responding prior to intervention implementation. Analogue assessment provides the opportunity to directly observe the students' behavior in a contrived setting that approximates the natural environment (Gold & Marx, 2006). The assessment situation can be standardized and designed to elicit the behaviors of interest in a far more efficient way than naturalistic observation. The method relies on the assumption that behavior in a contrived environment approximates what would occur naturally. In addition to observation, alternative methods include the students' responses to audio or videotaped scenarios and role-play enactments usually with a confederate child or adult. Most recently, researchers and clinicians have incorporated virtual reality simulations of feared situations to help in assessment, but few reports extend this to child samples. According to Mori and Armendariz (2001), analogue methods offer potential advantages such as tracking multiple behaviors simultaneously, accommodating variability across behavioral domains, ensuring the target behavior of interest, and being less intrusive than naturalistic observation.

Analogue methods have most commonly been used to assess fears, phobias, academic functioning, and social behavior. The *Behavioral Avoidance Test* (BAT) requires the student to enter a room that contains the feared object (snake, dog, the dark, etc., either real or fake) and to approach and interact in tasks that increase the anxiety potential. Behavioral measures of avoidance (proximity to the feared object, time spent in presence of object, etc.) and ratings of internal distress provide the assessment data. This can also be extended to include other situations that provoke intense anxiety, such as heights, enclosures, injections, and even school situations. These situations can be either contrived (i.e., dogs) or natural (i.e., elevators) but can be standardized across assessment time points for comparative purposes. Silverman and Serafini (1998) include the use of a graphical "fear" thermometer to obtain a subjective and relative rating of fear while in the contrived situation.

Reported some time ago, a unique approach was developed by Glennon and Weisz (1978) for the assessment of separation anxiety in preschoolers. Using the *Preschool Observation Scale of Anxiety* (POSA), observers recorded 30 indicators of anxious behavior as they watched a preschooler complete tasks from several cognitive assessments with and/or without the mother. The coding of anxious behaviors represents a detailed topography of how anxiety is exhibited in young children.

In terms of academic functioning, it is easy to see how a simulated educational or testing situation could be set up to assess a student's frequency of attentional shifts, off-task behaviors, out-of-seat movements, etc., all indicative of ADHD or other learning difficulties. Early assessment attempts included an analogue playroom setting with a movement grid across the floor to determine locomotor activity in hyperactive children. Direct assessment of movement patterns at a pre- and then post-assessment point would help to determine effects of treatment components on motor behavior. Barkley (1990) developed an ADHD coding system to be used in an analogue academic setting. A child would be placed alone in a playroom and asked to complete a packet of math problems within 15 min. Further, the child was instructed not to leave the table or touch the toys. Observers recorded via a one-way mirror the time the child was off task or out of seat and how often s/he vocalized and played with objects. This was revised into the *Restricted Academic Task* (*RAT*) by Fischer (1998) which standardized the coding system for interval recording of the following behaviors: engaged in task, off task, fidgeting, task-relevant vocalization, task-irrelevant vocalization, and out of seat. Fischer reports the use of this assessment probe as a way to help optimize medication dose for ADHD children and as an adjunct to parent and teacher reports of treatment outcomes. It may be more practical to videotape the child in the academic situation for later coding as well as for the child, treatment provider, and parent to have a visual record of behavioral change across time. The coding systems described are usually time consuming and complex requiring observer training and thus may be impractical for the school environment.

Children's social behavior might best be assessed using analogue methods to capture a description of the specific behaviors of interest and their functional relations. Shyness and social withdrawal can be observed in a contrived play setting in which familiar and then unfamiliar peers and/or adults can be included or in situations similar to those encountered every day. Behavior of interest might include shared play, verbal interactions, spontaneous comments, playing by self, or removal from others. The *Behavioral Assertiveness Test for Children* (*BAT-C*; Bornstein, Bellack, & Hersen, 1977) was developed for pre–post-assessment of children's social skills programs. The format includes social scenarios to which a child responds. The scenes requiring assertive behavior (accepting help, giving and receiving compliments and negative assertion) are introduced by a narrator, followed by a prompt from a confederate child or adult. The behaviors recorded include six categories of verbal behavior and four categories of nonverbal behavior in addition to overall assertiveness. Scenarios particular to a given child's social difficulties could be developed and used as an assessment probe prior to intervention and then as an outcome measure. A similar format was developed in the pre–post-assessment of

Script 1:	Interpersonal Conflict Situation
Narrator:	You are watching your favorite TV show. What is your favorite show? Okay You're watching___. John comes in and after a minute turns the channel.
John:	I don't like this program, it's for babies.
You respond:	
Script 2:	Interpersonal Conflict Situation
Narrator:	There is Eddie playing with a basketball that is yours. You go over and ask to have the ball because you want to play with another friend. Eddie gets mad.
Eddie:	I'm not done with the ball. I'm still playing, man. Just wait a half second and I'll give it to you.
You respond:	
Script 3:	Interpersonal Conflict Situation
Narrator:	You dropped a dollar a minute ago on the couch, and you just realized it. You go back to get the dollar and there is Ted with a dollar in his hand on the couch. You tell him you dropped the dollar and would like it back.
Ted:	It's mine. I found it and I'm not giving it back. Now get outta here!
You respond:	

Fig. 2.2 Sample role-play scripts

adolescent anger management training wherein the scenario and the prompts were typical antecedents to angry and aggressive outbursts for target youth (Feindler & Ecton, 1986). Responses to these scenarios were videotaped and later coded for behaviors specific to anger management training (Figs. 2.2 and 2.3).

Wakschlag and colleagues (Wakschlag et al., 2005, 2008) have developed the *Disruptive Behavior Diagnostic Observation Schedule (DB-DOS)*. Designed as an analogue method to accompany typical parent interviews, the DB-DOS is a 50-min structured laboratory observation involving both parent and examiner along with the child. Problems in both behavior regulation and anger modulation are elicited by performance tasks, and the target child's natural behavior is coded. Performance tasks may include simulations, tasks with the child alone, or tasks where the parental behavior is scripted to systematically elicit the full range of behaviors relevant to a particular diagnosis. The DB-DOS includes diagnostic observation, which is structured to allow for a wide range of clinically relevant behaviors to be observed, and clinical judgment may be used to rate behaviors on a continuum of atypicality, ranging from *normative variation* to *clinically concerning*. The DB-DOS demonstrates good inter-rater and test–retest reliability as well as strong predictive and concurrent validity . Their multi-informant, multi-method research has indicated that the DB-DOS is reliable and valid in terms of its utility for discriminating clinical levels of disruptive behavior in young children (McKinney & Morse, 2012). Other analogue assessments used in the examination of disruptive behaviors of older children include simulations such as a computer pinball competition with an alleged peer, to study cheating, responses to provocation, and aggressive behaviors.

Subject: _____ Rater: _____
Testing: _____
Date: _____

Irrelevant Comments	Hostile Comments	Inappropriate Requests	Appropriate Requests

In Pocket	Gesture	At Side	Positive Physical	Negative Physical

Duration of Scene: _____
Duration of eye contact: _____
Duration subject speech: _____
Ratio: _____

Loudness

1	2	3	4	5
too soft/ whisper		just right		too loud/ yelling

Overall global rating

1	2	3	4	5	6	7
very passive			*very assertive*			*very aggressive*

Fig. 2.3 Role-play coding sheet

Lastly, clinicians have reported on the use of an analogue paradigm to measure aspects of parent–child interaction and in particular child compliance to adult instructions. The *Compliance Test* (CT) was developed to determine interaction patterns between parents and their disruptive or noncompliant children. Usually, the parent and child are placed in a playroom situation with a variety of toys and containers. After a period of habituation, the parent issues a standard set of instructions related to task completion as well as cleanup, and observers note not only the child's compliance/noncompliance but can also record the parent's behaviors. The CT has been used to evaluate the outcomes of parent training programs and has shown good validity with other methods of noncompliance assessment (Filcheck, Berry, & McNeil, 2004). It would be easy to extend this paradigm for the assessment of teacher–child compliance issues in an educational setting. What might also be helpful in further understanding the variables that maintain children's disruptive behavior, the school clinician could easily observe the parent and child completing a simple task together (such as a puzzle) and then cleaning up. A wealth of information about compliance and reinforcement contingencies is available in a relatively short observation of the dyad in this analogue situation. Some have extended this to include watching and coding (*Parent–Adolescent Interaction Coding System*) a verbal interaction between parents and adolescents over a "hot topic" to get a fuller understanding of the communication dynamics with a conflicted family (Robin & Foster, 2002).

Since analogue situations are developed specifically for a particular assessment target and participant, it seems easily adapted to any age child. For the young child who may not be able to complete a questionnaire assessment or who is not yet able to self-reflect and accurately report on their experience, observation of natural behavior in a contrived setting might be the best possible assessment. When incorporating role-play scenarios or more simulated settings (i.e., the BAT), the reliability and validity of the assessment does depend on the child's capacity for mental representation. Since students are asked to respond "as if" they were in the natural environment, their understanding of and flexibility with pretense and imagination will influence their responses.

Some have written about the methodological limitations and the psychometric concerns with analogue assessment (Mori & Armendariz, 2001), and others continue to examine issues of reliability and validity (Filcheck et al., 2004; DiLorenzo & Michelson, 1983). Overall the results are mixed for role-play assessments; the psychometric outcomes depend on how much the behavior in the analogue situation reflects real behavior. Often what children say they would do and what they actually do in a real-world situation do not correspond. There are demand characteristics in contrived settings that may exert influence on the child's behavior. For example, most children know that the simulated feared environment (such as a darkened room) is made safer because of the person conducting the assessment. Further, since all analogue assessments only sample actual behavior, a question of adequate sampling arises. Do the chosen role-play scenarios or the compliance instructions represent enough of a range for a particular child to truly provide an accurate rating of the behaviors of interest? A recent study sought to examine the representativeness of parent–child analogue tasks usually used in the measurement of noncompliance. Rhule, McMahon, and Vando (2009) asked a community sample of mothers who were observed in 4 parent–child compliance tasks about their experience, and the majority rated the interaction as comparable to what would go on at home. The children however were young (4–6 years old) and might experience fewer behavioral constraints even in an analogue setting.

In general, analogue assessment methods have long been developed and employed in the assessment of a range of children's difficulties in both clinical and academic endeavors. Extremely flexible and able to be individualized, the use of simulated situations and/or role-play scenarios is recommended to help directly observe specific behaviors and their functional relations, to test clinical hypotheses, and to evaluate outcomes of intervention efforts. We suggest the use of analogue measures at least at pre- and posttreatment, but perhaps midway as an assessment probe as well to supplement questionnaire data. If the student's behavior is videotaped, a visual comparison across time will be instructive and rewarding for the student, their parents, and for the treatment provider. Lastly, these role-play techniques can easily be included in an initial interview with a youth and his/her parents to support the other information being gathered.

Self-Monitoring

This unique method of behavioral assessment involves a student's observation of their own behaviors and/or experiences and the recording of information on aspects of importance for intervention planning and evaluation. According to Silverman and Ollendick (2005), self-monitoring has often been viewed as a more efficient and easier way to accomplish the same goals as direct observations—that is, to identify and quantify symptoms and behaviors, to identify and quantify controlling variables, and to evaluate and monitor treatment outcome. The method is direct in that the data are gathered at the time of the occurrence; however, self-monitoring is far more subjective than other methods as the observer and observed is one and the same person. Self-monitoring can help to identify functional relationships impacting a student's problem behaviors in real time and across multiple contexts.

In general, the student records the occurrence of the target behavior or aspects of the behavior of interest (frequency, intensity, duration) or other variables hypothesized to influence the target behavior on some kind of data sheet, recording card, or recording device. Often the treatment provider will develop a specific form for record keeping which is turned in on some regular basis (i.e., daily, weekly, at each meeting). Just about any behavior that can be clearly defined can be monitored, and the format can be adjusted according the student's cognitive level. Data can be recorded either continuously from baseline to the end of an intervention program or at specified time as a sample of behavior. Most clinicians would agree that self-monitoring is a highly flexible and efficient method to gather data on low frequency, less observable behaviors and on internal experiences, especially thoughts and feelings. Cohen and colleagues (Cohen, Edmunds, Brodman, Benjamin, & Kendall, 2013) provide a number of specific suggestions for implementation of self-monitoring so that the student and treatment provider can work together to gather data to track target behaviors and associated variables, to plan and implement interventions, and to provide feedback and outcome data. They describe this type of collaborative empiricism, characteristic of current CBT approaches, in a case illustration of self-monitoring with an anxious 11-year-old boy (Cohen et al., 2013).

Clearly there are developmental considerations when designing a self-monitoring procedure. Often synonymous with self-recording and self-observation, this assessment method does depend upon the child's cognitive and emotional capacities. More complex recordings assume that the child has achieved a meta-cognitive level that involves the ability to think about one's own thinking. Further, learning to monitor one's own behavior (reactions, experiences) is a key requisite to self-regulation and affect regulation. By about age 8, children have an understanding of multiple emotions of varying intensities and of opposite valences and by about age 10 can invoke affect regulation strategies. Often these related thoughts and feelings are at the very core of interventions for anxious, angry, or depressed students. Daly and Ranalli (2006) have developed a unique method for helping students to record data on their behaviors even if they cannot read. Their creative development of "*Countoons*" (see Fig. 2.4) shows the flexibility of the self-monitoring approach,

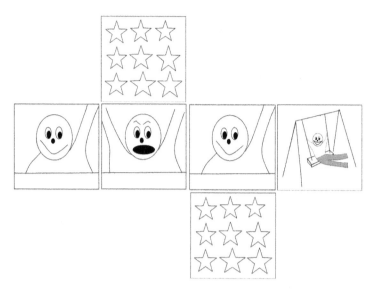

Fig. 2.4 A blank countoon for handraising versus yelling

and they offer detailed steps for the treatment provider to follow in the development of a Countoon strategy. Generally, younger children will need a simpler recording format, while older children are able to include more information and even expand on their experiences in a diary entry format.

There are a number of methodological limitations in the use of data collected via self-monitoring procedures. Self-monitoring is a behavior and as such is susceptible to a number of sources of reactivity and influence. Behavior change itself can result from the recoding of behavior as a student's attention is drawn to the variables of interest. This unfortunately inserts a level of inaccuracy in the data collection, but inadvertently can result in a prompt for an alternative behavior or newly acquired skill. For example, when recording an anger trigger on the Hassle log (see Fig. 2.5) often used in anger management protocols (Feindler, 2012), the student can then opt to invoke a newly learned alternative response (deep breath, walk away) and thus record a less intense anger experience. This renders self-monitoring an intervention strategy in addition to being an assessment method.

McGlynn and Rose (1998) suggest that the valence of the target behaviors to be monitored may impact accuracy and reactivity: negatively valenced behaviors might be recorded less accurately by students less motivated for treatment or concerned about consequences of reporting. Youth may not be accurate in monitoring their own behaviors, but they may still exhibit a desirable behavior change so choice of behaviors to self-monitor requires careful consideration.

Self-monitoring is certainly limited by the student's ability and level of motivation to understand and comply with the instructions and the procedures. Greater compliance is usually associated with the student's involvement in the design of the

Hassle Log

Name:________________ Date:________ Time:________

Where were you? ___Home ___School ___Outside Car/Bus ___Other

What happened: ___Teased ___Told to do something ___Someone stole from me
___Someone started a fight with me ___I did something wrong ___Other

Who was that somebody? ___Friend ___Sibling ___Another student ___Parent
___Teacher ___Another adult ___Therapist/Counselor ___Other

What did you do: ___Hit back ___Ran away ___Yelled ___Cried ___Ignored
___Broke something ___Was restrained ___Told adult ___Walked away calmly
___Talked it out ___Told friend

How did you handle yourself: ___Poorly ___Not so well ___OK ___Good Great

How angry were you: ___Burning mad ___Really angry ___Moderately angry
___Mildly angry ___Not angry at all

Notes:________________

Fig. 2.5 Hassle log example

data process: students that pick their own target behaviors and help to make up the data sheet (and PDA options can be quite useful) participate more eagerly in data collection. Checklists (see *Hassle Log*: Fig. 2.5) are often easier to complete and can be designed in such a fashion as to subtly teach the components of a CBT approach to treatment. In this data sheet, students first record setting events (i.e., "where are you?"), then record the triggering events ("What happened"), and then record their behavioral responses, feelings, and thoughts ("What did you do?"). This represents a written sequence of events upon which affect regulation and/or alternative responses can eventually be invoked. Pretreatment use of a self-monitoring strategy, often done to establish baseline levels of functioning, can also be used as an early compliance probe. Since many interventions for children and adolescents rely on completion of homework assignments, it is best to get an early assessment of compliance level. Radley and Ford (2013) have provided helpful guidelines for developing self-monitoring intervention for educators creating individual behavior change programs for specific youth.

Overall, it is evident that self-monitoring is a valid and relevant assessment method for intervention for a variety of child and adolescent behavior problems. The clear advantages include:

1. It is inexpensive, highly flexible, and completely individualized.
2. It can be adapted for all students regardless of developmental level.
3. It allows for continuous monitoring of fluctuations in behaviors of interest and in evaluating treatment outcome.
4. It can help to determine functional relationships and thus aid in case conceptualization and treatment formulation.
5. It provides immediate feedback on behaviors/variable of interest to the student and the treatment provider.

6. Data collection (and perhaps a visual graphing) can provide a clear picture of improvement that will be rewarding to all.
7. It can facilitate communication with both teachers and parents in an ongoing fashion.

Even with all the advantages of engaging a potentially problemed individual in self-monitoring strategies that have been outlined thus far, one rather significant obstacle to success necessitates acknowledgment: buy-in. Imperative to the success of this style of intervention is the likelihood that the student will actually engage in the process in a useful way. In this regard, there are two elements that must be considered when attempting to increase the chance that a student will buy-in to a self-monitoring intervention: *feasibility* and *utility*.

Many if not all of the "traditional" self-monitoring tools that have been researched and validated are pencil and paper style interventions. While on the surface this may seem trivial, the likelihood that an adolescent who is displaying externalizing or internalizing behaviors in school and whose primary concern is how he/she preserves social standing with a peer group, drawing attention to oneself by pulling a thought record out in the middle of class, may not make it to the list of priorities. In cases such as this, the utility of more technologically based tools may bear some consideration. Now, more than ever, students are inundated with a culture of immediate access to information and an excess of that information (Osit, 2008). To ignore the potential utility that engaging children and adolescents using devices they are *already* using in their daily lives seems almost neglectful. Several computer and smartphone-based apps have been developed throughout the last several years, some of which may be particularly useful in this capacity:

1. *CBT Pad*—a free, computer-based app that mimics the traditional thought record used in several CBT-style treatments. Individuals can customize the record to include precipitating events, thoughts triggered, consequences, challenges involved, and actions that followed. Each of these sections has further qualifiers that allow the student to give as much detail as necessary for who, what, where, and when the sought-after behaviors occurred. It also generates an ongoing chart/graph to easily identify patterns over time.
2. *Notepad*—this free iPhone app comes standard and is already installed on each device. For students who find that paper/pencil tools are invasive and call attention to them, use of this digital writing tool may eliminate arousal of suspicion from peer groups and increase adherence and likelihood that the data collected will be accurate and immediate.
3. *Panaganos*—smartphone app that includes a mood tracker with "what am I doing," "who is with me," "where am I" elements that can then chart out results over time by graph or by location. With GPS-enabled smartphones (which most are), triggering events recorded by location may add another element to pattern detection.
4. *DBT Diary Card*—though a steeper priced app, this integrative smartphone program is modeled after the tracking card used to monitor behaviors and urges to act throughout dialectical behavior therapy (DBT). With engaging visuals, the

app allows students to keep record of any target behavior including "urges" (the feeling preceding an impulsive or maladaptive action) and any alternative behaviors engaged in instead. Of note is that if the school psychologist or counselor working directly with the student also has a smartphone with this app, the two can connect, and the counselor will automatically be sent any self-monitoring data that the individual logs. This facet of the intervention not only has the potential to increase adherence, it also creates a sense of accountability that may impact continued and diligent use. Utility of this particular app should be considered strong with the more highly motivated self-monitorer.

Of course, should things like cell phone and computer use in school be an issue with either classroom or administrative policy, caution should be used before considering these options. Inviting the potential for more negative attention is not the goal. Additionally, as the world of apps is ever growing, be mindful of not using those that use "therapy" in either the title or the purpose. Several apps profess to be replacements for therapy or at the very least a helpful supplement to therapy. This is not the goal for use of self-monitoring in school. The goal is to simply have tools that are easily accessible to increase buy-in and adherence.

Other resources: As treatment manuals continue to be developed and worksheet incorporated for children, publishing websites have made materials more and more accessible. Readers are directed to Oxford University Press website: *Treatments That Work* for downloadable tools:

www.oup.com/us/companion.websites/umbrella/treatment/.../mforms/.

Examples include:

1. A *children's daily logbook* for school refusal treatment.
2. A *worry record* for treatment of youth anxiety.
3. A *feelings chart*. Practitioners can download these self-monitoring forms for particular children and/or settings or adapt them for specific interventions. Further forms are available for parent self-monitoring of their own responses to their children, and these might even be adapted for teachers as well.

Archival/Permanent Product Data

There are numerous sources of archival and continuous data available in any educational setting. These data are those that are routinely collected as a part of already existing programs and/or administrative policies and may easily be incorporated into any intervention effort. Baseline data is usually available for many weeks, even months and years prior to an intervention, and data will continue to be collected following any treatment program. These typical school records may include: absences, detentions, suspensions, demerits, expulsions, rule violations, class cuts, academic data (both local and statewide), grades in classes, homework completion, error rates, test scores, teacher evaluations, yearly reports, IEP data, nurses notes, fines or other response-cost measures from a behavior management system, etc. Such data are easily collected by teachers as well as by treatment providers and are both time and cost-efficient (Chafouleas, Christ, Riley-Tillman, Briesch, & Chanese, 2007). Any source of information that can be quantified can be charted across time for visual analysis of baseline stability and behavioral changes. For mental health personnel, we recommend keeping data on setting and keeping appointments, being on time, behavior during sessions (cooperation, compliance with tasks, verbal participation, eye contact, etc.), homework completion (i.e., self-monitoring or other task assignment), and contacts with family members and other professionals involved with the student. For some older students, there may also be community agencies involved with the target student who might be able to provide data that is already being collected, once permission has been obtained. Police and probation departments and other community organizations the student might be involved in (sports teams, scout clubs, etc.) might provide information about attendance and appropriate social behavior.

In an extremely large study across 2,500 elementary schools, McIntosh, Frank, and Spaulding (2010) examined the use of standardized *office discipline referrals* (*ODR*) to identify risk based on the time of year and the referral in order to determine responses to intervention. Although their data is promising in terms of efficient collection of archival data, the authors indicate that schools must adopt clear definitions for ODRs, use standardized ODR forms, and provide training of personnel in the use of this assessment. The eventual efficiency of such data collection must be weighed against the initial "costs" of implementation.

It might seem tempting to obtain archival data over the course of treatment as the data already exist and require no measures to be administered and scored. However, usually, archival data represents NOT student actual behavior, but rather a recording of an adult overseeing student behavior (teacher, administrator, parent, probation officer, etc.). As such, these data represent complex processes of student behavior (i.e., some rule infraction), observation and recording of consequent events, and a notation of some outcome. Caution in interpretation of such data sources is warranted. Student absence from school can be the result of multiple events and cannot be ascribed solely to the student's motivations. Since the working alliance is crucial to effective treatment, the student should be made aware that data from these sources may be collected and can be used in understanding the impact of treatment. In particular, we suggest collaborating with especially adolescents in obtaining data to inform and evaluate treatment.

Summary

In this chapter we have attempted to provide the practitioner with an overview of behavioral assessment principles and methods that are most suited to the assessment of student problem behaviors in the school environment. A general review of interviewing, self-report, self-monitoring, direct observation, analogue assessment, and the use of permanent product data has included examples of the methods as well as resources the practitioner can use to access the assessment tools and forms. Others have written extensively about evidence-based assessment protocols for various disorders (see, e.g., McKinney & Morse, 2012 for details about the assessment of disruptive behavior disorders) and provide step-by-step guidelines for baseline and repeated assessments. Most recently, Ebesutani and colleagues (2012) have responded to the burden of an ideal comprehensive assessment in terms of time and cost and have suggested a "real-world" protocol for the practitioner. The remainder of the chapters in this edited volume focus on school-based interventions for specific presenting problems and include a section on disorder-specific assessments.

References

Abidin, R. R. (1995). *Parenting stress index: Professional manual* (3rd ed.). Odessa, FL: Psychological Assessment Resources, Inc.

Althoff, R., Rettew, D., Ayer, L., & Hudziak, J. (2010). Cross informant agreement of the dysregulation profile of the Child Behavior Checklist. *Psychiatry Research, 178*, 550–555.

Barkley, R. (1990). *Attention deficit disorder: A handbook for diagnosis and treatment.* New York: Guilford.

Barkley, R. (2012). *Barkley functional impairment scale-children and adolescents (PFIS-CA)* (p. 166). New York: Guilford Press.

Barkley, A., & Murphy, K. (2006). *Attention-deficit hyperactivity disorder, third edition: A clinical workbook.* New York: Guilford.

Beck, A. T., & Steer, R. A. (1990). *Manual for the beck anxiety inventory.* San Antonio, TX: Psychological Corporation.

Beck, A. T., Steer, R. A., & Brown, G. (1996). *Beck depression inventory* (2nd ed.). San Antonio, TX: Harcourt.

Bornstein, M., Bellack, A., & Hersen, M. (1977). Social skills training for unassertive children: A multiple-baseline analysis. *Journal of Applied Behavior Analysis, 10*, 183–195.

Brunchmuller, K., Margaf, J., Suppiger, A., & Schneider, S. (2011). Popular or unpopular? Therapists' use of structured interviews and their estimation of patient acceptance. *Behavior Therapy, 42*, 634–643.

Chafouleas, S. M., Christ, T. J., Riley-Tillman, T. C., Briesch, A. M., & Chanese, J. A. M. (2007). Generalizability and dependability of direct behavior ratings to assess social behavior of preschoolers. *School Psychology Review, 36*(1), 63–79.

Chafouleas, S., Riley-Tillman, T. C., & Sassu, K. (2006). Acceptability and reported use of daily report cards among teachers. *Journal of Positive Behavior Interventions, 8*, 174–182.

Cohen, J., Edmunds, J., Brodman, D., Benjamin, C., & Kendall, P. (2013). Using self-monitoring: Implementation of collaborative empiricism in cognitive-behavioral therapy. *Cognitive and Behavioral Practice, 20*(4), 419–428. doi:10.1016/j.cbpra.2012.06.002.

Daly, P. M., & Ranalli, P. (2006). Using Countoons to teach self-monitoring skills. *Teaching Exceptional Children, 35*(5), 30–35.

DiLorenzo, T., & Michelson, L. (1983). Psychometric properties of the BAT-C. *Child and Family Behavior Therapy, 4*, 71–76.

Ebesutani, C., Bernstein, A., Chorpita, B., & Weisz, J. (2012). A transportable assessment protocol for prescribing youth psychosocial treatments in real-world settings: Reducing assessment burden via self report scales. *Psychological Assessment, 24*, 141–155.

Feindler, E. L. (2012). *TAME: Teen Anger Management Education.* Unpublished manuscript available from author.

Feindler, E. L., & Ecton, R. B. (1986). *Adolescent anger control: Cognitive-behavioral techniques.* New York: Pergamon.

Filcheck, H., Berry, T., & McNeil, C. (2004). Preliminary investigation examining the validity of the compliance test and a brief observational measure for identifying children with disruptive behavior. *Child Study Journal, 34.*

Fischer, M. (1998). Use of the Restricted Academic Task in DHD dose-response relationships. *Journal of Learning Disabilities, 31,* 608–612.

Glennon, B., & Weisz, J. (1978). An observational approach to the assessment of anxiety in young children. *Journal of Consulting and Clinical Psychology, 46,* 1246–1257.

Goodman, A., & Goodman, R. (2009). Strengths and difficulties questionnaire as a dimensional measure of child mental health. *Journal of the American Academy of Child and Adolescent Psychiatry, 48,* 400–403.

Gold, S., & Marx, P. (2006). Analogue and virtual reality assessment, chapter 4. In M. Hersen (Ed.), *Clinician's handbook of child behavioral assessment* (pp. 82–102). Burlington, MA: Elsevier Academic Press.

Haynes, S., & O'Brien, W. (2000). *Principles and practice of behavioral assessment.* New York: Kluwer/Plenum.

Johnston, C., & Mash, E. J. (1989). A measure of parenting satisfaction and efficacy. *Journal of Clinical Child Psychology, 18,* 167–175.

Kratchowill, T. (1985). Selection of target behaviors in behavioral consultation. *Behavioral Assessment, 7,* 49–61.

Lane, K. L., Little, M. A., Casey, A. M., Lambert, W., Wehby, J., Weisenbach, J. L., et al. (2009). A comparison of systematic screening tools for emotional and behavioral disorders. *Journal of Emotional and Behavioral Disorders, 17,* 93–105. doi:10.1177/1063426608326203.

Leyfer, O. T., Ruberg, J. L., & Woodruff-Borden, J. (2006). Examination of the utility of the Beck Anxiety Inventory and its factors as a screener for anxiety disorders. *Journal of Anxiety Disorders, 20,* 444–458.

McGlynn, F. D., & Rose, M. P. (1998). *Behavioral assessment: A practical handbook* (4th ed.). Needham Heights, MA: Allyn & Bacon.

McIntosh, K., Frank, J., & Spaulding, S. (2010). Establishing research-based trajectories of office disciple referrals for individual students. *School Psychology Review, 39,* 380–394.

McKinney, C., & Morse, M. (2012). Assessment of disruptive behavior disorders: Tools and recommendations. *Professional Psychology: Research and Practice, 43*(6), 641–649. doi:10.1037/a0027324.

McLeod, B., Jensen-Doss, A., & Ollendick, T. (2013). *Diagnostic and behavioral assessment in children and adolescents.* New York: Guilford Press.

Mori, L., & Armendariz, G. (2001). Analogue assessment of child behavior problems. *Psychological Assessment, 13,* 36–45.

Osit, M. (2008). *Generation text: Raising well-adjusted kids in an age of instant everything.* New York: Amazon.

Penney, S., & Skilling, T. (2012). Moderators of informant agreement in the assessment of adolescent psychopathology: Extension to a forensic sample. *Psychological Assessment, 24,* 386–401.

Phillips, M., & Gross, A. (2010). Children. Chapter 18. In D. Segal & M. Hersen (Eds.), *Diagnostic interviewing* (4th ed., pp. 423–441). New York: Springer.

Pritchett, R., Kemp, J., Wilson, P., Minnis, H., et al. (2011). Quick, simple measures of family relationships for use in clinical practice and research. A systemic review. *Family Practice, 28,* 172–187.

Radley, K., & Ford, B. (2013). Developing a self-monitoring intervention—2013. Retrieved October 28, 2013, from https://www.mcconference.net

Rhule, D. M., McMahom, R. J., & Vando, J. (2009). The acceptability and representativeness of standardized parent-child interaction tasks. *Behavior Therapy, 40,* 393–402.

Riley-Tillman, T. C., Kalberer, S. M., & Chafouleas, S. M. (2005). Selecting the right tool for the job: A review of behavior monitoring tools used to assess student response to interventions. *The California School Psychologist, 10*, 81–91.

Robin, A., & Foster, S. (2002). *Negotiating parent-adolescent conflict: A behavioral-family systems approach*. New York: The Guilford Press.

Salari, R., Terreros, C., & Sarkadi, A. (2012). Parenting scale: Which version should we use? *Journal of Psychopathology and Behavioral Assessment, 34*, 268–281.

Schlientz, M., Riley-Tillman, T., Walcott, C., Briesch, A., & Chafouleas, S. (2009). The impact of training on the accuracy of Direct Behavior Ratings (DBR). *School Psychology Quarterly, 24*(2), 73–83.

Silverman, W. K., & Ollendick, T. H. (2005). Evidence-based assessment of anxiety and its disorders in children and adolescents. *Journal of Clinical Child and Adolescent Psychology, 34*, 380–411. doi:10.1207/s15374424jccp3403_2.

Silverman, W., & Serafini, L. (1998). Assessment of child behavior problems: Internalizing disorders. Chapter 16. In A. Bellack & M. Hersen (Eds.), *Behavioral assessment: A practical handbook* (4th ed., pp. 342–360). New York: Allyn & Bacon.

Wakschlag, L., Briggs-Gowan, M., Hill, C., Danis, B., Leventhal, B., et al. (2008). Observational assessment of preschool disruptive behavior, part II: Validity of the Disruptive Behavior Diagnostic Observation Schedule (DB_DOS). *Journal of the American Academy of Child and Adolescent Psychiatry, 47*, 632–641.

Wakschlag, L., Leventhal, B., Briggs-Gowan, M., Danis, B., et al. (2005). Defining the "disruptive" in preschool behavior: What diagnostic observation can teach us. *Clinical Child and Family Psychology Review, 8*, 183–202.

Part II
Childhood Disorders

Chapter 3
Anxiety in Youth: Assessment, Treatment, and School-Based Service Delivery

Kristy A. Ludwig, Aaron R. Lyon, and Julie L. Ryan

Anxiety is a natural, protective, and normal part of childhood. Temporary fears are developmentally typical; however, fears and worries that persist and impair functioning may be indicative of an anxiety disorder (Muris, Merckelbach, Mayer, & Prins, 2000). Anxiety disorders are the most common mental health problem in children and youth and are a significant source of distress for those afflicted (Costello, Mustillo, Erkanli, Keeler, & Angold, 2003; Merikangas et al., 2011).

Untreated anxiety disorders are associated with poor school, social, and work functioning (Albano & Detweiler, 2001; Rapee, Schniering, & Hudson, 2009; Fergusson & Woodward, 2002; Ialongo, Edelson, Werthamer-Larsson, Crockett, & Kellam, 1996; McLoone, Hudson, & Rapee, 2006). Persistent, impairing, and untreated anxiety in childhood and adolescence tends to run a chronic course, with severe long-term consequences including difficulties in life-stage transitions, underemployment, substance abuse, suicidality, and comorbid psychiatric disorders (Bittner et al., 2007; Fergusson & Woodward, 2002; Gregory et al., 2007; Kendall, Safford, Flannery-Schroeder, & Webb, 2004; Kessler, 2003; Olfson et al., 2000; Pine, Cohen, Gurley, Brook, & Ma, 1998; Schneier, Johnson, Hornig, Liebowitz, & Weissman, 1992; Stein & Stein, 2008; Turner, Beidel, Dancu, & Keys, 1986; Wittchen, Lieb, Wunderlich, & Schuster, 1999).

Anxiety in youth can be difficult to detect, and as a result, many young people go without treatment. Unlike externalizing disorders, anxiety is often unrecognized by parents and teachers. Children and adolescents may not disclose their fears and

K.A. Ludwig, Ph.D. (✉) • A.R. Lyon, Ph.D.
Department of Psychiatry and Behavioral Sciences, University of Washington
School of Medicine, Seattle, WA, USA
e-mail: ludwik01@uw.edu; lyona@uw.edu

J.L. Ryan, Ph.D.
School of Psychology, Fairleigh Dickinson University, Teaneck, NJ, USA
e-mail: julieryanphd@gmail.com

© Springer Science+Business Media New York 2015
R. Flanagan et al. (eds.), *Cognitive and Behavioral Interventions in the Schools*, DOI 10.1007/978-1-4939-1972-7_3

worries and their distress is not always apparent or disruptive to those around them. For example, families and teachers may view shyness or social inhibition as part of normal development or may misattribute anxiety-driven perfectionism to healthy conscientiousness. Even with advances in the identification of mental health problems, the majority of young people needing mental health services do not receive them (Kataoka, Zhang, & Wells, 2002). Those who do receive care are most likely to do so in schools, making the educational setting a particularly crucial entry point for the identification and treatment of youth-based anxiety (Farmer, Burns, Phillips, Angold, & Costello, 2003; Lyon et al., 2013). Results of the National Comorbidity Survey found that fewer than 20 % of adolescents with anxiety disorders receive treatment (Merikangas et al., 2011). In addition, fewer than 20 % of those accessing mental health services receive empirically based interventions (Collins, Westra, Dozois, & Burns, 2004; Masia Warner, Fisher, Shrout, Rathor, & Klein, 2007). Social, interpersonal, or family problems are the most common reason for the receipt of mental health services in schools for youth of either gender; anxiety and adjustment issues are the second most common problem for female students (Foster & Connor, 2005).

Presenting Problems at Home and School

Anxiety is often experienced cognitively as perfectionistic preoccupations, worry, rumination, fears, and/or obsessive thoughts. Many people develop escape or avoidance patterns to manage anxiety symptoms. The associated avoidance and distress of anxiety can impair typical social interactions and development and interfere with academic performance. Anxious youth who refuse to participate in social activities or attend school may be miscategorized by parents or teachers as oppositional, lazy, or noncompliant. For example, a phobic second grader may refuse to go to recess because he is severely afraid of bees, or a senior in high school may not apply to college because she is too fearful to go to her school counselor to obtain the needed transcripts. While the problematic behavior may be overt (e.g., acting up to have to stay in during recess or not applying to college), the underlying fear and impairment is not always apparent. The list below provides guidelines for "red-flag" behaviors that might suggest the appropriateness for assessment of underlying anxiety symptoms:

Behaviors suggestive of anxiety more likely to be observed at home:

- Seeking excessive reassurance, asking the same questions repetitively, and/or asking a lot of "what if" questions.
- Demonstrating excessive avoidance (i.e., refuses to attend school, birthday parties, family gatherings, and other expected and age-appropriate activities).
- Unrealistic or impairingly high standards (e.g., nothing is good enough).
- Anticipatory anxiety where the child/adolescent worries days, weeks, or months in advance of events.
- Fears interfering with the child's and/or family's life; substantial time is spent managing or consoling a child who is upset.

- Excessive stress reactions that seem out of proportion to situations.
- Somatic complaints such as frequent headaches and stomachaches, often feeling too sick to attend school or social events.
- Sleep disruptions, including difficulty falling asleep and frequent nightmares.

Behaviors suggestive of anxiety more likely to be observed at school:

- Difficulty with concentration
- Avoiding reading aloud, raising hand, answering questions in class
- Not going to counselor or teacher with questions or problems related to homework, classes, schedule, bullying, or college process (may or may not have parent call school staff on their behalf)
- Not eating in front of others in cafeteria, in some cases avoiding the cafeteria entirely and going to classrooms or library during lunch
- Not using school bathrooms
- Appearing isolated and on the fringes of the group—e.g., sitting with a group of people in cafeteria or standing near a group at recess but not participating; may attend group/team meetings but will not participate (often more likely to participate in individual sports—cross country, swimming—and/or small clubs that are also attended by close friends)
- Regularly visiting the nurse or school counselor
- Excessive absences from school (even when excused by parent)
- Always early to class/school, experiences extreme anxiety, and/or will not go if late
- Avoids eye contact, may appear as being "stuck up" or socially awkward
- Resistant to taking more challenging classes when encouraged and academically capable
- Excessive time spent on homework and studying due to excessive concerns about poor performance
- Excessively checking grades or redoes assignments and asks same questions repeatedly to different or same people

Developmental Issues Impacting Diagnosis and Treatment

Ninety percent of all children report at least one fear and those fears often change over time (Pincus, 2012). In young children, fears may be associated with separation from caregivers or specific phobias. In school-age children, typical fears often focus on concerns surrounding health, safety, and competence. Teenagers' most frequent fears are commonly related to social interactions and the future. Clinical levels of anxiety tend to map onto this progression of typical fears in a manner consistent with child and adolescent cognitive developments (i.e., moving from concrete fears when they are young to more abstract fears as they grow older). For this reason, it is often more important to consider the process—rather than the content—of the fear when differentiating what is normative versus clinically salient.

For example, it is important to consider the frequency and intensity of the fear and worry, the amount of time spent focused on or recovering from the associated distress, and the level of interference to the child and family functioning when identifying clinical levels of anxiety. Typical fears will become less evident over time, whereas problematic fear and anxiety may change in content (i.e., fears associated with separation may move into fears associated with social situations) but increase in frequency, intensity, and impairment.

If parents and teachers are concerned about a child/adolescent, they should refer the child to a mental health clinician for a diagnostic evaluation and possible treatment. This may occur in either the school or community setting, depending on service availability. When detected early, targeted interventions are very helpful in providing young people with the tools and coping skills necessary to understand and effectively manage anxiety.

Assessment Considerations

The DSM-5 (American Psychiatric Association, 2013) allows for youth anxiety diagnoses of specific phobia, separation anxiety disorder, selective mutism, generalized anxiety disorder (GAD), social anxiety disorder (SAD), panic disorder (PD), agoraphobia, or other specified anxiety disorder/unspecified anxiety disorder. Despite the specific diagnosis, anxiety disorders are associated with cognitive, behavioral, and physiological reactions that interfere with functioning. Anxiety diagnoses differ from one another based on the focus of the anxiety. Despite high comorbidity among anxiety disorders, important diagnostic differences are evident. *Separation anxiety*, for instance, is associated with a fear of separation from a parent/caregiver during which children often worry about the safety and welfare of their parent. *Generalized anxiety disorder* (GAD) is associated with worries about health, family, future, and related physical and cognitive complaints (i.e., difficulty concentrating, muscle tightness, difficulty sleeping). Children experiencing GAD have difficulties with uncertainty and will often repeatedly seek reassurance to feel momentarily less anxious. For example, a child may continually pester their parent about the weather forecast and how it may impact their weekend beach plans. *Social anxiety*, or social phobia, is associated with a fear of social situations and evaluation by others. Children with social anxiety often avoid, or experience with great distress, social situations such as answering a question in class, attending birthday parties, inviting a friend to get together, and eating in the school cafeteria. *Panic disorder* involves a sudden onset of physical anxiety symptoms and a fear of them happening again in the future. Although many adolescents (and adults) experience panic attacks, it is the fear of having another attack and the avoidance of associated situations, substances, and places that lead to a diagnosis of panic disorder. A *specific phobia*, on the other hand, is an extreme and intense anxiety reaction related to a specific organism or situation (i.e. flying, heights, water, dogs, spiders, needles). *Agoraphobia* is when an individual experiences panic symptoms in a crowded place and fears they will not be able to escape. *Other specified anxiety disorder or unspecified anxiety disorder* is diagnosed when a child is experiencing anxiety that is clearly impairing but does not meet the full criteria for any anxiety disorder.

Diagnostic differentiation can be very challenging when assessing anxiety. Studies have estimated between 40 and 60 % of children with an anxiety disorder are diagnosed with more than one anxiety disorder (Benjamin, Costello, & Warren, 1990; Kashani & Orvaschel, 1990; Last, Strauss, & Francis, 1987). Anxiety disorders can co-occur with other anxiety disorders as well as with other common childhood mental health disorders, such as depression (Brady & Kendall, 1992). Some of the common conditions requiring a differential diagnosis are discussed below.

Attention-Deficit Hyperactivity Disorder (ADHD)

Attentional difficulties are often a symptom of anxiety. However, it is important to distinguish whether these difficulties are due to anxiety, attention-deficit hyperactivity disorder (ADHD), or both. In distinguishing anxiety symptoms from ADHD, it is important to thoroughly assess additional anxiety and ADHD symptoms. A sudden onset of inattention starting in middle school or inattention in one setting and not others could be more indicative of an anxiety disorder. Chapter 8 provides additional information on the assessment and treatment of ADHD in schools.

Autism Spectrum Disorders

In evaluating a child that "shies" away from social situations, it is important to distinguish a fear of negative evaluation from a lack of interest in making social connections. The latter may or may not be more *indicative* of an autism spectrum disorder (ASD). In addition, some young people on the spectrum are not interested in the variety of activities and topics that are engaging to their peers, and this may manifest as perseveration on a single area of interest. Unlike perseveration in OCD or other anxiety disorders, the function of which may be to relieve discomfort, children with ASD often perseverate on topics or activities because the perseveration is soothing or pleasurable. Although children with ASD often lack social skills, their skill deficits often differ from those with social anxiety. Skill deficits more common to ASD include speaking too loudly, speaking without inflection, and a lack of social reciprocity (e.g., not allowing the conversational partner a turn to speak) (see Chap. 10 for additional discussion and see Rogers & Vismara, 2008; Eldevik et al., 2009, for additional information).

Eating Disorders

Anxiety is commonly associated with eating disorders. If fear and avoidance of eating is primary and associated with excessive concerns about weight gain and/or control over body shape and weight, an eating disorder diagnosis may be warranted. An anxiety disorder may be present if anxiety symptoms exist prior to the onset of an eating disorder or if the scope of a child's or adolescent's anxiety extends beyond fears associated with eating, appearance, food, body shape, and weight gain (see Mash & Hunsley, 2005 or Keel & Haedt, 2008, for additional information on treatment and assessment of eating disorders).

Depression

Depression often accompanies anxiety. Evidence suggests that childhood anxiety disorders often precede depressive symptoms and disorders (Bittner et al., 2007; Pine et al., 1998). Symptoms such as attention difficulties, irritability, and difficulty sleeping are symptoms consistent with both anxiety and depression. (See Chap. 5 for further detailed information.)

Anxiety Disorders

Even across anxiety disorders many symptoms are similar. Specific symptoms including the content of the fears/worries and associated cognitions or behaviors may help distinguish among anxiety disorders and determine the presence of comorbidities. Worries and rumination, for instance, are more typical of GAD whereas obsessions or mental rituals are more typical of OCD. If worries and ruminations are focused on a specific topic (e.g., separating from a parent, social mistakes made the previous day), they may be indicative of an anxiety disorder other than GAD (i.e., separation anxiety or social anxiety). Finally, although trauma commonly results in anxiety, symptoms must result from—or increase following—a specific traumatic event to indicate the presence of PTSD .

Treatment and Case Conceptualization

Over the last 20 years, much has been learned about the diagnosis and treatment of anxiety disorders. Research has revealed the serious and stable course of anxiety disorders across the life span (Albano & Kendall, 2002). The resulting negative effects on long-term emotional development and functioning can be ameliorated and often prevented with effective anxiety treatment in childhood and adolescence (Saavedra, Silverman, Morgan-Lopez, & Kurtines, 2010; Kendall, Safford, Flannery-Schroeder, & Webb, 2004; Kendall & Southam-Gerow, 1996). Due to its documented efficacy and effectiveness, cognitive behavioral therapy (CBT) should be considered a first-line treatment for childhood anxiety disorders (Compton et al., 2004).

Case conceptualization of anxiety within a CBT model requires the identification of maladaptive and cyclical interactions between threat-laden thoughts, feelings, and behaviors (Demertzis & Craske, 2012). Children who attempt to relieve their fear and distress through avoidance or safety behaviors may become stuck in a cycle of momentary relief followed by increasing levels of anxiety, distress, and subsequent avoidance. CBT involves interventions that interrupt this problematic cycle by addressing anxiety-provoking thoughts, feelings, and behaviors. CBT typically consists of five primary components including psychoeducation, relaxation strategies, cognitive restructuring, exposure therapy, and relapse prevention (Albano & Kendall, 2002; Demertzis & Craske, 2012). For a detailed description of these components, please see Chaps. 13 and 14.

Regardless of the child's age, CBT is the most effective treatment for anxiety disorders. A significant challenge to implementing CBT for anxiety is the misconception that the child cannot handle the distress associated with the anxiety-provoking stimuli or situation. Psychoeducation regarding how the cycle of anxiety is maintained and the demonstration of exposure exercises can increase motivation for both the child and the parent. Similarly, psychoeducation for teachers may be important to the success of interventions delivered in a school setting (Ryan & Warner, 2012).

That being said, parental involvement is paramount for treatment success outside of the therapy room. While the intensity of parental involvement and choice of specific techniques may vary depending upon the child's age and developmental level, the overall strategies used in treatment are the same. Preschool-age children may have a more difficult time identifying their fearful thoughts and may benefit less from cognitive restructuring than older children. Younger children may also need more parental assistance during exposure than teenagers. Developmental adjustments aside, most children are likely to benefit from facing their fears in a structured and supported fashion. The following case study is an example of how CBT can be helpful with a school-age child with integral parental and teacher support.

Case Example

Clifford is a 7-year-old 1st grader who had great difficulty separating from his mother at school in the morning. He cried before school, complained about going to school, and resisted dressing and leaving the house. He said he was too scared to go to school and pleaded to stay home. Once at school, his mother would walk him to the classroom door; he would cry, hang on to her, and plead for her to stay. This often went on for up to an hour. Often, his mother would stay in school for most of the morning; or, when she was able to leave with the teacher's help, his mother would leave feeling drained and worried. Clifford's parents and teacher agreed it was important for Clifford and his parents to seek help from the school-based mental health counselor. The initial assessment revealed that Clifford also refused to attend drop-off birthday parties and play dates, would not go upstairs at his house without a parent or sibling, and refused to fall asleep in his room without a parent in the room. After he recovered from the morning drop-off at school, he was a leader among his peers, participated in class, and comfortably interacted with and was well liked by the other children in his class. At restaurants he ordered his own food and enjoyed meeting new kids and playing with them when he went with his mom to the park. The diagnostic assessment conducted using the parent version of the Anxiety Disorders Interview Schedule (ADIS) (Silverman & Albano, 1996) indicated that Clifford met the criteria for separation anxiety disorder. Treatment began with psychoeducation for Clifford, his parents, and his teacher about the relationship between his thoughts ("maybe something bad will happen to my mom when I'm at school"; "what if I need my mom when I'm at school and she is not here"), feelings (scared, panicked), and behaviors (do whatever possible to avoid having to be away from mom), relaxation strategies (deep breathing, progressive muscle relaxation), and the creation of a fear hierarchy in preparation for exposure. This was followed by some age-appropriate cognitive restructuring (e.g., *STOP*—recognizing when you are *S*cared, identify the *T*houghts that make you feel anxious, identify *O*ther things to think or do to feel less anxious, and *P*raise self for completing the steps; Chorpita, 2007) and coping thoughts (e.g., "I am scared but I can do this"; "it's only a false alarm in my body"; "brave is being afraid and doing it anyway") but moved quickly into conducting exposure associated with separation from his parents with the involvement of his classroom teacher. A recent study found that introducing exposure earlier in treatment resulted in reducing anxiety symptoms and associated impairment in fewer sessions (Gryczkowski et al., 2013).

Exposures to the distressing situations were sequenced to gradually increase the level of fear and distress Clifford experienced and to maximize the likelihood of his success. Exposure to separation at school began with Clifford's mom walking him to his classroom, having the teacher take his hand and help him stay in the classroom, while his mother quickly left regardless of his distressed reaction. In time, this was followed by having his mother walking Clifford to the classroom and having him walk into the classroom on his own, then to dropping him off in the car line with his teacher meeting him to walk him into school, and finally having his mom drop Clifford off in the car line and walking into school by himself. Once Clifford was going to school without difficulty, Clifford's parents gradually conducted exposure related to Clifford falling asleep on his own. They would stay in his bedroom with him for decreasing amounts of time and then sit outside the door for a designated period of time until finally Clifford could stay in his bed and fall asleep without his parents needing to be nearby. As Clifford had increasing success at different steps of his exposure ladder (hierarchy), he became increasingly brave in other areas of his life. Without having to address other fears directly, Clifford began wanting to go to play dates at the neighbor's house and then wanted to attend a drop-off birthday party. Throughout treatment, Clifford's parents and teachers were coached on how to respond most effectively to help Clifford overcome his anxiety. His parents and teacher were instructed to limit their reassurance, reinforce brave behavior with specific praise and tangible rewards, and convey confidence in Clifford's ability to handle the separation. At the conclusion of treatment, Clifford, his therapist, and his parents created a relapse prevention plan incorporating all the tools Clifford learned in treatment and a discussion on addressing any additional anxiety or associated distress in the future.

Delivering Evidence-Based Practices for Anxiety to Youth in Schools

Although the majority of school-based mental health interventions have focused on externalizing behaviors (Forman & Barakat, 2011; Hoagwood et al., 2007), schools provide important opportunities for the identification and treatment of internalizing problems. This is particularly true as many common anxiety-provoking stressors occur in the school environment (e.g., peer interactions, performance situations), and schools are one of the primary settings in which youth are likely to exhibit impairment (Ginsburg, Becker, Kingery, & Nichols, 2008). Moreover, schools provide access to youth who may not otherwise seek treatment in a traditional mental health specialty clinic (Adelman & Taylor, 1999; Weist, 1997; Anglin, 2003; Ryan & Warner, 2012). Incorporating mental health treatment into schools also has the added potential to decrease the stigma regarding mental illness. A meta-analysis of school-based mental health programs for low-income, urban youth revealed that programs targeting internalizing problems and those that had a universal focus were generally effective (Farahmand, Grant, Polo, & Duffy, 2011). This finding contrasted with school-based interventions for externalizing problems among the same population, which were found to be ineffective or, in some cases, iatrogenic. These results are consistent with a meta-analysis of school social work interventions, which found more positive effects for education-sector programs that addressed internalizing problems rather than externalizing problems (Franklin, Kim, & Tripodi, 2009).

Despite the existence of multiple intervention protocols with demonstrated efficacy for treating anxiety in youth (Silverman, Pina, & Viswesvaran, 2008), fewer well-researched interventions have been developed or adapted to address anxiety disorders in schools. Most of the interventions that have been researched in schools are delivered in group format. PracticeWise (www.practicewise.com) has developed a regularly updated, searchable Evidence-Based Services database (PWEBS) which synthesizes hundreds of randomized clinical trials of treatments for children's mental health problems to inform clinical decision making in children's mental health (PracticeWise, 2013). A variety of search parameters can be included, such as presenting problem, age, ethnicity, level of empirical support, and treatment setting. A search of PWEBS for effective anxiety treatments that have been tested in schools, and which demonstrate "Good Support or Better" outcomes (i.e., "Level 2"—see Chorpita & Daleiden, 2007 for specific criteria; Level 2 is similar to the American

Psychological Association's operationalization of a "probably efficacious" intervention Chorpita et al., 2002), indicated that 84 % of the treatments tested in the education sector have been group based. This finding contrasts sharply with more traditional clinic settings, where only 29 % of the interventions have been group based. This difference suggests that there may be characteristics of the school setting (e.g., large numbers of young people in requiring services and the need to adapt to the school schedule) that cause researchers and service providers to consider alternatives to individual service delivery.

Some of the most significant work related to the treatment of anxiety in schools and the implementation of effective interventions has been done in the context of child/adolescent trauma (Kataoka et al., 2011; Kataoka et al., 2003; Langley, Nadeem, Kataoka, Stein, & Jaycox, 2010). These interventions are discussed elsewhere in this volume (see Chap. 4). Below, we discuss additional approaches for delivering evidence-based interventions for youth anxiety in schools. Although a number of anxiety prevention programs have also been developed for use in schools (Lowry-Webster, Barrett, & Lock, 2003) and targeting test anxiety (Aydin & Yerin, 1994), those programs are not included as they are beyond the scope of this chapter and its focus on interventions for clinically significant anxiety in youth.

Manualized Treatment Protocols

The majority of anxiety interventions for youth have been tested in settings other than schools. Nevertheless, a number of well-articulated protocols are available that have been developed or adapted for and tested in the education sector. These include structured intervention protocols delivered to individuals or groups and school-based implementations of emerging modularized or "common elements" approaches to psychotherapy.

Group Manualized Treatments

Groups are the most common intervention modality for the effective treatment of anxiety in schools; multiple group treatment protocols have been developed—or, more commonly, adapted for existing interventions—and then tested in the education sector (see Table 3.1 for an overview). Masia Warner and colleagues (Fisher et al., 2004; Masia et al., 1999; Masia Warner et al., 2005; Masia Warner et al., 2007) developed the Skills for Academic and Social Success (SASS) protocol. This 12-session protocol was derived from the Social Effectiveness Therapy for Children (SET-C; Beidel et al., 1998) but was adapted to match the unique characteristics of the school setting (e.g., intervention timing, use of peers and teachers in addition to parents). The SASS intervention includes five core components: (1) psychoeducation, (2) realistic thinking, (3) social skills training, (4) exposure, and (5) relapse prevention. In one study of SASS versus an attention control, Masia Warner et al. (2007) found that 59 % of

Table 3.1 Research findings for group format anxiety interventions in schools

Researchers	Sample	Treatment conditions	Outcome measure(s)	Findings	Follow-up data
Constantino et al. (1994)	N=90 Hispanic/Latino children/adolescents (9–13 years) with symptoms of anxiety, conduct, or phobic disorders (randomized to two conditions)	(1) Group storytelling intervention (based on images from the Tell Me a Story, TEMAS)	Symptom Check List (SCL-90), Anxiety and Phobia Symptom scales	Between-group differences identified on anxiety and school conduct, but not depression	None
		(2) Movies and educational discussion of plots/content	Center for Epidemiologic Studies Depression Scale (CES-D)	Most effects were only significant for 6th graders (and not for 4th or 5th graders)	
			Connors' Teacher Behavior Rating Scale (BRS)		
Ginsburg and Drake (2002)	N=12 African American adolescents (14–17 years) with diagnosed DSM-IV anxiety disorders (randomized to two conditions)	(1) Group CBT	Anxiety Disorders Interview Schedule (ADIS) for DSM-IV Child Version Impairment ratings (0–8)	Fewer adolescents in the CBT group met diagnostic criteria at posttreatment than in the control condition and greater improvement on the SCARED	None
		(2) Anxiety Support Group	Self-Report for Childhood Anxiety Related Emotional Disorders (SCARED)		
			Social Anxiety Scale for Adolescents (SAS-A)		

(continued)

Table 3.1 (continued)

Researchers	Sample	Treatment conditions	Outcome measure(s)	Findings	Follow-up data
Manassis et al. (2010)	$N = 148$ (grades 3–5) who screened high on the MASC or CDI. Fifty-seven percent Caucasian (randomized to two conditions)	(1) 12-week group CBT group	Anxiety Disorders Interview Schedule	Participants in both conditions improved, but there was no added benefit for the CBT group.	1-year follow-up: nonsignificant trend toward fewer children meeting diagnostic criteria for an anxiety disorder on the Anxiety Disorders Interview Schedule
		(2) Structured, after-school condition	Children's Depression Inventory (CDI)		
			Multidimensional Anxiety Scale for Children (MASC)		
			Child Behavior Checklist (CBCL)		
Masia Warner et al. (2005)	$N = 35$ (13–17 years) with a diagnosis of Social Anxiety Disorder or another anxiety disorder. Participants were 83 % Caucasian (randomized to two conditions)	(1) Skills for Social and Academic Success (SASS)	ADIS Parent and Child Versions (ADIS-PC)	The majority of students in the treatment group (67 %) no longer met social phobia diagnostic criteria at follow-up vs. few from the wait-list condition (6 %). Adolescents in the treatment group also demonstrated greater reductions in social anxiety and avoidance and improved overall functioning.	9-month follow-up with a subset of the intervention group indicated that gains were maintained
		(2) Wait-list control	Severity rating		
			CDI		
			Children's Global Assessment Scale (CGAS)		
			Liebowitz Social Anxiety Scale for Children and Adolescents (LSAS-CA)		
			Loneliness Scale (LS)		
			SAS-A		
			Social Anxiety Scale for Adolescents: Parent Version (SAS-AP)		
			Social Phobia and Anxiety Inventory for Children (SPAI-C)		
			Social Phobic Disorders Severity and Change Form (SPDSCF)		

Masia Warner et al. (2007)	N = 36 (14–16 years) Primary diagnosis of Social Anxiety Disorder (randomized to two conditions)	(1) Skills for Social and Academic Success (SASS) (2) Attention Control (Educational Supportive Group)	ADIS Parent and Child Versions Severity Rating Beck Depression Inventory-II (BDI) CGAS Clinical Global Impressions Scale—Improvement (CGI-I) Parent and Adolescent Clinical Global Impressions Social Phobia and Anxiety Inventory for Children (SPAI-C) SAS-A SAS-AP	The majority of students in the treatment group (59 %) no longer met social anxiety disorder diagnostic criteria at follow-up vs. none from the wait-list condition. Superiority of the SASS condition was also evident on measures of social phobia severity, depression, and overall functioning.	6-month follow-up indicated that clinical improvements were maintained
Muris et al. (2002)	N = 30 (9–12 years) with elevated RCADS subscales or total scores (Twenty children were randomized to condition 1 or 2. An additional 10 children were recruited for the wait-list condition)	(1) Group CBT (2) Emotional Disclosure placebo (3) Wait list	Revised Children's Anxiety and Depression Scale (RCADS) State-Trait Anxiety Inventory for Children (STAIC) Trait Anxiety Scale	CBT was found to be superior to emotional disclosure and wait-list control at posttreatment for reductions of anxiety symptoms, train anxiety, and depression.	None

active-intervention participants no longer met criteria for social anxiety disorder following treatment, compared to 0 % in the control group.

Ginsburg and Drake (2002) adapted a cognitive behavioral therapy (CBT) group intervention for use in schools to treat anxiety disorders (excluding OCD and trauma) in African American adolescents aged 14–17. Adaptations were made to reduce session length and number and to make the protocol developmentally and culturally appropriate, but core CBT elements were retained including psychoeducation, relaxation, cognitive restructuring, and exposure. The authors reported using the protocol with a small group of students ($n = 12$) assigned to either the CBT intervention or an attention-support control. Results indicated that the CBT group demonstrated greater gains in symptom reduction and diagnostic status.

Other examples of group-based school interventions for youth anxiety include the Feelings Club group intervention (Manassis et al., 2010) and culturally specific anxiety interventions (Constantino et al., 1994).

Individual Manualized Treatments

A number of individually focused interventions for child and adolescent anxiety disorders have been developed and tested—although primarily outside of school settings—based on CBT principles and techniques. Even outside the school setting, no *well-established* interventions exist for youth anxiety using the criteria outlined by Chambless and Hollon (1998; Silverman et al., 2008); criteria include at least two independent, rigorous, group-designed experiments demonstrating superiority to a control or equivalence to an existing established treatment. Nevertheless, a variety of interventions have received strong empirical support and some interventions have been evaluated in the education sector, albeit in small-scale feasibility trials.

One widely researched youth anxiety CBT intervention, Coping Cat (CC), has been extensively tested in more traditional clinic settings (Kendall, 1994; Silverman et al., 2008). Although a recent, high-quality description of an effective method of training school-based clinicians in the CC model exists (Beidas et al., 2012), no studies have tested the protocol in schools. Similarly, an Australian adaptation of Coping Cat—Cool Kids—has a school version that has demonstrated feasibility for use in schools but has yet to be extensively tested (McLoone & Rapee, 2012). Overall, these studies and others suggest that the delivery of individual CBT for youth anxiety in schools, although promising, would benefit from additional study (Ginsburg et al., 2008).

Modular Interventions

Youth who experience anxiety frequently present with problems in other domains as well (e.g., depression, oppositional behavior) and such comorbidity appears to be associated with higher impairment in school functioning (Kendall, Brady, &

Verduin, 2001; Kendall, Kortlander, Chansky, & Brady, 1992; Mychailyszyn, Mendez, & Kendall, 2010). These findings underscore the need for interventions that can be responsive to the needs of diverse client populations, rather than single diagnoses. To address this reality, multiple authors have suggested that modular approaches to the organization and delivery of intervention content may be particularly appropriate for use in schools (Lyon, Charlseworth-Attie, Vander Stoep, & McCauley, 2011; Stephan, Wissow, & Pichler, 2010; Weist et al., 2009). Modular psychotherapy has been defined as involving "self-contained functional units [modules] that connect with other units, but do not rely on those other units for their own stable operations" (Chorpita, Daleiden, & Weisz, 2005). In this way, modular approaches have the potential to be more flexible than traditional manualized treatment protocols, which may be/are more compatible with the characteristics of the unpredictable school environment (Lyon et al., 2013). Recent evidence has demonstrated the superiority of a modular intervention to both standard-arranged manuals and usual care for youth receiving services in both clinic and school settings (Weisz et al., 2012).

Trials of modular interventions that were specific to schools for a full range of youth mental health problems have been described, and some researchers have examined the use of modular protocols for treating anxiety or internalizing problems (Stephan et al., 2010; Weist et al., 2009). Lyon and colleagues (2011) trained a small group of school-based clinicians to use a modular approach to treat children and adolescents with primary problems of anxiety or depression and found that participating clinicians were able to effectively select and use modules in the context of ongoing progress monitoring. Similarly, Becker, Becker, and Ginsberg (2012) described the use of a school-based modular approach that was specific to anxiety (including seven modules: psychoeducation, exposure, cognitive restructuring, contingency management, problem solving, relaxation, and relapse prevention). They found that trained practitioners delivered the exposure module most frequently with their clients, followed by psychoeducation and cognitive restructuring. Despite these promising findings, additional research is needed related to the effectiveness of modular approaches to augment existing feasibility studies.

Implementation and Service Delivery Issues

The identification and development of a number of practices that appear to have utility in the treatment of youth anxiety in schools is ongoing, but similar to other service delivery contexts, the routine use of these practices in schools is uncommon (Evans & Weist, 2004). It has been suggested that research devoted to understanding implementation processes in SBMH has lagged behind implementation research in the larger mental health field (Lyon, McCauley, & Vander Stoep, 2011). Nevertheless, recent studies indicate that many of the most significant implementation issues encountered in schools are similar to those in the broader literature. Forman and Bakarat (2011), for example, reviewed studies that implemented cognitive behavioral interventions for youth mental health in schools and found that the factors most frequently identified were organizational structure, program characteristics, fit with school goals, policies and program, training/technical assistance, and administrator support. Furthermore, they articulated three overarching characteristics of implementation initiatives related to success: (1) characteristics of the innovation being implemented (e.g., relative advantage over current practices), (2) characteristics of the implementer (e.g., attitudes/beliefs, knowledge), and (3) characteristics of the organization (e.g., organizational climate). These factors, interactions among them, and the specific importance of organization-level processes have been repeatedly echoed throughout the implementation literature (e.g., Aarons, Hurlburt, & Horwitz, 2011; Beidas & Kendall, 2010; Fixsen, Naoom, Blase, Friedman, & Wallace, 2005).

Summary

Anxiety disorders are the most common type of psychiatric disorder in childhood and can negatively impact functioning and development into adulthood. Although anxiety disorders are often less overt and observable than externalizing disorders, specific behaviors (outlined above) at home and school are indicative of anxiety symptoms. Diagnosis and treatment in childhood and adolescence can prevent the chronic course and negative long-term consequences associated with untreated anxiety. CBT has the most evidence for effective treatment results and is currently a first-line treatment for anxiety disorders in children and adolescents.

Given the large number of young people suffering with anxiety disorders, schools provide an optimal access point for the delivery of mental health treatment. As a place that the child's functioning can be assessed across contexts, schools are a particularly ideal setting for both identification and intervention. Research has indicated that school-based interventions (primarily groups) for anxiety disorders can be effective. This chapter highlighted the current research on group and individual approaches to the delivery of evidence-based interventions for the treatment of youth anxiety in schools and the need for continued research and practice focused on expanded implementation of effective practices across settings.

References

Aarons, G., Hurlburt, M., & Horwitz, S. (2011). Advancing a conceptual model of evidence-based practice implementation in child welfare. *Administration and Policy in Mental Health, 38,* 4–23.

Adelman, H. S., & Taylor, L. (1999). Mental health in schools and system restructuring. *Clinical Psychology Review, 19*(2), 137–163.

Albano, A. M., & Detweiler, M. F. (2001). The developmental and clinical impact of social anxiety and social phobia in children and adolescents. In S. G. Hofmann & P. M. DiBartolo (Eds.), *From social anxiety to social phobia: Multiple perspectives* (pp. 162–178). Needham Heights, MA: Allyn and Bacon

Albano, A. M., & Kendall, P. C. (2002). Cognitive behavioural therapy for children and adolescents with anxiety disorders: Clinical research advances. *International Review of Psychiatry, 14*(2), 129–134.

American Psychiatric Association. (2013). *Diagnostic and statistical manual of mental disorders, fifth edition (DSM-5)*. Washington, DC: American Psychiatric Publishing.

Anglin, T. M. (2003). *Mental health in schools: Programs of the federal government*. New York: Kluwer Academic/Plenum Publishers.

Aydin, G., & Yerin, O. (1994). The effect of a story-based cognitive behavior modification procedure on reducing children's test anxiety before and after cancellation of an important examination. *International Journal for the Advancement of Counselling, 17*(2), 149–161.

Becker, E. M., Becker, K. D., & Ginsburg, G. S. (2012). Modular cognitive behavioral therapy for youth with anxiety disorders: A closer look at the use of specific modules and their relation to treatment process and response. *School Mental Health, 4*(4), 243–253.

Beidas, R. S., & Kendall, P. C. (2010). Training therapists in evidence-based practice: A critical review of studies from a systems-contextual perspective. *Clinical Psychology: Science & Practice, 17*, 1–30.

Beidas, R. S., Mychailyszyn, M. P., Edmunds, J. M., Khanna, M. S., Downey, M. M., & Kendall, P. C. (2012). Training school mental health providers to deliver cognitive-behavioral therapy. *School Mental Health*, 1–10.

Beidel, D. C., Turner, S. M., & Morris, T. L. (1998). *Social effectiveness therapy for children: A treatment manual*. Charleston: Medical University of South Carolina.

Benjamin, R. S., Costello, E. J., & Warren, M. (1990). Anxiety disorders in a pediatric sample. *Journal of Anxiety Disorders, 4*(4), 293–316.

Bittner, A., Egger, H. L., Erkanli, A., Jane Costello, E., Foley, D. L., & Angold, A. (2007). What do childhood anxiety disorders predict? *Journal of Child Psychology and Psychiatry, and Allied Disciplines, 48*(12), 1174–1183.

Brady, E. U., & Kendall, P. C. (1992). Comorbidity of anxiety and depression in children and adolescents. *Psychological Bulletin, 111*(2), 244–255.

Chambless, D. L., & Hollon, S. D. (1998). Defining empirically supported therapies. [Review]. *Journal of Consulting and Clinical Psychology, 66*(1), 7–18.

Chorpita, B. F. (2007). *Modular cognitive behavioral therapy for childhood anxiety disorders*. New York: Guilford Press.

Chorpita, B. F., & Daleiden, E. L. (2007). *Biennial report: Effective psychosocial interventions for youth with behavioral and emotional needs*. Honolulu, HI: Child and Adolescent Mental Health Division, Hawaii Department of Health.

Chorpita, B. F., Daleiden, E. L., & Weisz, J. R. (2005). Modularity in the design and application of therapeutic interventions. *Applied and Preventive Psychology, 11*(3), 141–156.

Chorpita, B. F., Yim, L. M., Donkervoet, J. C., Arensdorf, A., Amundsen, M. J., McGee, C., et al. (2002). Toward large-scale implementation of empirically supported treatments for children: A review and observations by the Hawaii Empirical Basis to Services Task Force. *Clinical Psychology: Science and Practice, 9*, 165–190.

Collins, K. A., Westra, H. A., Dozois, D. J., & Burns, D. D. (2004). Gaps in accessing treatment for anxiety and depression: Challenges for the delivery of care. [Review]. *Clinical Psychology Review, 24*(5), 583–616.

Compton, S. N., March, J. S., Brent, D., Albano, A. M., Weersing, V. R., & Curry, J. (2004). Cognitive-behavioral psychotherapy for anxiety and depressive disorders in children and adolescents: An evidence-based medicine review. *Journal of the American Academy of Child & Adolescent Psychiatry, 43*(8), 930–959.

Constantino, G., Malgady, R. G., & Rogler, L. H. (1994). Storytelling through pictures: Culturally sensitive psychotherapy for Hispanic children and adolescents. *Journal of Clinical Child Psychology, 23*(1), 13–20.

Costello, E. J., Mustillo, S., Erkanli, A., Keeler, G., & Angold, A. (2003). Prevalence and development of psychiatric disorders in childhood and adolescence. *Archives of General Psychiatry, 60*(8), 837–844.

Demertzis, K. H., & Craske, M. G. (2012). Cognitive-behavioral therapy for anxiety disorders in primary care. *Primary Psychiatry.* Retrieved from primarypsychiatry.com.

Eldevik, S., Hastings, R. P., Hughes, J. C., Jahr, E., Eikeseth, S., & Cross, C. (2009). Meta-analysis of early intensive behavioral intervention for children with autism. *Journal of Clinical Child & Adolescent Psychology, 38*(3), 439–450.

Evans, S. W., & Weist, M. D. (2004). Implementing empirically supported treatments in the schools: What are we asking? *Clinical Child and Family Psychology Review, 7*(4), 263–267.

Farahmand, F. K., Grant, K. E., Polo, A. J., & Duffy, S. N. (2011). School-based mental health and behavioral programs for low-income, urban youth: A systematic and meta-analytic review. *Clinical Psychology: Science and Practice, 18*(4), 372–390.

Farmer, E. M., Burns, B. J., Phillips, S. D., Angold, A., & Costello, E. J. (2003). Pathways into and through mental health services for children and adolescents. *Psychiatric Services, 54*(1), 60–66.

Fergusson, D. M., & Woodward, L. J. (2002). Mental health, educational, and social role outcomes of adolescents with depression. *Archives of General Psychiatry, 59*(3), 225–231.

Fisher, P. H., Wasian Warner, C., & Klein, R. G. (2004). Skills for social and academic success: A school-based intervention for social anxiety disorder in adolescents. *Clinical Child and Family Psychology Review, 7,* 241–249.

Fixsen, D. L., Naoom, S. F., Blase, K. A., Friedman, R. M., & Wallace, F. (2005). *Implementation research: A synthesis of the literature.* Tampa, FL: University of South Florida, Louis de la Parte Florida Mental Health Institute, The National Implementation Research Network.

Forman, S. G., & Barakat, N. M. (2011). Cognitive-behavioral therapy in the schools: Bringing research to practice through effective implementation. *Psychology in the Schools, 48*(3), 283–296.

Foster, E. M., & Connor, T. (2005). The public costs of better mental health services for children and adolescent. *Psychiatric Services, 56,* 50–55.

Franklin, C., Kim, J. S., & Tripodi, S. J. (2009). A meta-analysis of published school social work practice studies: 1980-2007. *Research on Social Work Practice, 19*(6), 667–677.

Ginsburg, G. S., Becker, K. D., Kingery, J. N., & Nichols, T. (2008). Transporting CBT for childhood anxiety disorders into inner-city school-based mental health clinics. *Cognitive and Behavioral Practice, 15*(2), 148–158.

Ginsburg, G. S., & Drake, K. L. (2002). School-based treatment for anxious African-American adolescents: A controlled pilot study. *Journal of the American Academy of Child and Adolescent Psychiatry, 41,* 768–775.

Gregory, A. M., Caspi, A., Moffitt, T. E., Koenen, K., Eley, T. C., & Poulton, R. (2007). Juvenile mental health histories of adults with anxiety disorders. *American Journal of Psychiatry, 164*(2), 301–308.

Gryczkowski, M. R., Tiede, M. S., Dammann, J. E., Brown Jacobsen, A., Hale, L. R., & Whiteside, S. P. (2013). The timing of exposure in clinic-based treatment for childhood anxiety disorders. *Behavior Modification, 37*(1), 113–127.

Hoagwood, K. E., Serene Olin, S., Kerker, B. D., Kratochwill, T. R., Crowe, M., & Saka, N. (2007). Empirically based school interventions targeted at academic and mental health functioning. *Journal of Emotional and Behavioral Disorders, 15*(2), 66–92.

Ialongo, N., Edelson, G., Werthamer-Larsson, L., Crockett, L., & Kellam, S. (1996). Social and cognitive impairment in first-grade children with anxious and depressive symptoms. *Journal of Clinical Child Psychology, 25*(1), 15.

Kashani, J. H., & Orvaschel, H. (1990). A community study of anxiety in children and adolescents. *American Journal of Psychiatry, 147*(3), 313–318.

Kataoka, S., Jaycox, L. H., Wong, M., Nadeem, E., Langley, A., Tang, L., et al. (2011). Effects on school outcomes in low-income minority youth: Preliminary findings from a community-partnered study of a school-based trauma intervention. *Ethnicity and Disease, 21*(3 Suppl 1), 71–77.

Kataoka, S. H., Stein, B. D., Jaycox, L. H., Wong, M., Escudero, P., Tu, W., et al. (2003). A school-based mental health program for traumatized Latino immigrant children. *Journal of the American Academy of Child and Adolescent Psychiatry, 42*(3), 311–318.

Kataoka, S. H., Zhang, L., & Wells, K. B. (2002). Unmet need for mental health care among US children: Variation by ethnicity and insurance status. *American Journal of Psychiatry, 159,* 1548–1555.

Keel, P. K., & Haedt, A. (2008). Evidence-based psychosocial treatments for eating problems and eating disorders. *Journal of Clinical Child & Adolescent Psychology, 37*(1), 39–61.

Kendall, P. C. (1994). Treating anxiety disorder in youth: Results of randomized clinical trial. *Journal of Consulting and Clinical Psychology, 62*(10).

Kendall, P. C., Brady, E. U., & Verduin, T. L. (2001). Comorbidity in childhood anxiety disorders and treatment outcome. *Journal of the American Academy of Child and Adolescent Psychiatry, 40*(7), 787–794.

Kendall, P. C., Kortlander, E., Chansky, T. E., & Brady, E. U. (1992). Comorbidity of anxiety and depression in youth: Treatment implications. *Journal of Consulting and Clinical Psychology, 60*(6), 869–880.

Kendall, P. C., Safford, S., Flannery-Schroeder, E., & Webb, A. (2004). Child anxiety treatment: Outcomes in adolescence and impact on substance use and depression at 7.4-year follow-up. *Journal of Consulting and Clinical Psychology, 72*(2), 276–287.

Kendall, P. C., & Southam-Gerow, M. A. (1996). Long-term follow-up of a cognitive-behavioral therapy for anxiety-disordered youth. *Journal of Consulting and Clinical Psychology, 64*(4), 724–730.

Kessler, R. C. (2003). The impairments caused by social phobia in the general population: Implications for intervention. *Acta Psychiatrica Scandinavica. Supplementum, 417,* 19–27.

Langley, A. K., Nadeem, E., Kataoka, S. H., Stein, B. D., & Jaycox, L. H. (2010). Evidence-based mental health programs in schools: Barriers and facilitators of successful implementation. *School Mental Health, 2*(3), 105–113.

Last, C. G., Strauss, C. C., & Francis, G. (1987). Comorbidity among childhood anxiety disorders. *Journal of Nervous and Mental Disease, 175*(12), 726–730.

Lowry-Webster, H. M., Barrett, P. M., & Lock, S. (2003). A universal prevention trial of anxiety symptomology during childhood: Results at 1-year follow-up. *Behaviour Change, 20*(01), 25–43.

Lyon, A. R., Charlseworth-Attie, S., Vander Stoep, A., & McCauley, E. (2011). Modular psychotherapy for youth with internalizing problems: Implementation with therapists in school-based health centers. *School Psychology Review, 40*(4), 569–581.

Lyon, A. R., Ludwig, K., Vander Stoep, A., Gudmundsen, G., & McCauley, E. (2013). Patterns and predictors of mental healthcare utilization in schools and other service sectors among adolescents at risk for depression. *School Mental Health, 5,* 155–165.

Lyon, A. R., McCauley, E., & Vander Stoep, A. (2011). Toward successful implementation of evidence-based practices: Characterizing the intervention context of counselors in school-based health centers. *Report on Emotional and Behavioral Disorders in Youth, 11,* 19–25.

Manassis, K., Wilansky-Traynor, P., Farzan, N., Kleiman, V., Parker, K., & Sanford, M. (2010). The feelings club: Randomized controlled evaluation of school-based CBT for anxious or depressive symptoms. *Depression and Anxiety, 27*(10), 945–952.

Mash, E. J., & Hunsley, J. (2005). Evidence-based assessment of child and adolescent disorders: Issues and challenges. *Journal of Clinical Child & Adolescent Psychology, 34*(3), 362–379.

Masia Warner, C., Fisher, P. H., Shrout, P. E., Rathor, S., & Klein, R. G. (2007). Treating adolescents with social anxiety disorder in school: An attention control trial. *Journal of Child Psychology and Psychiatry, and Allied Disciplines, 48*(7), 676–686.

Masia Warner, C., Klein, R. G., Dent. H. C., Fisher, P. H., Alvir, J., Albano, A. M., et al. (2005). School-based intervention for adolescents with social anxiety disorder: Results of a controlled study. *Journal of Abnormal Child Psychology, 33,* 707–722.

Masia, C., Beidel, D. C., Albano, A. M., Rapee, R. M., Turner, S. M., Morris, T. L., et al. (1999). Skills for academic and social success. Available from Carrie Masia Warner, PhD, New York University School of Medicine, Child Study Center.

McLoone, J., Hudson, J. L., & Rapee, R. M. (2006). Treating anxiety disorders in a school setting. *Education and Treatment of Children, 29*(2), 219–242.

McLoone, J. K., & Rapee, R. M. (2012). Comparison of an anxiety management program for children implemented at home and school: Lessons learned. *School Mental Health, 4*(4), 231–242.

Merikangas, K. R., He, J. P., Burstein, M., Swendsen, J., Avenevoli, S., Case, B., et al. (2011). Service utilization for lifetime mental disorders in U.S. adolescents: Results of the National Comorbidity Survey–Adolescent Supplement (NCS-A). *Journal of the American Academy of Child and Adolescent Psychiatry, 50*(1), 32–45.

Muris, P., Meesters, C., & van Melick, M. (2002). Treatment of childhood anxiety disorders: A preliminary comparison between cognitive-behavioral group therapy and a psychological placebo intervention. *Journal of Behavior Therapy and Experimental Psychiatry, 33*(3), 143–158.

Muris, P., Merckelbach, H., Mayer, B., & Prins, E. (2000). How serious are common childhood fears? *Behaviour Research and Therapy, 38*(3), 217–228.

Mychailyszyn, M. P., Mendez, J. L., & Kendall, P. C. (2010). School functioning in youth with and without anxiety disorders: Comparisons by diagnosis and comorbidity. *School Psychology Review, 39*(1), 15.

Olfson, M., Guardino, M., Struening, E., Schneier, F. R., Hellman, F., & Klein, D. F. (2000). Barriers to the treatment of social anxiety. *American Journal of Psychiatry, 157*(4), 521–527.

Pincus, D. (2012). *Growing up brave: Expert strategies for helping your child overcome fear, stress, and anxiety*: Little Brown and Company, New York.

Pine, D. S., Cohen, P., Gurley, D., Brook, J., & Ma, Y. (1998). The risk for early-adulthood anxiety and depressive disorders in adolescents with anxiety and depressive disorders. *Archives of General Psychiatry, 55*(1), 56–64.

PracticeWise. (2013). *Evidence-based services database*. Satellite Beach, FL: PracticeWise.

Rapee, R. M., Schniering, C. A., & Hudson, J. L. (2009). Anxiety disorders during childhood and adolescence: Origins and treatment. *Annual Review of Clinical Psychology, 5*, 311–341.

Rogers, S. J., & Vismara, L. A. (2008). Evidence-based comprehensive treatments for early autism. *Journal of Clinical Child & Adolescent Psychology, 37*(1), 8–38.

Ryan, J. L., & Warner, C. M. (2012). Treating adolescents with social anxiety disorder in schools. *Child and Adolescent Psychiatric Clinics of North America, 21*(1), 105–118.

Saavedra, L. M., Silverman, W. K., Morgan-Lopez, A. A., & Kurtines, W. M. (2010). Cognitive behavioral treatment for childhood anxiety disorders: Long-term effects on anxiety and secondary disorders in adulthood. *Journal of Child Psychology and Psychiatry, 51*(8), 924–934.

Schneier, F. R., Johnson, J., Hornig, C. D., Liebowitz, M. R., & Weissman, M. M. (1992). Social phobia. Comorbidity and morbidity in an epidemiologic sample. *Archives of General Psychiatry, 49*(4), 282–288.

Silverman, W. K., & Albano, A. M. (1996). *The anxiety disorders interview schedule for children for DSM-IV (Child and parent versions)*. San Antonio, TX: Psychological Corporation.

Silverman, W. K., Pina, A. A., & Viswesvaran, C. (2008). Evidence-based psychosocial treatments for phobic and anxiety disorders in children and adolescents. *Journal of Clinical Child and Adolescent Psychology, 37*(1), 105–130.

Stein, M. B., & Stein, D. J. (2008). Social anxiety disorder. *The Lancet, 371*(9618), 1115–1125.

Stephan, S. H., Wissow, L., & Pichler, E. (2010). Utilizing common factors and practice elements to improve mental health care by school-based primary care providers. *Report on Emotional and Behavioral Disorders in Youth, 10*, 81–86.

Turner, S. M., Beidel, D. C., Dancu, C. V., & Keys, D. J. (1986). Psychopathology of social phobia and comparison to avoidant personality disorder. *Journal of Abnormal Psychology, 95*(4), 389–394.

Weist, M. D. (1997). Expanded school mental health services: A national movement in progress. In T. H. Ollendick & R. J. Prinz (Eds.), *Advances in clinical child psychology* (Vol. 19, pp. 319–352). New York: Plenum.

Weist, M., Lever, N., Stephan, S., Youngstrom, E., Moore, E., Harrison, B., et al. (2009). Formative evaluation of a framework for high quality, evidence-based services in school mental health. *School Mental Health, 1*(4), 196–211.

Weisz, J. R., Chorpita, B. F., Palinkas, L. A., Schoenwald, S. K., Miranda, J., Bearman, S. K., et al. (2012). Testing standard and modular designs for psychotherapy treating depression, anxiety, and conduct problems in youth: A randomized effectiveness trial. *Archives of General Psychiatry, 69*(3), 274–282.

Wittchen, H.-U., Lieb, R., Wunderlich, U., & Schuster, P. (1999). Comorbidity in primary care: Presentation and consequences. *Journal of Clinical Psychiatry, 60*(suppl 7), 29–36.

Chapter 4
Trauma, PTSD, and Secondary Trauma in Children and Adolescents

Robert W. Motta

Description of the Problem

Trauma and posttraumatic stress disorder (PTSD) in children and adolescents refer to reactions to extremely frightening and threatening events. For those who are interested in learning about PTSD and those subclinical trauma reactions referred to as acute stress disorders, there is often a tendency to go to the latest version of the Diagnostic and Statistical Manual of the American Psychiatric Association (DSM-5, 2013) where one encounters a list of symptoms such as intrusive thoughts, negative alterations in cognition and mood, and alterations in arousal and reactivity. The DSM-5 introduces a PTSD subtype for children 6 years and younger which requires avoidance or intrusive thoughts, rather than both, and thereby simplifies the diagnosis of young children. The problem with this approach to defining PTSD and trauma reactions is that the DSM provides a skeletal, and in many ways a distorted view, of what PTSD actually is, especially as seen from the viewpoint of practicing school and clinical psychologists. A major issue in trauma reactions, regardless of the age of the trauma victim, is an alteration of one's self-view and a change in how the environment is perceived. These changes from prior levels of functioning are so profound that they tend to overshadow most of the specific DSM listed symptoms. The alteration in a child's or adolescent's perspective of themselves and their environments are characteristically in the more negative and pessimistic direction than they were before being traumatized (e.g., Ellis, 2005).

Children, adolescents, and adults who are traumatized often feel a sense of alienation from themselves and others. In addition, they often develop a fairly negative

R.W. Motta, Ph.D., A.B.P.P. (✉)
Department of Psychology, Hofstra University, Hempstead, NY, USA
e-mail: Robert.W.Motta@hofstra.edu

© Springer Science+Business Media New York 2015
R. Flanagan et al. (eds.), *Cognitive and Behavioral Interventions in the Schools*, DOI 10.1007/978-1-4939-1972-7_4

view of themselves and a wary, suspicious stance toward their environment. For example, the child who has been physically abused will often have a diminished sense of self perhaps brought on by the belief that they have behaved badly in order to have warranted such abuse. This view can transform a child's perspective into believing that they are a bad person, not just a person who behaves poorly. The declining sense of self-regard will often lead a youngster into asocial and antisocial activities, and the negative feedback that eventuates from these actions perpetuates and validates the negative sense of self (e.g., Evans, Ehlers, Mezey, & Clark, 2007). From this, it should be apparent that PTSD is not simply a disorder characterized by a menu of symptoms but that it is also a pervasive and often persistent alteration of one's self-view and a wary take on their environment.

A related concept that involves trauma in children and adolescents is the diagnosis of secondary traumatization (e.g., Motta, 2012). Secondary trauma has been given far less attention than has PTSD, and yet it is among the more common problems that can afflict the young. Secondary trauma of childhood typically encompasses negative psychological experiences that are due to a child having a close and extended relationship with someone who has been traumatized. The traumatized individual could be a parent, guardian, relative, or anyone else with whom the child is emotionally close. The prototypical example is presented by Rosenheck and Nathan (1985) and involved the 10-year-old son of a Vietnam veteran. This child had an unusually close relationship with his father and the father's emotional life. Unfortunately the father was experiencing PTSD as a result of his war experience and the child began to acquire the father's depressive and anxious affect and moodiness, along with a wariness of others and a tendency toward isolation. In a related investigation, Parsons, Kehle, and Owen (1990) compared childhood social and emotional functioning as viewed by Vietnam era veterans with PTSD to similar veterans without PTSD. Overall, it was found that the children of veterans with PTSD were seen as having substantially more social and emotional difficulties marked by an inability to initiate and maintain relationships and by negative effect. The children of veterans with PTSD were also seen as having a greater lack of self-control and more aggressive, delinquent, and hyperactive behaviors.

While secondary trauma has not been extensively studied in children, there are a number of situations in which it has been found to occur in adult samples. It has been reported to take place in families living with a traumatized family member (Catherall, 1992), in partners of those who have been sexually abused (Nelson & Wampler, 2000), in wives of combat veterans with PTSD (Waysman, Mikulincer, Solomon, & Weisenberg, 1993), in young adult children of Vietnam veterans with PTSD (Suozzi & Motta, 2004), in wives of police officers (Dwyer, 2005), in grandchildren of Holocaust survivors (Kassai & Motta, 2006; Kellerman, 2001; Perlstein & Motta, 2012), and in family members of those with a serious illness (Boyer et al., 2002; Libov, Nevid, Pelcovitz, & Carmony, 2002; Lombardo, 2005).

Epidemiology

The vast majority of epidemiological studies on PTSD have been done with adult samples; however, there are available studies referring to PTSD rates in children and adolescents. For example, terrorized communities in Cambodia during the era of the Khmer Rouge atrocities and rampages revealed that virtually 100 % of children and adolescents displayed symptoms similar to those seen in PTSD. After 3 years the rate was down to still troubling 50 % (Kinzie, Sack, Angell, Mason, & Ben, 1986). A study of sexually abused foster care children and adolescents revealed PTSD rates of 60 % (Dubner & Motta, 1999). These rates are remarkably high especially in light of the fact that fewer than 10 % of adults who have been traumatized meet the criteria for PTSD as described in the DSM.

Given that traumatized parents negatively impact children, it is important to examine adult PTSD rates. Nearly one in four (24.5 %) of Iraq and Afghanistan war veterans have received a PTSD diagnosis by the Veterans Health Administration. A commonly reported statistic is that approximately 7 % of individuals have PTSD in the general population and 19 % of Vietnam War veterans are current PTSD cases (Dohrenwend et al., 2006). Females generally develop PTSD at a higher rate than males. In addition to younger age increasing one's vulnerability, the existence of preexisting psychological problems also predicts an increased probability of developing PTSD (Breslau, Chilcoat, Kessler, Peterson, & Lucia, 1996). Female children who have witnessed serious interpersonal conflict among adults in the home and those from abusive and emotionally non-supportive home environments are seriously at risk for developing secondary trauma and PTSD reactions. What follows below are typical cases of secondary trauma and PTSD.

Case Examples

Case #1

The first case highlights the symptoms and behavioral characteristics that are commonly seen in cases of childhood secondary traumatization. At the time of this event, Larry was 5 years old and had five siblings. His intact family was sitting at home when approximately 50 bullets hit the house. A number of police officers had cornered a deranged man who had threatened them with a shotgun, which turned out to be empty. The fusillade of bullets from the police officers killed the man but also hit the house behind him and thoroughly traumatized the parents and the older children who were sitting at home watching television. Larry really did not know what to make of what was happening. He interpreted the events as rocks being thrown against the house. He did not grasp that there were bullets hitting the house or that he and his family members were lucky to be alive. As a result, he did not have the intense fear that typically precipitates PTSD. His parents and the older teenage siblings, however, were horrified and fully realized that luck was the only factor that prevented them from being injured or killed.

He witnessed extreme upset among his family members, their sleeplessness, their anxiety, their depression, and their growing distrust and insecurities, and he began to react. He started having nightmares about being attacked by monsters and was unable to sleep. He became sullen, moody, withdrawn, and irascible. He developed nocturnal enuresis and began failing at school. His teachers described an increasing tendency to isolate himself from others, a general moodiness and withdrawal, and difficulties with concentration. Nothing seemed to console Larry. He was reacting not to a traumatic event, but to his family's responses, to their upset, and to the overall disruption in the home. He cried in response to his mother's unhappiness and to his father's now frequent emotional outbursts. Larry was traumatized by the emotional reaction of those with whom he was emotionally bonded and upon whom he relied for guidance and support. He was showing classic symptoms of secondary traumatization.

Larry entered into counseling and made significant progress. Given that a major issue for him was that of secondary trauma, i.e., the emotional upset of his family, parental counseling significantly benefitted him. Overall, his therapy followed a CBT and exposure framework. For example, Larry was often asked to recount the events that took place, in detail. This form of exposure through imagery was supplemented with efforts to reframe his thinking from seeing the shooting event as a common occurrence to a highly unusual one. Attempts were also made to reframe his thoughts in the direction of positive changes and adjustments being made by his family. It was clear that this child's emotional adjustment was directly tied to that of his parents and siblings. Stability and relative normalcy eventually returned to the home and Larry continued to improve and eventually reverted to his old spontaneous and fun loving self. In school his grades began to improve and he showed a notable improvement in the quality of his social interactions. While he continues to have occasional nightmares and startle reactions, overall he is markedly improved.

Case #2

Case 2 is a more typical PTSD case that occurred in response to a rape which took place in the first year of college but is unfortunately typical of such events seen in high schools. Janet was a highly athletic, academically talented, and extroverted teen who was accepted to a fairly selective university in California. She had also been accepted by the Naval Academy but chose this particular private university because it had a renowned swimming program and swimming was the area in which she excelled. One night she accepted an invitation to a fraternity house Halloween party where the alcohol was flowing heavily. At some point during the revelry, she was pulled into a room and raped by two competitive swimmers from her school.

Janet hid this horrific event from her parents because she was ashamed and felt that she displayed bad judgment in going to the party. However, her parents saw an inexplicable and dramatic change in her. She began transforming from an exuberant, athletic, honors student into a depressed, angry, rebellious, substance-abusing teen that her parents no longer recognized. Rather than being proud of her accomplishments she now felt sullied, diminished, and undesirable. Her primary emotional states were anger, depression, and anxiety. She developed a pervasive sense that the world is a dangerous place where one's safety and security are never assured. Janet had changed in profound ways. She now had a critical and negative view of herself and the motivations of others. She felt intensely threatened and vulnerable. Janet's radically negative transformation of her self-view and her equally pessimistic views of the environment are common outcomes of those suffering from PTSD.

Janet refused to take court action because the process of reliving what happened was too much for her to manage. She did identify the two rapists to the administration of her school and they were dismissed from that university, but without her testimony, no further action could be taken. Janet pursued psychotherapy and drug abuse counseling. The cognitive-behavioral focus of her therapy was aimed at altering her self-blaming thoughts and negative self-evaluations. She has made tremendous strides and is now a more mature person who gives rape-counseling seminars at local high schools. Overall, Janet has made a good recovery. She is a serious and focused individual and seems more emotionally seasoned than her years would dictate.

Case #3

This is not the case of an individual, but rather, a case of group trauma. The current author and his assistant recently held a meeting of Long Island, New York, residents who endured the ravages of Hurricane Sandy, which struck in October 2012. This hurricane devastated numerous seaside homes and did extensive damage to many other residences. What is of particular interest about this affected group of individuals was the variation in response to the trauma. The majority of those present at the meeting were seriously traumatized and spoke of the nightmarish experience of being in a home without lights and without heat or drinking water, often in subfreezing temperatures, for periods of weeks. As might be expected, there were many reports of nightmares, intrusive images during waking hours, and a profound suspiciousness of community and state leaders who promised relief. Little relief came, even after 3 months. Many reported that they had changed from a religious, community oriented individual to something of a wary, suspicious survivor. However, there were a few in the group of 25 who reported no PTSD symptoms and, in fact, had a relatively positive stance of having the opportunity to build a new home. This highlights the fact that adults and children differ significantly in their ability to cope with trauma.

Many of the participants observed that their children seemed far more troubled by their parents' besieged responses to the hurricane, than to the hurricane itself. Some even reported that the children enjoyed the storm! From this one might surmise that the children were suffering from secondary trauma in that their exposure to the emotional upset of their parents had a more negative emotional impact than the storm itself. While systematic studies have not been carried out with groups within the schools, it seems reasonable to assume that getting children together to discuss their experiences would be a form of graded exposure and could lessen the anxiety and emotional upset that many of the children feel. It is important to assure children that normalcy and balance will return to their households and that their family can and will cope with this natural disaster. School psychologists and other mental health personnel can play an important role in facilitating such discussions.

Historical Roots

Reactions to trauma situations have been known and described for centuries. They have been alluded to as far back as Homer's Iliad and noted in literary heroes and heroines, including Shakespeare's Henry IV (Trimble, 1985). Samuel Pepys diary in 1666 contains quotations of sleeping difficulty and night terrors in response to the Great Fire of London (Daly, 1983). During the American Civil War (1861–1865), trauma reactions were noted to occur in the absence of physical injury, and these reactions included irritability, rapid heart rate, and increased arousal. The condition became known as Da Costa's Syndrome, named after the American physician who described them. The condition was also referred to as Soldiers' Irritable Heart or Irritable Heart Syndrome, perhaps in reference to the fact that the heart rate was elevated and the condition seemed to have more of an emotional than physiological etiology. Similar emotional reactions have occurred as a result of railway accidents during the uncertain development of our rail system. These responses became known as "railway spine" due to a belief that the trauma reactions had a neurological basis (Trimble, 1981).

Terms such as "shell shock" and "rape trauma syndrome" also appear to be descriptive of the symptoms of PTSD. However, it was not until the publication of the Third Edition of the Diagnostic and Statistical Manual of Mental Disorders (3rd ed.; DSM III; American Psychiatric Association (APA), 1980) that PTSD became an officially recognized disorder. The DSM III alluded to traumatic events that were "beyond the range of normal human experience." The Vietnam War was a driving force in the inclusion of PTSD in the DSM. The criterion that the trauma experience should be beyond the range of normal human encounters was subsequently dropped when it was found that relatively common stressors such as car accidents, life threatening illness, and child abuse could also precipitate PTSD.

Assessment: Role of Clinical Observation

Assessment is commonly accepted to mean the use of measures, usually paper and pencil measures, to evaluate a particular psychological characteristic. There are no measures specifically designed to measure secondary trauma in childhood, although measures of secondary trauma do exist for adults (e.g., Motta, Hafeez, Sciancalepore, & Diaz, 2001). There are also a number of measures of PTSD in children and adolescents and these will be described below. An important point to consider is that PTSD is most often assessed not by scales, but by a clear-eyed process of clinical observation of PTSD characteristics. These characteristics include a falling off from a previous level of functioning; a tendency toward sullenness, isolation, anhedonia, irritability, sleeplessness and nightmares; and a tendency for these symptoms to persist for an extended time.

Among the more important characteristics of PTSD, which are included in the DSM-5 is the previously mentioned alteration in the sense of self and in the perception of one's environment. Perhaps the simplest way of encapsulating the change is to state that a child, an adolescent, or an adult who has been traumatized is far more pessimistic than they were before the trauma. Traumatized children come across as sullen, moody, and withdrawn. They show a lack of interest in many of the activities they once enjoyed, they tend to avoid close friendships and contacts, and they seem to be preoccupied. Herman (1992), in a classic examination of traumatized children who had been buried underground inside a school bus, noted many of the above characteristics in addition to what she referred to as "foreshortened future." By this she meant that many of the children could not view their future selves. They had no expectation of leading a long life. The lack of expectancy of continued living and the negative view of themselves and their world all reflect a pessimism that typically was not previously there.

Those who are traumatized, regardless of the nature of the trauma, see their world as lacking in possibilities they might desire. In fact, they often have few desires per se (e.g., Terr, 1983). The traumatized person sees their world as a negative place that is not only devoid of possibilities, but even if there were incentives in the world, there would be a lack of interest in them. This bleak stance reflects the negative view of the future, the self, and the world as initially descried in the CBT model of depression by Beck, Shaw, Rush, and Emery (1979). In the previous examples, the rape victim transformed from an exuberant, enthusiastic student, into a depressed, acting out, substance abuser. The young boy whose house had been hit by bullets became withdrawn, angry, and moody. People traumatized by Hurricane Sandy see themselves as having changed in a negative way. These outcomes are very common in trauma. Rape victims, torture victims, traumatized war veterans, natural disaster survivors, and many other survivors of varied traumas have a negative sense of self and a philosophically somber view of the world and any future that might be out there.

One of the particular problems in dealing with traumatized children is that PTSD and secondary traumatization can often mimic depressive and anxiety reactions.

From a differential diagnosis perspective, the difference between common anxiety reactions, depression, and PTSD is that PTSD often is characterized by an identifiable event that caused extreme fear, startle reactions, threatening nightmares, prolonged sleeplessness, and avoidance of any stimuli that remind the traumatized individual of the traumatic event. Anxiety and depressive reactions are usually not associated with sudden fear-producing and life-threatening events.

Assessment Measures: Secondary Trauma

As noted above, diagnosis of secondary trauma is usually through clinical observation. The secondary trauma measures that do exist are usually designed to assess secondary trauma in therapists. One such scale is the Secondary Trauma Stress Scale (STSS: Bride, Robinson, Yegidis, & Figley, 2004). The scale shows good psychometric characteristics but has two relative weaknesses. First, it is designed specifically for therapists and therefore does not have defensible application to other populations, particularly children. The second problem is that it lacks empirically derived cutoff scores that are based on standardized measures. The same strengths and weakness are revealed in the Traumatic Stress Institute Belief Scale (TSI; Pearlman, 1996), the Compassion Satisfaction and Fatigue Test (CSFT, Figley & Stamm, 1996), and the Compassion Fatigue Scale-Revised (CFS-R; Adams, Boscarino, & Figley, 2006). The Professional Quality of Life (ProQOL; Stamm, 2010) has been used with varied populations but it is not specifically a measure of secondary trauma and, again, lacks empirically based cutoff scores. These issues are addressed by the Secondary Trauma Scale (STS; Motta et al., 2001) in that the measure is applicable across a wide range of populations including community samples, therapists, students, etc. It is designed specifically to assess secondary trauma and also has cutoff scores such that a given score on the STS is associated with levels of anxiety and depression. Like the scales mentioned above, however, it is not applicable to children.

Assessment Measures: PTSD

Regarding childhood PTSD itself, a sampling of measures will be reviewed. One such inventory is the Children's PTSD Inventory (Saigh et al., 2000). This scale assesses emotional reactivity to trauma situations and also assesses re-experiencing, avoidance and numbing, increased arousal, significant impairment in functioning, and a diagnosis category. The scale shows good psychometric characteristics in terms of inter-rater reliability, internal consistency, and content validity. The samples used in the development of this scale included children and adolescents from 6 to 17 years of age.

Solid internal consistency and overall strong validities and reliabilities have been reported for the Clinician-Administered PTSD Scale for Children and Adolescents

(CAPS-CA; Nader et al., 1996) and the PTSD module of the Diagnostic Interview for Children and Adolescents—Revised (DICA-R; Reich, Leacock, & Shanfeld, 1994). Whereas information regarding inter-rater reliability has not been presented for the Childhood PTSD Interview of the CAPS-CA, these scales do show strong internal consistency.

An inherent difficulty in assessing childhood trauma reactions is the child's reluctance to openly discuss their trauma experiences. The emotional or modified Stroop procedure has proven to be helpful in overcoming this reluctance. Stroop (1935) found that when a color word such as "red" is printed in red ink, one can more quickly name the ink color than when the word "red" is printed in a non-congruent color such as green. Here the task of saying "green" when the underlying word is red, takes longer because there is interference between the desire to name the color and the meaning of the word.

Using a similar approach, the modified or emotional Stroop uses trauma relevant words which are printed in colors and the requirement is to name the colors in which the words are printed. For example, a person who was traumatically injured in a car accident will take longer to name the color in which the word "pain" is printed than the color in which the word "rain" is printed. Also, the response time to naming the color of "pain" would be longer for the person who had an accident in comparison to one who had not. The modified Stroop has been used in investigations of secondary trauma, PTSD, anxiety, depression, and other disorders.

An area where the modified Stroop has been found to be particularly useful is in the assessment of PTSD due to childhood sexual abuse. In one such study (Dubner & Motta, 1999), three groups of foster care children, ages 8–17, were utilized: sexually abused, physically abused, and non-abused. The children were shown a variety of words that were either relevant or not relevant to their abuse. So, for example, sexually abused children were timed in naming the colors in which 50 words related to their abuse, e.g., "naughty," "touch," etc. It was found that the color naming times of sexually abused children of words relevant to such abuse was significantly longer than to words that were not abuse related. Similarly, sexually abused children took significantly longer to name such words than those who were physically abused or those who were not abused. Paper and pencil measures of trauma, anxiety, and intrusive cognitions did not differentiate the physical and sexually abused groups but the modified Stroop measures did so.

The value of the Stroop procedure in assessing traumatized children is that it is fairly impervious to attempts to minimize or cover-up traumatic incidents such as sexual abuse. The drawback of the procedure is that different stimulus words need to be developed for each type of trauma. For example, the stimulus words relevant to sexual abuse would not be similar to those for physical abuse. Another drawback is that there are no cutoff scores that the clinician can use that would help in making diagnostic decisions. As a result it becomes necessary to do comparisons of response latencies between those who are suspected of having been traumatized and those who are not.

Aside from the standardized measures mentioned above, school psychologists can often arrive at a PTSD diagnosis through a knowledge of the child's trauma experiences, their behavior within the schools, and the use of standard childhood anxiety and depression inventories such as the Revised Childhood Manifest Anxiety Scale-2 (RCMAS-2; Reynolds & Richmond, 2008) and the Children's Depression Inventory (CDI-2; Kovacs, 2010).

Therapeutic Interventions

Before describing therapeutic interventions for PTSD and secondary trauma, an important caveat must be considered for anyone who attempts to treat this disorder, whether in children, adolescents, or adults. Avoidance of stimuli that have any similarity to the trauma situation is one of the DSM diagnostic criteria of PTSD. The significance of this is that the closer a therapist gets to the relevant material that forms the basis of PTSD, the more likely it is that person being treated will engage in avoidance maneuvers. Children and adolescents may become reticent when questioned about the trauma or may simply deny that any such trauma has taken place. Adults often respond by terminating treatment when the therapist attempts to have the person confront their trauma situation. Lack of attention to the important issue of avoidance will often lead to failure among novice therapists and seasoned therapists as well. The motivation to avoid discussing or revisiting trauma material is so strong that the majority of traumatized individuals will not seek help in the first place and will resist any suggestion of therapy. A critical piece of trauma therapy is developing a trusting relationship and then moving forward cautiously and not overwhelming the trauma victim with anxiety. This ability to know when to move forward and how quickly to advance is a skill that takes time and patience to acquire.

Another important issue in treating PTSD is that, despite the menu of symptoms listed in the DSM-5, alleviating the avoidance symptoms is frequently only a first step. Adolescents and adults with PTSD often have problems of social isolation, substance abuse, and relationship problems. While substance abuse is not a common problem with children, they too suffer from withdrawal and isolation and have academic deficiencies. These problems must be addressed in a comprehensive treatment of this disorder, and a failure to do so results in incomplete or unsuccessful treatment. Therefore, once some of the more prominent symptoms of PTSD have subsided, there may then be a need for interventions such as social skills retraining, academic remediation, and, when necessary, substance abuse interventions. In summary, treating PTSD involves the critical step of establishing a trusting relationship, moving forward with care so the client does not become overwhelmed and avoid therapy, and then making efforts to undo some of the collateral damage in academic and social relationship spheres.

There is virtually no research on the comparative efficacy of treatment for secondary traumatization. In fact, the literature does not report specific approaches of any kind that are used with secondary trauma exclusively. As indicated earlier, those experiencing secondary or vicarious trauma have symptoms similar to those of primary trauma victim but usually of a lesser intensity. Therefore, therapeutic approaches with secondary trauma center around supportive counseling and strategies oriented toward the alleviation of anxiety and depression.

While there are over 400 different forms of psychotherapy, and advocates of each of these types might claim that they can be effective in treating PTSD, some of the more common forms of therapy include cognitive-behavioral therapy (CBT), psycho-pharmacology, exposure therapy, anxiety management training, and stress management techniques (Foa & Meadows, 1997). Behavioral approaches such as relaxation training and in vivo desensitization are among the more common approaches with children. CBT, while also used with children, is more commonly used with adolescents and adults as this form of treatment has been supported by a large number of sound empirical studies. Virtual Reality procedures have also been used with all age groups as has Eye Movement Desensitization and Reprocessing (EMDR; Shapiro, 2001). Finally, drugs are commonly used in treating PTSD and these will be described below. It is most important to restate that regardless of the form of therapy that is implemented, without a trusting and mutually respectful relationship, and this is especially true with children, little of therapeutic value will take place.

Cognitive Behavior Therapy

Cognitive behavior therapy (CBT) is a generic descriptor that includes exposure therapy and therapeutic approaches designed to alter dysfunctional patterns of thinking and behaving. Exposure therapy essentially involves inducing children, adolescents, and adults to confront and not avoid situations that remind them of their trauma experiences. So, for example, a traumatized child might be encouraged to openly discuss instances of abuse. An adolescent might be encouraged to openly discuss an assault. A combat veteran might be asked to describe their trauma situations in great detail and to re-experience associated painful emotions or to view and listen to real or simulated firefights and other combat scenarios. Exposure can be in vivo, where one re-exposes oneself to actual trauma situations in the hope that fear reactions will eventually extinguish, or imaginal, where guided imagery assists in revisiting the trauma situation in great detail.

CBT for PTSD or secondary trauma involves altering ones thoughts and beliefs with regard to trauma situations and encouraging individuals to confront the trauma, whether in small steps or all at once (sometimes referred to as flooding or implosive therapy). The beliefs that are addressed are of the nature "I can't handle this, it is too much for me" or the view that "I cannot overcome my reactions to trauma; nothing will ever change" and "Mom is late. Maybe she was killed in a car accident." Thoughts such as these lead to negative emotional states such as elevated anxiety and depression, and it is often helpful to work with children to consider more likely alternatives to their negativistic and fatalistic thinking.

At times, therapies are combined. For example, cognitive therapy is combined with exposure therapy or exposure therapy is done within a group format (e.g., Foa et al., 1999; Sutherland, Mott, Williams, Teng, & Ready, 2012).

Similarly, cognitive therapy might be used with a traumatized child and that child's parents in order to deal with commonly occurring negative interpersonal sequelae resulting from, for example, an abuse incident (Fredman, Monson, & Adair, 2011). Negative interpersonal consequences may be avoidance of adults or overly aggressive or sexualized behavior with peers.

Manualized forms of CBT are common, and while they were designed for adults, they are often adopted for use with children. One example is Cognitive Processing Therapy (CPT; Resick, 2001). An initial session involves brief psychoeducation addressing the nature of CPT and PTSD. The next two sessions involve writing and reading about the nature of the traumatic event and why one believes it happened. For children, drawings can be helpful, because these can provide a vehicle for communication. Here, attempts are made to identify problematic beliefs about the event and to learn how these beliefs affect the individual's thoughts and feelings. Emphasis is placed on how thoughts and feelings are connected. In children, concrete verbiage must be used, e.g., "So Mary, can you see how thinking bad thoughts can make you feel scared?" Additional sessions are dedicated to learning to challenge one's self-statements and assumptions and to eventually modify dysfunctional and maladaptive beliefs. Remaining sessions involve challenging overgeneralizations about oneself (I'm a bad person because of what happened) and others (You can't trust anybody) and developing more objective ways of perceiving one's environment (Alvarez et al., 2011).

While CPT clearly emphasizes a cognitive viewpoint of PTSD, it could be argued that the majority of other forms of CBT focus upon exposure and reprocessing of trauma material in order to reduce the high levels of anxiety that trauma situations generate. Examples here might include a teen that has been raped being helped to discuss the details of what happened during the rape including the fear, helplessness, and the eventual feelings of hopelessness that the rape generated. By revisiting this disturbing event within the safe and secure confines of the therapist's office, the fear is lessened and a more objective perspective is developed. This process of exposure must take place at a place that can be tolerated by the child or adolescent, and it is possible to conduct such sessions within the schools. An assignment can be given, for example, for the child to construct a written narrative of their life including the trauma incident. The child is then asked to reread and review this narrative (e.g., Ruf et al., 2010). There is no substitute for therapist sensitivity and skill in determining how quickly or slowly one should progress. No therapy manual can be of much assistance in determining how much the client can tolerate before avoidance maneuvers begin.

Recent Research on Exercise as a Trauma Intervention

There is an evolving area of research that loosely falls into the behavioral or CBT domains in treating PTSD, and this is the role of exercise. One of the first studies to specifically evaluate aerobic exercise as an intervention for PTSD involved a small sample of adults who had experienced tragic death of a relative or friend, sexual or physical assault, severe auto accident, combat, serious illness, injury, or disease (Manger & Motta, 2005). Results of this study showed that aerobic exercise alone resulted in significant reductions in PTSD, anxiety, and depression. Follow-up studies were conducted with adolescents and children most of whom had suffered some form of abuse (Diaz & Motta, 2008; Newman & Motta, 2007). These studies again demonstrated significant reduction in PTSD and related symptoms.

It is unknown as to why aerobic exercise would have such positive effects but it is speculated that this may be due to the well-researched impact of aerobic exercise in reducing anxiety (Motta, McWilliams, Schwartz, & Cavera, 2012). Given that PTSD is often comorbid with anxiety, reduction of anxiety might be associated with the lessening of PTSD symptoms.

Regardless of the type of intervention, once the initial steps of anxiety reduction and enhanced coping are achieved, the focus of therapy then moves to addressing more general social, academic, employment, substance abuse, and family functioning issues. When progress is made in these areas, then children, adolescents, and adults are encouraged to reevaluate themselves and their view of the future with the hope of developing more positive perspectives.

Virtual Reality and EMDR

Among the various forms that exposure therapy may take, Virtual Reality therapy (VR) is an exposure-based approach that has been used in the treatment of PTSD. When employing VR, headgear is worn that allows participants to look around and as they do so, the scenery changes as if they were actually scanning the environment. The need for specialized equipment renders VR impractical in many school districts, and thus, VR often necessitates external referral. A good deal of the research with VR in children has centered on those with developmental delays and helping these children overcome perceived life challenges (e.g., Salem, Gropack, Coffin, & Godwin, 2012). After an initial burst of enthusiasm for VR, a fading of interest occurred. This may have been due to the expense of the equipment and the even greater cost of developing the software underlying the electronic scenery. As technology has advanced, prices have been reduced, but VR is still a somewhat inconvenient procedure to employ, especially if one is treating a variety of traumas. Another issue that has reduced enthusiasm for the VR procedure is that there is not an abundance of evidence that VR works any better than other forms of exposure. Its real value in treating war-related PTSD is that re-exposing someone to actual war scenarios is, in most cases, neither possible nor desirable. In all, VR does play a role in treating trauma and PTSD especially when other forms of exposure are not possible.

Like Virtual Reality therapy, Eye Movement Desensitization and Reprocessing (EMDR; Shapiro, 2001) has also been used in the treatment of PTSD and has been shown in meta-analyses to be useful in treating traumatized children (Rodenburg,

Benjamin, Carlijn, Meijer, & Stams, 2009). Typically traumatized clients engaged in therapist-directed lateral eye movements, alternate finger tapping, or listening to bilateral auditory tones, and while doing this, they also imagine their unique trauma in detail. This dual process of imagining the trauma while engaged in one of the above activities is said to allow trauma memories to now be processed in an area that is more readily accessible and, thereby, treatable. Thus, it would appear that an information processing model is the basis of this form of intervention (Shapiro, 2001).

A number of researchers (e.g., Herbert et al., 2000) report that there is no evidence to support the information processing model and that what accounts for the ostensible efficacy of EMDR is simply exposure. It is argued that because clients are asked to imagine the trauma situation in detail as part of the EMDR procedure, the exposure rather than the inferred information processing, accounts for the change.

Drug Treatment for PTSD and Secondary Trauma

Two caveats are offered before discussing pharmacological treatments. First, there is seldom any sound justification for choosing medication to treat trauma reactions in children and adolescents, without first thoroughly exploring nonmedical interventions. Adverse side effects and an overdependence on medication are among the risks of such usage. Nevertheless, medications are increasingly used and therefore merit coverage in this chapter. Second, while there is research on the use of medications in treating trauma reactions and PTSD in adults, there is little such research for drug use with childhood and adolescent trauma, and there is no research in treating secondary trauma pharmacologically. For these reasons, medications for PTSD in childhood and adolescence should only be considered in extreme cases involving behavior disorders or potential suicidality.

Psychopharmacological treatment for PTSD typically center on an alleviation of the symptoms but are not considered a primary means of treating this disorder. The evidence base for drug treatment is most supported in studies of selective serotonin reuptake inhibitors (SSRI's). Two medications, Sertraline (Zoloft) and Paroxetine (Paxil), have FDA approval for treatment of PTSD (Brady et al., 2000).

Mood stabilizers are preferred in situations where there is a bipolar disorder that is comorbid with PTSD, especially in situations where SSRI's are found to precipitate mania. Carbamazepine (Tegretol), Divalproex (Depakote), Lamotrigine (Lamictal), and Topiramate (Topamax) are common mood stabilizers. All such medications should be used with care due to potentially serious side effects such as agranulocytosis (severe lowering of white blood count), liver toxicity, skin rash, sedation, and dizziness, among others.

Antipsychotics have also been used to treat PTSD and they impact the dopaminergic and serotonergic systems. Risperidone (Risperdal) is one such medication. These drugs have been used when a psychotic disorder is comorbid with PTSD and, regrettably, have often been used to treat childhood behavior disorders. The unconscionable use of these medications in young people may be due to the huge sums spent by the pharmaceutical industry to promote them.

When anxiety accompanies PTSD symptoms, Benzodiazepines can be used but must be used with discretion. Two problems emerge with these medications and they are addiction and disinhibition. Examples of these drugs include Lorazepam (Ativan), Clonazepam (Klonopin), and Alprazolam (Xanax).

Although psychopharmacological treatment has a place in dealing with the complex and debilitating symptoms of PTSD, it is best to view their role as adjuncts to psychotherapeutic approaches. This is especially the case when dealing with children. Behavioral and cognitive-behavioral approaches should be the first form of intervention. Psychotherapeutic methods emphasize the fact that the traumatized person, whether child, adolescent, or adult, must eventually learn to function in their world and to view that world and themselves in a more objective and positive light.

Summary

Childhood and adolescent PTSD and secondary traumatization bring with them a unique set of emotional torments. Aside from their debilitating symptoms, these disorders often precipitate a negative, suspicious, and diminished sense of self and a dark view of the present and future. PTSD contains within its diagnostic criteria the especially problematic feature of avoidance. This tendency to avoid thoughts, feelings, and images that remind the PTSD sufferer of their trauma significantly interferes with treatment. While many of those who suffer emotional disturbance refuse treatment as a way of denying their problems, PTSD is the only disorder that has this feature as one of its diagnostic criteria. For this reason childhood and adolescent therapists who treat PTSD must have a delicate and sensitive appreciation of avoidance tendencies and must learn to tread lightly when dealing with relevant therapeutic issues. Manualized treatments can help the therapist develop an empirically based treatment framework, but the relationship between the child and the mental health worker is probably most important (Wampold, 2001).

Secondary traumatization adds an additional layer of complexity in that trauma reactions can and do spread contagiously to others, including offspring, therapists, and anyone else who has close and extended contact with the trauma victim. While no such studies have been done, it is not unreasonable to suggest that secondary traumatization is one of the primary sources of trauma reactions in children. Therapists who treat trauma reactions in young people must not only have excellent capabilities and awareness of their own vulnerability but must also function as something of disease control specialists. They must intervene to stem the spread of this disorder to others through the process of secondary traumatization. A further challenge for therapists is that while new assessment approaches to secondary trauma are beginning to emerge, research on effective therapeutic approaches are virtually nonexistent.

Cognitive behavior therapy, including exposure therapy, is probably the most empirically supported form of treatment of childhood and adolescent trauma.

Psychotherapeutic intervention should be the first line of treatment, while pharmacological approaches may have some role in suppression of trauma symptoms. Of course, the avoidance and negativism that is characteristic of PTSD results in both psychotherapy and pharmacotherapy often being unavailable to the trauma victim. Some recent findings suggest that the alternative approach of aerobic exercise can be an effective method of dealing with trauma reactions. Its typical role in the child's school days makes it an ecologically sound form of intervention.

The important inclusion of PTSD in the Diagnostic and Statistical Manual of Mental Disorders starting in 1980 has brought about more treatment funding and other resources for dealing with this disorder, and because of this, diagnostic and treatment approaches have continued a slow but continuing advance. Therefore, it is reasonable for both therapists and researchers to have at least guarded optimism for future effective interventions for treating this disorder in children and adolescents. Progress is clearly being made but there are many hurdles to be overcome in treating this particularly life-altering and self-negating form of emotional distress.

References

Adams, R. E., Boscarino, J., & Figley, C. R. (2006). Compassion fatigue and psychological distress among social workers: A validation Study. *American Journal of Orthopsychiatry, 76*, 103–108.

Alvarez, J., McLean, C., Haris, A. H. S., Rosen, C. S., & Ruzek, J. I. (2011). The comparative effectiveness of cognitive processing therapy for male veterans treated in a VHA posttraumatic disorder residential rehabilitation program. *Journal of Consulting and Clinical Psychology, 79*(5), 590–599.

American Psychiatric Association. (1980). *Diagnostic and statistical manual of mental disorders* (3rd ed.) Washington, DC: American Psychiatric Association.

American Psychiatric Association. (2013). *Diagnostic and statistical manual of mental disorders* (5th ed.). Washington, DC: American Psychiatric Association.

Beck, A., Rush, J., Shaw, S., & Emery, G. (1979). *Cognitive therapy of depression*. New York: Guilford.

Boyer, B., Bubel, D., Jacobs, S. R., Knolls, M., Harwell, V. D., Goscicka, M., et al. (2002). Posttraumatic stress in women with breast cancer and their daughters. *The American Journal of Family Therapy, 30*, 328–338.

Brady, K., Pearlstein, T., Asnis, G. M., Baker, D., Rothbaum, B. O., Sikes, C. R., et al. (2000). Efficacy and safety of sertraline treatment of posttraumatic stress disorder: A randomized controlled trial. *Journal of the American Medical Association, 282*(14), 1837–1844.

Breslau, N., Chilcoat, H. D., Kessler, R. C., Peterson, E. L., & Lucia, V. C. (1996). Vulnerability to assaultive violence: Further specification of the sex difference in post-traumatic stress disorder. *Psychological Medicine, 29*, 813–821.

Bride, B. E., Robinson, M. M., Yegidis, B., & Figley, C. R. (2004). Development and validation of the Secondary Traumatic Stress Scale. *Research on Social Work Practice, 14*, 27–35.

Catherall, D. R. (1992). *Back from the brink: A family guide to overcoming traumatic stress*. New York, NY: Bantam Books.

Daly, R. J. (1983). Samuel Pepys and posttraumatic stress disorder. *British Journal of Psychiatry, 143*, 64–68.

Diaz, A. B., & Motta, R. W. (2008). The effects of an aerobic exercise program on posttraumatic stress disorder symptom severity in adolescents. *International Journal of Emergency Mental Health, 191*, 49–59.

Dohrenwend, B. P., Turner, J. B., Turse, N. A., Adams, B. G., Koenen, K. C., & Marschall, R. (2006). The psychological risks of Vietnam for U.S. veterans: A revisit with new data and methods. *Science, 313*, 979–982.

Dubner, A. E., & Motta, R. W. (1999). Sexually and physically abused foster care children with PTSD. *Journal of Consulting and Clinical Psychology, 67*, 367–373.

Dwyer, L. A. (2005). *An investigation of secondary trauma in police wives.* Unpublished doctoral dissertation, Hofstra University, Hempstead, NY.

Ellis, A. (2005). *The myth of self-esteem.* New York: Prometheus Books.

Evans, C., Ehlers, A., Mezey, G., & Clark, D. M. (2007). Intrusive memories in perpetrators of violent crime: Emotions and cognitions. *Journal of Consulting and Clinical Psychology, 75*, 134–144.

Figley, C. R., & Stamm, B. H. (1996). Psychometric review of Compassion Fatigue Self Test. In B. H. Stamm (Ed.), *Measurement of stress, trauma, and adaptation* (pp. 129–130). Lutherville, MD: Sidran.

Foa, E. B., Dancu, C. V., Hembree, E. A., Jaycox, L. H., Meadows, E. A., & Street, G. P. (1999). A comparison of exposure therapy, stress inoculation training, and their combination for reducing posttraumatic stress disorder in female assault victims. *Journal of Consulting and Clinical Psychology, 67*, 194–200.

Foa, E. B., & Meadows, E. A. (1997). Psychosocial treatments for posttraumatic stress disorder: A critical review. *Annual Review of Psychology, 48*, 449–480.

Fredman, S. J., Monson, C. M., & Adair, K. C. (2011). Implementing cognitive-behavioral conjoint therapy for PTSD with the newest generation of veterans and their partners. *Cognitive and Behavioral Practice, 18*(1), 120–130.

Herbert, J., Lilienfeld, S., Montgomery, R., O'Donohue, W., Rosen, G., & Tolin, D. (2000). Science and pseudoscience in the development of eye movement desensitization and reprocessing. *Clinical Psychology Review, 20*(8), 945–971.

Herman, J. (1992). *Trauma and recovery.* New York: Basic Books.

Kassai, S. C., & Motta, R. W. (2006). An investigation of the spread of potential Holocaust-related secondary traumatization to the third generation. *International Journal of Emergency Mental Health, 8*, 35–47.

Kellerman, N. (2001). Psychopathology in children of Holocaust survivors: A review of the research literature. *Israeli Journal of Psychiatry and Related Sciences, 38*, 36–46.

Kinzie, J. D., Sack, W. H., Angell, R. H., Mason, S. M., & Ben, R. (1986). A tree year follow-up of Cambodian young people traumatized as children. *Journal of the American Academy of Child and Adolescent Psychiatry, 25*, 370–376.

Kovacs, M. (2010). *Children's depression inventory* (2nd ed.). North Tonawanda, NY: Multi-Health Systems.

Libov, B. G., Nevid, J. S., Pelcovitz, D., & Carmony, T. M. (2002). Posttraumatic stress symptomatology in mothers of pediatric cancer survivors. *Psychology and Health, 19*, 501–511.

Lombardo, M. (2005). *Secondary trauma in individuals exposed to a person with a serious medical illness.* Unpublished doctoral dissertation, Hofstra University, Hempstead, NY.

Manger, T. A., & Motta, R. W. (2005). The impact of an exercise program on posttraumatic stress disorder, anxiety, and depression. *International Journal of Emergency Mental Health, 7*, 49–57.

Motta, R. W. (2012). Secondary trauma in children and school personnel. *Journal of Applied School Psychology, 28*(3), 256–269.

Motta, R. W., Hafeez, S., Sciancalepore, R., & Diaz, A. B. (2001). Discriminant validation of the Secondary Trauma Scale. *Journal of Psychotherapy in Independent Practice, 24*, 17–24.

Motta, R. W., McWilliams, M. E., Schwartz, J. T., & Cavera, R. S. (2012). The role of physical exercise in reducing childhood PTSD, anxiety, and depression. *Journal of Applied School Psychology, 28*(3), 224–238.

Nader, K. O., Kriegler, J. A., Blake, D. D., Pynoos, R. S., Newman, E., & Weathers, F. W. (1996). *Clinician-Administered PTSD Scale for Children and Adolescents for (DSM-IV).* Boston, MA: National Center for PTSD, Boston Veterans Administration Medical Center.

Nelson, B. S., & Wampler, K. S. (2000). Systemic effects of trauma in clinic couples: An exploratory study of secondary trauma resulting from childhood abuse. *Journal of Marital and Family Therapy, 26,* 171–184.

Newman, C. J., & Motta, R. W. (2007). The effect of aerobic exercise on childhood PTSD, anxiety, and depression. *International Journal of Emergency Mental Health, 9*(2), 133–158.

Parsons, J., Kehl, T. J., & Ownn, S. V. (1990). Incidence of behavior problems among children of Vietnam war veterans. *School Psychology International, 11,* 253–259.

Pearlman, L. A. (1996). Psychometric review of TSI Belief Scale, revision L. In B. H. Stamm (Ed.), *Measurement of stress, trauma, and adaptation* (pp. 415–417). Lutherville, MD: Sidran.

Perlstein, R., & Motta, R. W. (2012). An investigation of potential Holocaust-related Secondary Trauma in the third generation. *Traumatology.* doi:10.1177/153765612449659.

Reich, W., Leacock, N., & Shanfeld, C. (1994). *Diagnostic interview for Adolescents-Revised (DICA-R).* St. Louis, MO: Washington University.

Resick, P. A. (2001). *Cognitive processing therapy: Generic version.* St. Louis, MO: University of Missouri, St Louis.

Reynolds, C. R., & Richmond, B. O. (2008). *Revised child manifest anxiety scale* (2nd ed.). Torrance, CA: Western Psychological Associates.

Rodenburg, R., Benjamin, A., Carlijn, D., Meijer, A. M., & Stams, G. J. (2009). Efficacy of EMDR in children: A meta analysis. *Clinical Psychology Review, 29*(7), 599–606.

Rosenheck, R., & Nathan, P. (1985). Secondary traumatization in children of Vietnam veterans with posttraumatic stress disorder. *Hospital and Community Psychiatry, 36,* 538–539.

Ruf, M., Schauer, M., Neuner, F., Catani, C., Schauer, E., & Elbert, T. (2010). Narrative exposure therapy for 7- to 16 year olds: A randomized controlled trial with traumatized refugee children. *Journal of Traumatic Stress, 23,* 437–445.

Saigh, P. A., Yaski, A. E., Oberfield, R. A., Green, B. L., Halamandaris, P. V., Rubenstein, J. N., et al. (2000). The Children's PTSD Inventory: Development and reliability. *Journal of Traumatic Stress, 13*(3), 369–380.

Salem, Y., Gropack, S. J., Coffin, D., & Godwin, E. M. (2012). Effectiveness of a low-cost virtual reality system for children with developmental delays: A preliminary randomized single-blind controlled trial. *Physiotherapy, 98*(3), 189–195.

Shapiro, F. (2001). *EMDR: Eye Movement Desensitization and Reprocessing: Basic principles, protocols and procedures* (2nd ed.). New York: Guilford Press.

Stamm, B. H. (2010). *The concise ProQOL manual* (2nd ed.). Pocatello, LD: ProQOL.org.

Stroop, J. R. (1935). Studies of interference in serial verbal reactions. *Journal of Experimental Psychology, 28*(6), 643–662.

Suozzi, J. R., & Motta, R. W. (2004). The relationship between combat exposure and the transfer of trauma-like symptoms to offspring of veterans. *Traumatology, 10,* 17–37.

Sutherland, R. J., Mott, J. S., Williams, W., Teng, E. J., & Ready, D. J. (2012). A pilot study of a 12-week model of group-based exposure therapy for veterans with PTSD. *Journal of Traumatic Stress, 25*(2), 150–156.

Terr, L. C. (1983). Chowchilla revisited: The effects of psychic trauma four years after a school bus kidnapping. *American Journal of Psychiatry, 140,* 1543–1550.

Trimble, M. R. (1981). *Post-traumatic neurosis: From railway spine to whiplash.* New York: Wiley.

Trimble, M. R. (1985). Post-traumatic stress disorder: History of a concept. In C. R. Figley (Ed.), *Trauma and its wake: The study and treatment of post-traumatic stress disorder.* New York: Bruner/Mazel.

Wampold, B. E. (2001). *The great psychotherapy debate: Models, methods, and findings.* Mahwah, NJ: Lawrence Erlbaum Associates, Inc.

Waysman, M., Mikulinger, M., Solomon, Z., & Weisenberg, M. (1993). Secondary traumatization among wives of posttraumatic combat veterans: A family topology. *Journal of Family Psychology, 7,* 104–118.

Chapter 5
Depression

Janay B. Sander, Jenny Herren, and Jared A. Bishop

The symptoms of depression can be manifested in several ways, most often presenting as a sad or depressed mood but also as irritability or a loss of interest in activities (anhedonia). Suicidal ideation in depressed youths is of particular concern as it is a particularly common symptom in this population (Rohde, Beevers, Stice, & O'Neil, 2009). Importantly, depression is one of the most commonly occurring mental health disorders in children and adolescents. Up to 17 % of females may experience a depressive episode that meets diagnostic criteria by the time they reach age 20, with the peak point incidence of clinical depression near 5 % in 16-year-old females (Rohde et al., 2009). Youth in high-risk communities, including non-Caucasian ethnic groups (Rohde et al., 2009) and youths from poverty-stricken areas are at even greater risk for depressive symptoms (Riolo, Nguyen, Greden, & King, 2005). In low-risk community samples, between 8 % and 20 % of children aged 11–18 may be experiencing depressive symptoms (Diamantopoulou, Verhulst, & van der Ende, 2011). While both male and female youth experience clinical depression, females have a typically higher prevalence rates for the disorder at the onset of adolescence.

In school settings, the symptoms of children and adolescents with depression (i.e., sadness, difficulty concentrating, insomnia, and low energy) often can interfere with academic performance. This compounds stress and academic difficulties (Rohde et al., 2009). If a child or adolescent is struggling in school due to depression, it could potentially become an educational service to provide intervention for that student. Depression is recognized as one form of disability or emotional disturbance that may qualify a student for special education and related services. Federal regulations of the

J.B. Sander, Ph.D., H.S.P.P. (✉) • J.A. Bishop, M.A.
Department of Educational Psychology, Ball State University, Muncie, IN, USA
e-mail: jbsander@bsu.edu; jabishop@bsu.edu

J. Herren, Ph.D.
Judge Baker Children's Center & Harvard University, Boston, MA, USA
e-mail: jennyherren@gmail.com

© Springer Science+Business Media New York 2015
R. Flanagan et al. (eds.), *Cognitive and Behavioral Interventions in the Schools*, DOI 10.1007/978-1-4939-1972-7_5

Individuals With Disabilities Education Act (IDEA), 20 United States Code § 1400 (2004), Part A Sec. 300.8 (c) (4) (i) include the words "pervasive mood of unhappiness or depression" in the definition of an emotional disturbance. In summary, the presence of depression is very relevant to schools and for some students is a condition that may warrant consideration for protection and services as a disability. For other students depressive symptoms may interfere in a less impairing way with school functioning. Cognitive behavioral approaches that adhere to evidence-based practices and methods, in particular, are very compatible with the structure and culture of schools (Christner, Forrest, Morley, & Weinstein, 2007).

Prevention and Early Intervention

Given the prevalence and impact of depression on youth functioning, including academic performance, school-based, research-supported interventions for depressed children and adolescents are a needed service. Mental health services to address depression in schools could take the form of a universal, targeted, or intensive intervention within the schools' continuum of educational programs. Prevention programs for depression, as well as early intervention to address low levels of symptoms of depression, are highly recommended (Gillham, Jaycox, Reivich, Seligman, & Silver, 1990; Gillham, Hamilton, Freres, Patton, & Gallop, 2006; Rohde, Stice, & Gau, 2012). Many of the prevention programs for youth depression include CBT elements. Several prevention program outcomes that have been examined and published by researchers are addressed in following sections.

Assessment

Evidence-based academic interventions are the expectation in school settings. With that in mind, using formal assessment and evidence-based psychosocial intervention approaches in schools is highly recommended. Assessment tools that are consistent with evidence-based practice would include empirically supported assessment methods and using data to inform interventions (D'Angelo & Augenstein, 2012). At the same time, however, efficiency and cost are important considerations (Ebesutani, Bernstein, Chorpita, & Weisz, 2012). There are several purposes of assessment in relation to youth depression. In school settings, the use of evidence-based interventions is emphasized, and assessment should also reflect the same approach (Jensen-Doss, 2011). For educational purposes, obtaining a diagnosis of depression may not be required as much as identifying students who may have impairments in functioning due to depressive symptoms, and often these students are already identified by schools as having other educational concerns (Maag & Swearer, 2005).

In schools in particular, the use of norm-referenced rating scales (self, parent, and teacher reports) is recommended (Maag & Swearer, 2005). These are preferred due to the established validity and reliability information, combined with an objective way to document symptoms via scores. These measures are also commonly adopted for outcome measures in randomized controlled trials of depression interventions with youths, so these have been accepted by the scientist practitioner literature in general. Diagnostic interviews are very time consuming, and may not be as efficient for use in school settings unless it is for a small number of students considered at high risk of having a depressive disorder. For schools in general, symptom documentation with the use of norm-referenced rating scales and symptom inventories would be more efficient for most purposes. These methods fit with school culture of assessment and monitoring student progress using scores in general, unless a formal diagnosis of depression is required.

Assessment data should be used to identify symptoms but also to inform ongoing interventions, such as when a student may either require more intensive interventions or may no longer need the intervention due to symptom remission. For adolescents, the youth self-report is recommended as a key assessment component, as parents and teachers may not have as accurate a perspective of the youth's internal experience (Weisz, McCarty, & Valeri, 2006). See Table 5.1 for a list of depression assessment tools that have been reported in published treatment outcome research and used in meta-analytic studies (see Maag, Swearer, & Toland, 2009; Mychailyszyn, Brodman, Read, & Kendall, 2012; Weisz et al., 2006). Some of these measures are available for no charge to download, such as the Mood and Feelings Questionnaire (Angold, Costello, Messer, & Pickles, 1995; see http://devepi.duhs.duke.edu/mfq.html).

Table 5.1 Measures of depression and potential application in schools

Measure name	Original citation[a]	Recommended uses			
		Screening	Pre-intervention	Progress monitoring	Outcomes
Automatic Thoughts Questionnaire	Hollon and Kendall (1980)	X	X		X
Beck Depression Inventory for Youth (BDI-Y)	Beck, Beck, and Jolly (2003)	X	X		X
Beck Depression Inventory, Second Edition (BDI-2)	Beck, Steer, and Brown (1996)	X	X	X	X
Brief Impairment Scale	Bird et al. (2005)	X	X		X
Center for Epidemiologic Studies Depression Scale (CES-D)	Radloff (1977)	X	X	X	X
Child Behavior Checklist (CBCL), (includes parent, teacher, or youth self-reports)	Achenbach and Rescorla (2001)	X	X		X

(continued)

Table 5.1 (continued)

Measure name	Original citation[a]	Recommended uses			
		Screening	Pre-intervention	Progress monitoring	Outcomes
Children's Attributional Style Questionnaire— Revised	Kaslow and Nolen-Hoeksema (1991)	X	X	X	X
Children's Depression Inventory, 2nd edition (CDI-2)	Kovacs (2010)	X	X	X	X
Children's Depression Rating Scale, Revised	Poznanski et al. (1984)	X	X	X	X
Dysfunctional Attitude Scale	Weissman (1979)	X	X	X	X
Hopelessness Scale for Children	Kazdin, Rodgers, and Colbus (1986)	X	X		X
Mood and Feelings Questionnaire (MFQ), short and long forms	Angold et al. (1995)	X	X	X	X
Revised Hamilton Rating Scale for Depression	Warren (1994)	X	X	X	X
Reynolds Adolescent Depression Scale	Reynolds (1986)	X	X	X	X
Reynolds Child Depression Scale	Reynolds (1989)	X	X	X	X
Schedule for Affective Disorders and Schizophrenia for School-Aged Children (K-SADS)	Ambrosini and Dixon (2000)		X		X
Self-Report Coping Scale	Causey and Dubow (1992)	X	X		X
Suicidal Ideation Questionnaire	Reynolds (1988)	X	X		X

[a]These measures have been used in studies that have been published much more recently than the original citation

Interventions

A number of manualized depression interventions with promising and/or well-established efficacy are available for therapist use. Many of these interventions have been applied or adapted to school settings. Table 5.2 provides a summary of select manuals that are designed to treat depression. One of the most widely studied interventions

Table 5.2 Examples of manualized CBT interventions for youth depression

Manual	Therapy format	Primary CBT components
ACTION (Stark, Struesand, Krumholz, & Patel, 2010)	Age range: 9–14	Psycho-education; goal setting; behavioral activation; coping skills and emotion regulation skills training; problem solving skills; cognitive restructuring; improvement in self-schema; mood monitoring; interpersonal skills; homework
	Format: group	
	Number of sessions: 20, plus 2 individual meetings	
	Duration: 11 weeks, 60 min meetings	
	Other: Parent training component available; booster sessions following therapy	
Coping with Depression for Adolescents (CWD-A) (Clarke, Lewinsohn, & Hops, 1990)	Age range: 14–18	Assertiveness; relaxation skills; cognitive restructuring; mood monitoring; pleasant activity scheduling; communication and conflict-resolution techniques; problem solving skills; homework
	Format: group	
	Number of sessions: 16	
	Duration: 8 weeks; 2 h meetings	
	Other: parent intervention component; booster sessions following therapy	
Modular Approach to Therapy for Children with Anxiety, Depression, Trauma, and Conduct Problems (MATCH-ADTC) (Chorpita & Weisz, 2009)	Age range: 8–13	Psycho-education; mood monitoring; goal setting; problem solving skills; behavioral activation; relaxation; interpersonal skills; cognitive restructuring; cognitive coping; homework
	Format: individual	
	Number of sessions: varies	
	Duration: varies	
	Other: flexible to address comorbidity, if needed	
Primary and Secondary Control Enhancement Training (PASCET) (Weisz, Gray, Bearman, Southam-Gerow, & Stark, 2005)	Age range: 8–15	Teaches primary and secondary control coping methods; goal setting; behavioral activation; coping skills; problem solving skills; relaxation; cognitive restructuring; cognitive coping; homework
	Format: individual	
	Number of sessions: 10–15+	
	Duration: 50 min, length varies	
Penn Resiliency Program (PRP) (Gillham, Jaycox, Reivich, Seligman, & Silver, 1990; Gillham, Hamilton, Freres, Patton, & Gallop, 2006)	Age range: 8–15	Psycho-education; cognitive restructuring; assertiveness and negotiation; coping strategies; graded task and social skills training; decision making; problem solving skills; interpersonal skills; homework
	Format: group	
	Number of sessions: 12–24 depending on duration	
	Duration: 60 min sessions over 24 meetings or 90 min sessions over 12 meetings	
Stress-busters (Asarnow & Scott, 1999)	Age range: 8–12	Social skills; problem solving training; goal setting; relaxation skills; psycho-education of emotional spirals; pleasant activity scheduling; cognitive restructuring and coping; cognitive and behavioral strategies for reversing negative emotional spirals; homework
	Format: group	
	Number of sessions: ten	
	Duration: 90 min sessions over 5 weeks	
	Other: family education sessions	

(continued)

Table 5.2 (continued)

Manual	Therapy format	Primary CBT components
TADS (Curry, et al., 2005)	Age range: 12–17	Psycho-education; mood monitoring; goal setting: increasing pleasant activities; problem solving; cognitive restructuring; social interaction; assertion; communication and compromise; relaxation; affect regulation; homework; maintenance
	Format: individual	
	Number of sessions: 15–18 plus boosters	
	Duration: 60 min for 12 weeks (acute phase) followed by 18 weeks of continuation and maintenance	
	Other: family CBT component, modular depending on client needs, booster sessions following therapy	

is the Coping with Depression for Adolescents (CWD-A; Clarke, Lewinsohn, & Hops, 1990), which is available for free download (see http://www.kpchr.org/research/public/acwd/acwd.html). Other manuals are available from the authors or from the publisher of the manual. While these treatments vary in length, duration, and format, they are all based upon CBT principles and contain similar therapy components.

Chorpita and Daleiden (2009) report that the most common therapy strategies, or "practice elements," for treating childhood depressed mood include cognitive, psychoeducational–child, maintenance/relapse prevention, activity scheduling, problem solving, and self-monitoring. Rather than discussing each manual separately, we will focus on describing these commonly used CBT approaches for children. Brief descriptions of which elements are within the available manualized interventions are included in Table 5.2.

The first therapy element typically found in depression manuals is psycho-education for the child, which establishes the foundation for therapy. Typically, a cognitive behavioral model of depression is presented to teach a child about the relation between thoughts, feelings, and behaviors and how depression is maintained. Manuals may present this information in different ways. For instance, some manuals discuss the downward and upward spirals of depression (Asarnow & Scott, 1999; Clarke et al., 1990; Curry et al., 2005), whereas others do not. A typical goal of psychoeducation in CBT protocols is to help children understand that behaviors and thoughts influence emotions, and you can improve your mood by doing and thinking differently. PASCET (Weisz, Sandler, Durlak, & Anton, 2005) exemplifies this concept by using "ACT" (Primary Control) and "THINK" (Secondary Control) skills as ways children can change their mood. Children also learn about the structure of the intervention and the importance of therapeutic homework.

Activity scheduling or behavioral activation is another frequent practice element. The goal of this therapy strategy is to increase the amount and quality of pleasant activities the child engages in on a weekly and daily basis. Youth with depression, especially with anhedonia, tend to withdraw and do not engage in pleasurable activities or tend to select activities that are not reinforcing. Most manuals encourage children and adolescents to identify a number of activities they can engage in on a weekly basis, including more physical activities. Treatment manuals may also focus on demonstrating this skill in vivo in session as well as how to manage when children are "stuck" and "don't feel like doing anything."

Problem solving is another therapy strategy common to depression manuals. Children and adolescents who are depressed tend to feel helpless and hopeless and often have a difficult time handling problems. Problem solving teaches children an active, systematic approach to managing problems. Different protocols have various acronyms to help children remember the steps of problem solving, such as "5 P's" (Stark, Struesand, Krumholz, & Patel, 2010), "STEPS" (Chorpita & Weisz, 2009; Weisz, Gray, Bearman, Southam-Gerow, & Stark, 2005), and "RIBEYE" (Curry et al., 2005). Each of these procedures help children to brainstorm various solutions, evaluate each solution by thinking of the pros and cons, choose a solution to try, and use self-reinforcement (e.g., praise, pat on the back).

Not surprisingly, a major component of the CBT model is identifying and changing negative thinking to improve one's mood (Beck, 2011). A case conceptualization provides a guiding framework to tailor treatment to a child's individual needs and creates an understanding of the client's uniqueness, as well as their cognitive patterns. Case conceptualizations evolve over time and should be refined throughout treatment as a therapist gains a better understanding of the client. Each manual presents various methods for helping children and/or adolescents identify negative thoughts and change them into more positive thoughts. For instance, CWD-A (Clarke et al., 1990; Rohde, Lewinsohn, Clarke, Hops, & Seeley, 2005) uses a C-A-B method to help youth identify the Consequence (e.g., noticing when the youth is feeling down), Activating event (e.g., what situation triggered the low mood), and Belief (e.g., the thoughts that led from the activating event to the consequences). The therapist then helps the adolescent develop an alternative belief using Socratic questioning (e.g., What is another way to look at the situation? What would you tell your best friend?). Many manuals also incorporate techniques to manage cognitive rumination, such as "Changing the Channel" found in PASCET (Weisz, Gray et al., 2005).

Self-monitoring and maintenance relapse prevention are also common approaches. Typical CBT for depression incorporates self-monitoring throughout treatment. Practice or homework is assigned outside of the session and mood monitoring is used to determine the effects of various strategies. Given that depression is a recurrent disorder, maintenance and relapse prevention are included in many depression intervention protocols. In addition to preparation at the conclusion of therapy, many protocols incorporate "booster" sessions to help promote continued use of skills and monitor progress (Clarke et al., 1990; Curry et al., 2005; Stark et al., 2010).

Overall, these CBT programs for treating depression in youth involve a combination of behavioral and cognitive strategies. The principles for these strategies are common across treatment manuals; however, the presentation of the skills and the amount of time dedicated to each skill will vary for each protocol. Other variations to the manuals that therapists should consider include the format of the intervention (individual vs. group), duration and length of sessions, developmental appropriateness, incorporation of other practice elements (e.g., communication training, interpersonal skills), availability of the manual (e.g., free vs. cost), training required, and caregiver involvement.

Obstacles to Implementing CBT Depression Intervention in Schools

While schools are recognized as an important setting to deliver mental health services (Atkins, Hoagwood, Kutash, & Seidman, 2010), there are a number of roadblocks that should be considered when implementing manualized depression programs in schools. Lack of support from school administrators and staff can be a fundamental barrier. Although there is a strong desire for practitioners to do therapy in schools, specifically CBT, administrators often do not want student achievement to be adversely impacted by their spending time out of the classroom to receive an intervention. Several strategies can be used to ease this concern and gain support from staff.

First, it can be helpful to provide education around the prevalence of depression and its negative impact on students' academic performance, as well as about the therapy itself to resolve any misperceptions about depression or the need for therapy. As examples, the practitioner can educate staff about how a quietly depressed student may not necessarily appear to be in distress, especially in a classroom with 25 other adolescents, but that this "internalizing" of symptoms can mask the extent of a child's impairment. Another important educational point is that the irritability associated with depression may often be misperceived as oppositional behavior. Sharing information with school staff in general about depression may help build awareness about how depressive symptoms can interfere at school. Therapists should also emphasize the goal of CBT is to help students learn to improve and manage their mood through acquiring "toolbox" of skills that they can use in and outside of the classroom. Once the teacher or administration is in support of allowing screenings, prevention, or interventions for depression in the school, the next barrier is related to logistics.

Teacher support is important for ongoing therapy success if students may often miss class in order to participate in therapy. The first negotiation will be about times the child can attend therapy during the school day. Schools may have a dedicated "intervention" time, when tiered academic or other interventions (i.e., speech therapy, occupational therapy, or counseling services) are permitted. It is helpful for clinicians to recognize that the schools have specific educational priorities, and in some schools it is required that students spend a certain number of minutes per day on specific academic areas, such as reading. Being flexible to accommodate the school's other constraints is essential. Therapy may need to move or rotate through class periods, for example, to make sure the student does not miss the same class each week and is not absent from core content, especially if the student is struggling academically.

Next, it is essential that students are not penalized (e.g., receiving a zero on a missed quiz, not receiving instruction on the homework assignment) for attending therapy. If the sessions are occurring during the school day, obtaining permission and meeting with a student's teachers prior to the initiation of therapy can be very helpful to discuss the rationale for the intervention, and how it will benefit the student. It is also important to discuss classroom concerns and any potential obstacles around the child missing class. The clinician must also be respectful of the school's pressures and constraints and be willing (and sometimes creative) to find a solution. If students are not formally recognized as in need of mental health services, either through special education, school-wide screenings, or other documentation of depression symptoms, it may not be feasible to provide therapy during the school day at school. In these situations, offering before- or after-school sessions may be feasible. Lunch schedules may be very short, but this may also be an option.

Other obstacles in the school environment may present threats to the validity of intervention being delivered. Despite being time-limited, most manualized interventions have a specific number of sessions and recommended duration of session (e.g., 45 min, 90 min), which may not fit with the typical school schedule. This can present therapeutic challenges if the therapist has to break up the material or reduce content covered. Therapists should do their best to minimize the impact of missing academic instruction while trying to be adherent to and preserve the validity of the intervention. Working with students during specials (physical education, music, or art) or electives and rotating meeting times so that the child does not miss one class repeatedly can be helpful ways to address this concern.

Additionally, some manualized programs include parental involvement for the standardized delivery of the intervention. Parent participation may be challenging in the school setting if parents are not able to take time off from work during the school day or are otherwise unable or unwilling to participate in therapy. Therapists may find more success in increasing caregiver participation if they are flexible around scheduling and work with the school around other community programs to pool resources for sibling care, for example. While implementation of manuals in the schools presents some obstacles, the benefits of school delivery are many. Several published manualized interventions were designed for and tested in the school system (Asarnow, Scott, & Mintz, 2002; Gillham et al., 2007; Lewinsohn, Clarke, Hops, & Andrews, 1990; Stark et al., 2010).

Developmental Considerations

In general, the CBT components will be more behavioral in emphasis with younger clients, such as early elementary age, and more balanced, or with more cognitive components as clients reach mid- to late adolescence. In addition, parent and/or environmental (school/teacher) components will be more important with elementary age clients relative to secondary education settings (grades 6–12). There may also be additional peer relationship and interpersonal considerations for adolescents relative to children.

Case Illustration

In order to illustrate how this type of therapy may be used in the schools, we present a case of a child who participated in a CBT intervention group for depression at school. Identifying information has been altered to protect the identity of this individual and her family. This child received the manualized ACTION intervention (Stark et al., 2010).

"Stephanie" was a 10-year-old Caucasian female in the 4th grade in a suburban elementary school. Stephanie was identified through a school-wide screening for emotional concerns. After the screening, clinicians conducted follow-up interviews with the children who had elevated symptoms. Based upon a structured K-SADS diagnostic interview with her and her mother, she met criteria for major depressive disorder (MDD). The school was supportive of her receiving therapy during the school day as part of a special program once it was clear that she had clinical depression.

She lived in an intact family with an older sister and younger brother. Stephanie was in a regular education classroom most of the time but was identified as having a math disability and is receiving special education services. The onset of Stephanie's depression started around the beginning of the school year. Prior to school starting, she had a close friend move away, which was particularly difficult for her. She was struggling academically and described herself as "stupid" because she received special education services.

Developing a case conceptualization is important in the treatment of depression. For Stephanie, it was initially hypothesized that she had a helpless core belief of "I am inadequate." She identified thinking "I'm stupid" and frequently compared herself to her high-achieving older sister. Social comparison seemed paramount for Stephanie, which frequently resulted in interpersonal difficulties with her friends and siblings. Her depression appeared to have been precipitated by the loss of her primary social support (i.e., move of her best friend) and the start of a new school year. Additionally, her depressive symptoms, including irritability and social withdrawal, were impacting her current relationships and straining her remaining social network. Friendships were important to Stephanie and she desired to make new friends.

She also demonstrated a number of strengths. Stephanie was already using a number of positive coping strategies, such as playing her guitar, and was involved in sports. She had very supportive parents, who described her as caring and sensitive. Based upon this conceptualization, treatment goals were aimed at targeting Stephanie's negative beliefs about her inadequacy, reconnecting with and establishing new sources of social support, and increasing her positive coping strategies to deal with life stressors.

Given that Stephanie was already having difficulties in school and was receiving special education services, it was important to minimize the amount of core academic content she had to miss for therapy. The therapist worked with the school staff to primarily schedule meetings during elective times with a rotating schedule. The therapist also had consent to discuss Stephanie's progress with the school and provided psychoeducation to Stephanie's teachers about her depression and the importance of her being able to make up any academic instruction she missed due to attending therapy sessions. Collaboration with the teachers and school psychologist was essential in this case in order to set Stephanie up for success. Because this intervention was delivered in the school setting during school hours, parental involvement was fairly limited. The therapist met with the caregivers in person at the outset of treatment to explain the treatment model and provide education about depression in children. The therapist also checked in with the parents over the phone every few weeks to see how things were progressing from the parent perspective, reinforce the use of skills at home, and address any concerns.

Stephanie was in a group with three other girls in the 4th and 5th grades who were also experiencing a depressive disorder. The initial treatment sessions focused on group rapport building, psychoeducation about cognitive model, mood monitoring, and increasing engagement in positive activities. When presented with the cognitive model, Stephanie immediately made the connection between missing her best friend and feeling sad. The therapist helped Stephanie identify that when she thinks about her friend being so far away, she feels quite sad. However, if Stephanie focused on getting to talk with her on the phone, her mood improved. To make this more salient, the therapist had Stephanie rate her mood on a "mood meter" scale from 0 to 10 (where 0 is totally completely down and 10 is feeling terrific) when she focused on each thought, and then rate her corresponding mood level.

Pleasant event scheduling and behavioral activation were also introduced early in treatment. Introduction of behavioral activation was done in vivo. That is, the therapist induced a mildly negative mood and then had all group participants engage in a quick, fun activity, such as freeze tag. Stephanie reported her mood improved from a 4 to a 10! She quickly started applying this skill in her life. For instance, Stephanie reported that she had an argument with a friend and read a book to feel better. It is important to help clients to identify positive activities that are mood boosting for them and get them to regularly engage in these activities outside of treatment.

As part of the group intervention, the therapist met individually with each client to develop personal treatment goals. Stephanie identified two treatment goals, which were to feel better about missing her mother when she travels for work and to get along better with peers. The next few meetings focused on sharing of treatment goals, application of coping strategies, and the introduction and application of problem solving. Stephanie seemed to really grasp the concept of doing something to change her mood and reported using many coping strategies, such as watching a movie and dancing, to improve her mood.

At this point in therapy, Stephanie's depressed mood seemed to be mostly triggered by interpersonal difficulties with peers or her family. During these meetings, she reported having negative thoughts about her relationships, such as "She doesn't want to be my friend anymore" and "They hate me." As Stephanie shared these beliefs, the therapist adjusted her case conceptualization to include a core belief about being unlovable. Her social evaluation concerns continued to extend into group as Stephanie refused to share her goals with the group and experienced negative thoughts about how the group would perceive her goals. Over the course of several meetings, the therapist helped make the skills most relevant for Stephanie by helping her apply systematic problem solving to difficulties related to her peers. She related particularly well to another group member who was experiencing teasing at school. As Stephanie felt more supported by and connected to the group, she initiated sharing her goals with the group and heard only positive feedback from her peers. This experience also served to highlight for her how her negative assumptions were inaccurate! As these mid-treatment sessions progressed, Stephanie continued to open up about interpersonal difficulties with her family and peers and reported engaging in problem solving and behavioral activation outside of session. Stephanie also became a strong group member and offered support and suggestions to other members when they were upset. This shift in interpersonal connectedness with the therapist and group seemed to increase her engagement and willingness to try the strategies being taught.

Throughout the second half of treatment, Stephanie was engaged in the therapeutic process and added her own topics to the agenda in the group, shared progress on her goals, and was open about her negative beliefs. Stephanie rose to the challenge and was able to "talk back" to her negative thoughts, which was referred to as the Muck Monster. Toward the end of therapy, Stephanie was not having interference from negative thoughts. The therapist also worked with her on building a self-map highlighting her strengths to promote a positive self-schema. This component of treatment was especially crucial for Stephanie. The therapist gathered positive comments from her teachers and parents for her to add to the self-map. Stephanie loved hearing all the positive things her teachers and parents had to say! The last few sessions were spent preparing Stephanie and her fellow group members for their graduation from the group, maintaining gains and use of skills, as well as celebrating their progress. At posttreatment, a diagnostic interview was readministered to Stephanie and her caregiver. Stephanie no longer met the criteria for MDD and reported no symptoms in the clinical range. All her initial symptoms were very much improved.

Other Practice Considerations

Therapy for depression in schools includes several important features. Fitting sessions within the school schedule and those educational constraints is essential. Finding creative and flexible solutions to allow the client to attend the most enjoyable classes, as part of experiencing pleasant activities, is also recommended. Next, the relationship with peers in class, or with the teachers, may be impaired due to the depressive symptoms. This may become an important treatment goal.

Finally, it is important for clinicians to incorporate a variety of learning strategies to create experiences for the child to facilitate change in therapy, not just talk about the ideas in an academic sense (Stark, Arora, & Funk, 2011). Good therapy will include teaching skills so that the client really learns and can apply the techniques. For example, planning a fun activity and using a mood meter to capture the child's feelings before and after the fun activity are more meaningful as experiential learning than assigning fun activities as homework alone. It is important for the therapist to be flexible in the delivery method of the therapeutic skills and content and adjust according to how the child seems to best take in that information or skill.

Research

There are several meta-analytic synthesis investigations of depression prevention and intervention studies. Two are of particular interest and relevance due to the focus on children and adolescents. One meta-analysis focused specifically on prevention. This study by Stice, Bohon, Shaw, Marti, and Rohde (2009) incorporated 32 different depression prevention programs (from 1980 to 2008) from 47 different trials, allowing for calculation of 60 different effect sizes. Depression prevention programs did reduce risk for depression with small effect sizes ($r = .11$ to $.14$), which is encouraging since these were prevention or early intervention studies (Stice et al., 2009). Most of the programs included had a cognitive behavioral foundation. As summarized by Stice and colleagues, the programs with the most promise in terms of positive intervention effects included the Coping with Stress program (Clarke & Lewinsohn, 1995) and the Blues Program (Stice, Burton, Bearman, & Rohde, 2007). Other prevention programs have had mixed reports of effects overall, including the Penn Prevention Program and the Penn Resiliency Program (Gillham et al., 1990, 2006). The authors urged researchers to continue contributing to school-based targeted intervention and prevention research to replicate findings from promising programs and examine additional moderators of program outcomes.

Another meta-analysis about treatment outcomes is by Weisz and his colleagues (2006), which synthesized psychosocial therapy outcomes for depression in children and adolescents, including CBT and other approaches. Researchers analyzed outcomes of 35 different studies that included 44 different treatments from published and non-published studies (1980–2004). The overall mean effect size was .35, considered a small to medium effect. All in all, psychotherapy was recommended as a treatment option for depressed youths. In terms of offering CBT as highly beneficial over other psychotherapy approaches, it remains unclear. It does appear that CBT did produce positive effects and was considered a viable option based on analysis of the available treatment studies, so is a reasonable empirically supported treatment at this time, but it is not the only approach that may be effective (Weisz et al., 2006).

In addition to trials that were completed at the time of the meta-analyses above, there are two recently developed depression early intervention programs of note. One is the Positive Thoughts and Action (PTA) Program. PTA is a CBT-based group program tailored for adolescents and their parents, delivered in school settings (McCarty, Violette, Duong, Cruz, & McCauley, 2013). The PTA yielded moderate effect sizes ($d = .36$) for lowering depressive symptoms at the end of the program and was evaluated using a randomized control trial design. This program was delivered at school, once per week for 12 weeks. It is also important to note that Interpersonal Therapy for Adolescents (IPT-A) has been shown to an effective intervention for adolescents with depression; however, given its primary interpersonal focus, it is outside the scope of this chapter but is nonetheless considered an effective intervention (see Mufson, Dorta, Olfson, Weissman, & Hoagwood, 2004).

Concluding Comments

In conclusion, it is highly recommended that clinicians offer CBT for depressed youths in school settings. The availability of manualized programs, some of which are free for public use, allow for portability of empirically supported treatment methods to clinicians with training in CBT. These programs could be offered during the school day if there is flexibility in scheduling or after school. The available evidence-based literature includes several programs that have been successfully delivered in school settings. With that said, it is also essential that clinicians adhere to the school constraints and adjust or accommodate for school scheduling with the youth participants to mitigate stress from missing core content. As outlined earlier, data-driven assessment and treatment monitoring is particularly beneficial in school settings. In summary, the literature is clearly urging clinicians to provide more CBT in school settings to address youth depression. An array of programs, including the prevention/early intervention and more targeted, intensive CBT interventions, have empirical support for their positive effects with children and adolescents. As the field of psychology adjusts to the constraints and demands within educational settings, hopefully these programs will be more readily available to youths in need of them.

References

Achenbach, T. M., & Rescorla, L. A. (2001). *Manual for the ASEBA school-age forms and profiles.* Burlington: University of Vermont, Center for Children, Youth and Families.

Ambrosini, P. J., & Dixon, J. F. (Eds.). (2000). *Schedule for Affective Disorders and Schizophrenia for School-Age Children (6-18 yrs.). KIDDIE-SADS (K-SADS) Present State and Lifetime Version, K-SADS IVR (Revision of K-SADS).* Unpublished manuscript, Drexel University College of Medicine, Philadelphia.

Angold, A., Costello, E. J., Messer, S. C., & Pickles, A. (1995). Development of a short questionnaire for use in epidemiological studies of depression in children and adolescents. *International Journal of Methods in Psychiatric Research, 5*(4), 237–249.

Asarnow, J. R., & Scott, C. V. (1999). *A combined cognitive–behavioral family education intervention for depression in children.* Unpublished manuscript. University of California at Los Angeles.

Asarnow, J. R., Scott, C. V., & Mintz, J. (2002). A combined cognitive–behavioral family education intervention for depression in children: A treatment development study. *Cognitive Therapy and Research, 26*(2), 221–229.

Atkins, M. S., Hoagwood, K. E., Kutash, K., & Seidman, E. (2010). Toward the integration of education and mental health in schools. *Administration and Policy in Mental Health and Mental Health Services Research, 37*(1–2), 40–47. doi:10.1007/s10488-010-0299-7.

Beck, J. S. (2011). *Cognitive therapy: Basics and beyond* (2nd ed.). New York: Guilford Press.

Beck, J. S., Beck, A. T., & Jolly, J. B. (2003). *Beck youth inventories.* San Antonio, TX: Psychological Corporation.

Beck, A. T., Steer, R. A., & Brown, G. K. (1996). *Beck depression inventory–2nd edition manual.* San Antonio, TX: The Psychological Corporation.

Bird, H. R., Canino, G. J., Davies, M., Ramirez, R., Chavez, L., Duarte, C., et al. (2005). The Brief Impairment Scale (BIS): A multidimensional scale of functional impairment for children and adolescents. *Journal of the American Academy of Child and Adolescent Psychiatry, 44*, 699–707. doi:10.1097/01.chi.0000163281.41383.94.

Causey, D., & Dubow, E. (1992). Development of a self-report coping measure for elementary school children. *Journal of Clinical Child Psychopathology Review, 21*(1), 47–59.

Chorpita, B. F., & Daleiden, E. L. (2009). Mapping evidence-based treatments for children and adolescents: Application of the distillation and matching model to 615 treatments from 322 randomized trials. *Journal of Consulting and Clinical Psychology, 77*(3), 566–579. doi:10.1037/a0014565.

Chorpita, B. F., & Weisz, J. R. (2009). *Modular approach to therapy for children with anxiety, depression, trauma, or conduct problems (MATCH-ADTC).* Satellite Beach, FL: Practicewise, LLC.

Christner, R. W., Forrest, E., Morley, J., & Weinstein, E. (2007). Taking cognitive-behavior therapy to school: A school-based mental health approach. *Journal of Contemporary Psychotherapy, 37*(3), 175–183.

Clarke, G. N., & Lewinsohn, P. M. (1995). *Adolescent coping with stress class*. Portland, OR: Kaiser Permanente for Health Research.

Clarke, G. N., Lewinsohn, P. M., & Hops, H. (1990). *Adolescent coping with depression course.* The therapist manual and the adolescent workbook may be downloaded for free from the Internet at http://www.kpchr.org/acwd/acwd.html

Curry, J. F., Wells, K. C., Brent, D. A., Clarke, G. N., Rohde, P., Albano, A. M., et al. (2005). *Treatment of Adolescents with Depression Study (TADS) cognitive behavior therapy manual: Introduction, rationale, and adolescent sessions*. Duke University Medical Center. The therapist manual may be downloaded for free from the Internet at https://trialweb.dcri.duke.edu/tads/tad/manuals/TADS_CBT.pdf

D'Angelo, E. J., & Augenstein, T. M. (2012). Developmentally informed evaluation of depression: Evidence-based instruments. *Child and Adolescent Psychiatric Clinics of North America, 21*(2), 279–298. doi:10.1016/j.chc.2011.12.003.

Diamantopoulou, S., Verhulst, F. C., & van der Ende, J. (2011). Gender differences in the development and adult outcome of co-occurring depression and delinquency in adolescence. *Journal of Abnormal Psychology, 120*(3), 644–655. doi:10.1037/a0023669.

Ebesutani, C., Bernstein, A., Chorpita, B. F., & Weisz, J. R. (2012). A transportable assessment protocol for prescribing youth psychosocial treatments in real-world settings: Reducing assessment burden via self-report scales. *Psychological Assessment, 24*(1), 141–155. doi:10.1037/a0025176.

Gillham, J. E., Hamilton, J., Freres, D. R., Patton, K., & Gallop, R. (2006). Preventing depression among early adolescents in the primary care setting: A randomized controlled study of the Penn Resiliency Program. *Journal of Abnormal Child Psychology, 34*, 203–219.

Gillham, J. E., Jaycox, L. H., Reivich, K. J., Seligman, M. E. P., & Silver, T. (1990). *The Penn Resiliency Program*. Unpublished manual, University of Pennsylvania, Philadelphia.

Gillham, J. E., Reivich, K. J., Freres, D. R., Chaplin, T. M., Shatté, A. J., Samuels, B., et al. (2007). School-based prevention of depressive symptoms: A randomized controlled study of the effectiveness and specificity of the Penn Resiliency Program. *Journal of Consulting and Clinical Psychology, 75*(1), 9–19. doi:10.1037/0022-006x.75.1.9.

Hollon, S. D., & Kendall, P. C. (1980). Cognitive self-statements in depression: Development of an automatic thoughts questionnaire. *Cognitive Therapy and Research, 4*, 383–397.

Individuals with Disabilities Education Act (IDEA) of 2004, 20 U.S.C. § § 1400–1415.

Jensen-Doss, A. (2011). Practice involves more than treatment: How can evidence-based assessment catch up to evidence-based treatment? *Clinical Psychology: Science and Practice, 18*(2), 173–177. doi:10.1111/j.1468-2850.2011.01248.x.

Kaslow, N. J., & Nolen-Hoeksema, S. (1991). *Children's attributional style questionnaire—revised: Psychometric examination*. Unpublished Manuscript, Emory University School of Medicine.

Kazdin, A. E., Rodgers, A., & Colbus, D. (1986). The Hopelessness Scale for Children: Psychometric characteristics and concurrent validity. *Journal of Consulting and Clinical Psychology, 54*(2), 241–245.

Kovacs, M. (2010). *Children's Depression Inventory 2*. New York: Multi-Health Systems.

Lewinsohn, P. M., Clarke, G. N., Hops, H., & Andrews, J. (1990). Cognitive-behavioral treatment for depressed adolescents. *Behavior Therapy, 21*(4), 385–401.

Maag, J. W., & Swearer, S. M. (2005). Cognitive-behavioral interventions for depression: Review and implications for school personnel. *Behavioral Disorders, 30*(3), 259–276.

Maag, J. W., Swearer, S. M., & Toland, M. D. (2009). Cognitive-behavioral interventions for depression in children and adolescents: Meta-analysis, promising programs, and implications for school personnel. In M. J. Mayer, J. E. Lochman, & R. Van Acker (Eds.), *Cognitive-behavioral interventions for emotional and behavioral disorders: School-based practice* (pp. 235–265). New York, NY: Guilford Press.

McCarty, C. A., Violette, H. D., Duong, M. T., Cruz, R. A., & McCauley, E. (2013). A randomized trial of the positive thoughts and action program for depression among early adolescents. *Journal of Clinical Child and Adolescent Psychology, 42*(4), 554–563. doi:10.1080/15374416.2013.782817.

Mufson, L. H., Dorta, K. P., Olfson, M., Weissman, M. M., & Hoagwood, K. (2004). Effectiveness research: Transporting interpersonal psychotherapy for depressed adolescents (IPT-A) from the lab to school-based health clinics. *Clinical Child and Family Psychology Review, 7*(4), 251–261.

Mychailyszyn, M. P., Brodman, D. M., Read, L., & Kendall, P. C. (2012). Cognitive-behavioral school-based interventions for anxious and depressed youth: A meta-analysis of outcomes. *Clinical Psychology: Science and Practice, 19*(2), 129–153. doi:10.1111/j.1468-2850.2012.01279.x.

Poznanski, E. O., Grossman, J. A., Buchsbaum, Y., Banegas, M., Freeman, L., & Gibbons, R. (1984). Preliminary studies of the reliability and validity of the Children's Depression Rating Scale. *Journal of the American Academy of Child Psychiatry, 23*(2), 191–197. doi:10.1097/00004583-198403000-00011.

Radloff, L. S. (1977). A CES-D scale: A self-report depression scale for research in the general population. *Applied Psychological Measurement, 1*, 385–401.

Reynolds, W. M. (1986). *Reynolds adolescent depression scale*. Odessa, FL: Psychological Assessment Resources.

Reynolds, W. M. (1988). *Suicidal ideation questionnaire: Professional manual*. Odessa, FL: Psychological Assessment Resources.

Reynolds, W. M. (1989). *Reynolds Child Depression Scale*. Odessa, FL: Psychological Assessment Resources.

Riolo, S. A., Nguyen, T., Greden, J. F., & King, C. A. (2005). Prevalence of depression by race/ethnicity: Findings from the National Health and Nutrition Examination Survey III. *American Journal of Public Health, 95*(6), 998–1000. doi:10.2105/AJPH.2004.047225.

Rohde, P., Beevers, C. G., Stice, E., & O'Neil, K. (2009). Major and minor depression in female adolescents: Onset, course, symptom presentation, and demographic associations. *Journal of Clinical Psychology, 65*(12), 1339–1349. doi:10.1002/jclp.20629.

Rohde, P., Lewinsohn, P. M., Clarke, G. N., Hops, H., & Seeley, J. R. (2005). The adolescent coping with depression course: A cognitive-behavioral approach to the treatment of adolescent depression. In E. D. Hibbs & P. S. Jensen (Eds.), *Psychosocial treatments for child and adolescent disorders: Empirically based strategies for clinical practice* (2nd ed., pp. 219–237). Washington, DC: American Psychological Association.

Rohde, P., Stice, E., & Gau, J. M. (2012). Effects of three depression prevention interventions on risk for depressive disorder onset in the context of depression risk factors. *Prevention Science, 13*(6), 584–593. doi:10.1007/s11121-012-0284-3.

Stark, K. D., Arora, P., & Funk, C. L. (2011). Training school psychologists to conduct evidence-based treatments for depression. *Psychology in the Schools, 48*(3), 272–282. doi:10.1002/pits.20551.

Stark, K. D., Streusand, W., Krumholz, L. S., & Patel, P. (2010). Cognitive-behavioral therapy for depression: The ACTION treatment program for girls. In J. R. Weisz & A. E. Kazdin (Eds.), *Evidence-based psychotherapies for children and adolescents* (2nd ed., pp. 93–109). New York, NY: Guilford Press.

Stice, E., Burton, E., Bearman, S., & Rohde, P. (2007). Randomized trial of a brief depression prevention program: An elusive search for a psychosocial placebo control condition. *Behaviour Research and Therapy, 45*(5), 863–876. doi:10.1016/j.brat.2006.08.008.

Stice, E., Shaw, H., Bohon, C., Marti, C., & Rohde, P. (2009). A meta-analytic review of depression prevention programs for children and adolescents: Factors that predict magnitude of intervention effects. *Journal of Consulting and Clinical Psychology, 77*(3), 486–503. doi:10.1037/a0015168.

Warren, W. L. (1994). *Revised Hamilton rating scale for depression*. Torrance, CA: Western Psychological Services.

Weissman, A. (1979). The dysfunctional attitude scale: A validation study. (Doctoral dissertation, University of Pennsylvania, 1979). *Dissertation Abstracts International, 40*, 1389b–1390b.

Weisz, J. R., Gray, J. S., Bearman, S. K., Southam-Gerow, M., & Stark, K. D. (2005). *Primary and Secondary Control Enhancement Training Program: Therapists manual* (2nd ed.). Unpublished manuscript, Harvard University.

Weisz, J. R., McCarty, C. A., & Valeri, S. M. (2006). Effects of psychotherapy for depression in children and adolescents: A meta-analysis. *Psychological Bulletin, 132*(1), 132–149. doi:10.1037/0033-2909.132.1.132.

Weisz, J. R., Sandler, I. N., Durlak, J. A., & Anton, B. S. (2005). Promoting and protecting youth mental health through evidence-based prevention and treatment. *American Psychologist, 60*(6), 628–648. doi:10.1037/0003-066X.60.6.628.

Chapter 6
Transdiagnostic Behavioral Therapy for Anxiety and Depression in Schools

Brian C. Chu, Alyssa Johns, and Lauren Hoffman

Transdiagnostic Behavioral Therapy for Anxiety and Depression in Schools

Anxiety and unipolar depression are among the most common disorders affecting children and adolescents (Costello, Egger, & Angold, 2005). Anxiety disorders, such as generalized anxiety disorder (GAD), social phobia (SOP), separation anxiety disorder (SAD), and panic disorder (PD), are associated with cognitive, physiological, and emotional distresses and confer significant impairment across home, school, and social domains (Roblek & Piacentini, 2005). As a group, anxiety disorders affect between 6 and 18 % of youth (Woodward & Fergusson, 2001) and can contribute to significant and lasting impairment in social adjustment, academic functioning, and family relationships (Langley, Bergman, McCracken, & Piacentini, 2004; Ludwig, Lyon, & Ryan, Chap. 3). Major depressive disorder (MDD) can be diagnosed in as many as 20 % of teens in any given year (Lewinsohn, Hops, Roberts, Seeley, & Andrews, 1993), and its acute episodes (with intensive depressive symptoms lasting nearly every day for at least 2 weeks) are likely to be recurrent and associated with significant long-term outcomes (Lewinsohn, Clarke, Seeley, & Rohde, 1994; Sander, Herren, & Bishop, Chap. 5).

B.C. Chu, Ph.D. (✉)
Department of Clinical Psychology, Graduate School of Applied and Professional Psychology, Rutgers University, Piscataway, NJ, USA

Graduate School of Applied and Professional Psychology, Rutgers, The State University of New Jersey, 152 Frelinghuysen Road, Piscataway, NJ, 08854, USA
e-mail: brianchu@rci.rutgers.edu

A. Johns, Psy.M. • L. Hoffman, Psy.M.
Department of Clinical Psychology, Graduate School of Applied and Professional Psychology, Rutgers University, Piscataway, NJ, USA
e-mail: alyssjohns@gmail.com; lhoffman919@gmail.com

© Springer Science+Business Media New York 2015   101
R. Flanagan et al. (eds.), *Cognitive and Behavioral Interventions in the Schools*, DOI 10.1007/978-1-4939-1972-7_6

The co-occurrence of anxiety and depression disorders within individuals may be even more vital to understand. Anxiety and depression co-occur frequently, with 69 % of anxious youth diagnosed with depression and up to 75 % of depressed youth diagnosed with an anxiety disorder (Angold, Costello, & Erkanli, 1999; Merikangas et al., 2010). Youth with co-occurring anxiety and depression often present with greater symptom severity and overall impairment than youth with either disorder alone (O'Neil, Podell, Benjamin, & Kendall, 2010) and may signal higher rates of psychopathology in later adolescence and adulthood (Feehan, McGee, & Williams, 1993). The impact of comorbidity on treatment outcomes is still being investigated. While some report minimal impact of comorbidity on treatment outcome (Kendall, Brady, & Verduin, 2001; Rhode, Clarke, Lewinsohn, Seeley, & Kaufman, 2001), others have identified worse outcomes for youth diagnosed with anxiety and depression comorbidity (O'Neil & Kendall, 2012; Rapee et al., 2013). Clinical wisdom, however, has identified increased comorbidity as a therapeutic challenge that requires flexibility and ingenuity on the part of the clinician.

A "transdiagnostic" treatment approach is one approach for addressing multiple clinical problems at the same time using a unified treatment conceptualization and focused set of treatment techniques. Transdiagnostic interventions draw from a unifying theoretical model and target core, shared processes that underlie problems across diagnostic classes (Ehrenreich-May & Chu, 2013; Taylor & Clark, 2009). By focusing on joint underlying mechanisms, transdiagnostic protocols produce robust, generalizable outcomes across multiple clinical problems (Chu, 2012). A good transdiagnostic treatment must not only provide a strong conceptual match for multiple treatment goals, but the strategies employed must be flexible enough to account for diverse problems (Ehrenreich-May & Chu, 2013). Transdiagnostic treatments can be distinguished from "eclectic" forms of therapy as eclectic therapy encourages an "ad hoc" selection of treatment strategies based on week-to-week client presentation. Transdiagnostic interventions work to identify a core set of mechanisms that underlie multiple clinical problems and then target these problems using a focused set of core interventions (Ehrenreich-May & Chu, 2013).

The current chapter describes one such transdiagnostic treatment approach that uses behavioral activation and exposure exercises to simultaneously address mood and anxiety problems that co-occur in the preteen and teenage years. This transdiagnostic approach has been developed in school settings and piloted using some school personnel as therapists to optimize its eventual implementation in school settings. Developing psychosocial treatments for schools has several advantages, including permitting access of evidence-based treatment to a wide range of youth who may otherwise not seek mental health care due to financial, logistical, or other family barriers (Weissman, Antinoro, & Chu, 2008). In this chapter, we highlight developmental issues to consider when selecting youth for this program and professional and systems issues that impact the program's implementation. Case studies are also provided.

Assessing Anxiety and Mood Problems in the Schools

A multi-source, multi-domain assessment strategy is recommended for assessing anxiety and mood disorders in preteens and adolescents (Chu, 2008; Silverman & Ollendick, 2005). A comprehensive evaluation of the youth's psychosocial functioning requires a diversified assessment strategy including diagnostics status, symptoms, and impairment across home, social, academic, health, and family life. Multiple perspectives (e.g., parent, teacher, youth, coach) are critical because different adults are exposed to the child across activities during the day, and the youth's functioning may vary. This is particularly important for internalizing problems, like depression and anxiety, where youth may be reluctant to self-disclose distress and may appear different at home and at school (Silverman & Ollendick, 2005). Conducting psychosocial assessments in a school setting comes with certain advantages and challenges, depending on whether the assessor is an outside consultant hired by the school or is a part of the school's internal child study team, special education department, or district-level school psychologist. We refer you to other chapters in this volume that have discussed this topic comprehensively (Feindler & Liebman, Chap. 2; Ludwig et al., Chap. 3; Sander et al., Chap. 5).

Addressing Anxiety and Mood with Exposure-Based Behavioral Activation

Attempting to address complex symptom and functional impairment across anxiety and mood disorders requires a comprehensive but robust and efficient approach. The customary evidence-based treatment approach typically has therapists rank order treatment goals and target one problem at a time (Barlow, Allen, & Choate, 2004). This approach is risky for clients who may drop out of treatment before receiving necessary components. This serial approach may also require high levels of therapist training in multiple treatment interventions (Barlow et al., 2004). A transdiagnostic approach that employs a smaller set of interventions designed to target core mechanisms may be more efficient and effective than treating disorders in a sequential manner (Barlow et al., 2004; Ehrenreich, Goldstein, Wright, & Barlow, 2009).

Two main intervention strategies comprise our transdiagnostic intervention: behavioral activation (BA) and in vivo exposure. BA is a brief, solution-focused intervention which aims to change the contextual factors that maintain or exacerbate depression symptoms (Coffman, Martell, Dimidjian, Gallop, & Hollon, 2007). Behavioral strategies for depression have traditionally emphasized pleasant activity scheduling in order to increase opportunities for enjoyment and enhance sensitivity to natural reinforcement (Lewinsohn & Graf, 1973). Reconceptualized BA, as recently developed by Jacobson and colleagues (Jacobson, Martell, & Dimidjian, 2001), emphasizes the specific role of avoidance in withdrawn and isolative behavior.

This model posits that avoidant behavior that follows a distressing event is reinforced as it reduces immediate levels of distress (Jacobson et al., 2001). Continued avoidance maintains a cycle of withdrawal and inactivity that perpetuates difficulty accessing positive, antidepressant sources of reinforcement (Jacobson et al., 2001). BA treatment thus involves using an idiographic functional assessment process to identify avoidant behavioral patterns and cultivate more adaptive approach behaviors (Addis & Martell, 2004; Jacobson et al., 2001).

Avoidance is thought to play a very similar role in the maintenance of anxiety disorders (Chu, Skriner, & Staples, 2014; Craske & Mystkowski, 2006; Foa & McNally, 1996). The primary targets for exposure in anxiety treatment are avoidant responses triggered by feared stimuli. Consistent with the BA approach, these avoidant responses reduce distress associated with escape and are thus negatively reinforced (Foa & McNally, 1996; Mineka & Zinbarg, 2006). Exposure treatment involves the creation of fear hierarchies and the use of problem solving and imaginal/in vivo exposures to practice approach behaviors. The goals of exposure treatment match those of BA, which are to expand behavioral repertoires, reduce passivity, and change avoidance patterns (Ferster, 1973).

To date, research on BA has produced promising findings for the treatment of depression in adults (see Table 6.1). BA has compared favorably to antidepressant medication in moderate to severe depression (Dimidjian et al., 2006) and in non-clinical adult anxiety (Chen, Liu, Rapee, & Pillay, 2013) and is expanding in its application to treat depressed patients with comorbid diagnoses such as anxiety, PTSD, substance use, obesity, and cancer (Dimidjian, Barrera, Martell, Munoz, & Lewinsohn, 2011). Downward extensions of BA to youth populations is relatively recent, but uncontrolled pilot studies and open trials have provided initial support, mostly for depressed adolescents (Chu, Colognori, Weissman, & Bannon, 2009; McCauley, Schloredt, Gudmundsen, & Martell, 2011; Ritschel, Ramirez, Jones, and Craighead, 2011; Weersing, Rozenman, Maher-Bridge, & Campo, 2012). Manassis and colleagues (2010) have developed an integrative cognitive behavioral therapy for anxiety and depression designed for primary school settings (grades 3–6), but symptom outcomes were not significantly better for the CBT program over the control at either posttreatment or 1-year follow-up.

Description of Group Behavioral Activation Therapy

The extant evidence, combined with the broader evidence base supporting integrative cognitive behavioral therapy for youth anxiety and depression (David-Ferdon & Kaslow, 2008; Silverman, Pina, & Viswesvaran, 2008), led us to extend the BA approach across diagnostic categories in a youth population. Group Behavioral Activation Therapy (GBAT; Chu et al., 2009) distills the most potent components of behavioral therapy into a single protocol. GBAT was originally developed in school settings and has been evaluated in open trials and a recent wait list-controlled randomized clinical trial (Chu, Crocco, Esseling, Areizaga, Staples, & Skriner, 2014).

Table 6.1 Empirical support for contemporary behavioral activation (BA) for anxiety and depression

Study	Sample	Design	Treatment	Posttreatment results	Follow-up results
Chen et al. (2013)	49 individuals experiencing excessive worry	Wait list-controlled Randomized Clinical Trial	BA (8-week) treatment for worry	Significantly greater reduction on worry and depression compared to wait list. No significant differences occurred for anxiety or stress symptoms.	4-week follow-up BA group showed continued improvement in life functioning
Chu et al. (2009)	Five youth (ages 12–14) with primary anxiety and/or depression	Open trial	Group BA (BA+exposures)	75 % of treatment completers did not meet diagnostic criteria for their principal or secondary diagnosis at posttreatment.	No follow-up
Chu, Crocco et al. (2014)	35 youth (ages 12–14) with primary anxiety or depression	Wait list-controlled Randomized Clinical Trial	Group BA (BA+exposures)	GBAT participants showed better overall functioning (Clinical Global Impairment) than wait list, greater remission of principal diagnosis at the trend level, and significantly better remission in secondary diagnosis.	15-week follow-up supported longer-term efficacy of GBAT; 100 % remission rate in mood disorders; most symptom measures showed improvement
Chu, Hoffman et al. (2013)	Five youth (ages 12–13) with elevated anxiety or depression symptoms, bullying victims	Open trial	Group BA for Bullying	3 out of 5 youth experienced remission in their principal diagnosis and remission in most comorbid diagnoses.	No follow-up

(continued)

Table 6.1 (continued)

Study	Sample	Design	Treatment	Posttreatment results	Follow-up results
Dimidjian et al. (2006)	242 adults (ages 18–60) with Major Depression	Randomized Clinical Trial: Cognitive Therapy, antidepressant medication, pill placebo	BA (approx. 24 sessions over 16 weeks)	BA comparable to antidepressant medication and more efficacious than cognitive therapy among moderately to severely depressed adults.	No follow-up
Manassis et al. (2010)	145 youth (grades 3–6) with internalizing symptoms	Randomized Clinical Trial, activity control	12-week group cognitive behavioral program	Internalizing symptoms decreased with cognitive behavioral therapy.	Further decrease at follow-up
McCauley et al. (2011)	17-year-old male with Major Depression	Single case description	BA (12-week, 14 sessions)	No significant clinical reductions in depressive symptoms.	No follow-up
Ritschel et al. (2011)	6 youth (ages 14–17) with Major Depression	Open trial	BA for teens	4 out of 6 no longer met criteria for Major Depression.	No follow-up
Weersing et al. (2008)	2 teens with anxiety and depression	Single case description	BA and exposure (8-week treatment)	Steady improvement across all symptom domains.	Decrease in anxiety and depression symptoms at 6-months follow-up

GBAT is completed in 10 weekly, hour-long sessions but can be delivered flexibly to accommodate school schedules and can be extended to increase in vivo exposure dosage. The first five sessions teach four core BA principles: (a) psychoeducation of anxiety and depression; (b) idiographic functional assessment of problem behavior, focusing on avoidance; (c) approach-oriented problem solving; and (d) graded exposures and behavioral activation. Graded exposures are embedded throughout treatment (as early as session 3) to provide group members with as much experiential practice time as possible.

The SKILLS acronym, taught in sessions 1 through 5, communicates the core skills (see Table 6.2). The first principle, "S" (*See where I'm stuck*), cues group members to conduct a self-assessment and determine the domains they would like to improve (e.g., school, friendships, family relationships, extracurriculars). The second skill, "K" (*Keep active and keep approaching*), teaches members the value of approach behaviors over avoidance. Group members complete a Goals Ladder while learning the "I" principle (*Identify goals I want to achieve*). The "L" principle (*Look for ways to accomplish my goals*) includes teaching TRAP (Trigger, Response, Avoidance Pattern) and TRAC (Trigger, Response, Alternative Coping or Active Choices) skills (Addis & Martell, 2004). TRAP and TRAC help group members dissect the patterns that perpetuate distress and generate alternatives to avoidant behavior.

Table 6.2 Major intervention strategies included in GBAT and GBAT-B

Common strategies	GBAT	GBAT-B
Psychoeducation (anxiety/depression): nature of anx/dep, distress, treatment approach	1	1
Self-assessment/goal setting: contingency management (building and applying reward plan)	2	2
Psychoeducation (bullying): legal definitions of bullying, different forms of bullying, school-specific policies	n/a	3
Building Social Network: identify current social contacts, discuss various kinds of social support, brainstorm ways to build social network	n/a	4
Assertiveness: teach communication styles, practice assertiveness	n/a	5
Support seeking: seek help from friends, family, school personnel	n/a	6
Behavioral activation (tracking): tracking and identifying link between events and mood	3	7
Functional assessment: identifying idiographic distress loops (TRAP)	4	8
Behavioral activation and problem solving: assigning rewarding activities or conducting idiographic problem solving after functional assessment (TRAC)	5	9
In vivo exposures	6–9	10–14
Self-assessment and relapse prevention	10	15
Common CBT skills not emphasized in GBAT		
Relaxation: progressive relaxation, breathing retraining	n/a	n/a
Cognitive restructuring: identifying and challenging negative thinking	n/a	n/a

TRAP helps group members identify specific triggers that lead to problematic avoidance responses. For example, a student who is dreading a quiz in school may try to stay home from school. This avoidance "works" to alleviate distress in the short term but leads to negative consequences in the future (poor attendance, falling behind in school work). TRAC helps remind the youth to identify (through problem solving) more active choices to address problems. Group members are encouraged to favor solutions that solve the immediate problem even if it is distressing in the short run. The second "L" (*Lasting Change*) corresponds to the BA principle of barrier identification and problem solving to overcome barriers. The final principle, "S" (*See what's worked*), focuses group members on reassessing their progress in reaching their goals.

Sessions 6 through 9 focus on exposure tasks (imaginal, in vivo) and behavioral experiments (role-plays, practice runs for homework). However, the number of sessions can be extended to increase the number of exposures students receive. The group selects one or two "lead" members each session to conduct an in vivo exposure. The group leaders help each lead member select an item off of his/her "challenge hierarchy" to practice in session. Items of a challenge hierarchy might include avoiding homework, tutoring, or seeking help from a teacher, if one is having difficulty in math class. Another item might focus on a student who isolates herself from friends after an argument instead of pursuing greater communication. Each item is rated (e.g., "0" not at all to "10" extremely) for the level of distress it causes and the degree of avoidance the student uses.

To conduct an in vivo exposure, one group member is identified as the "lead" member, and the remaining members become the supporting cast. The purpose of exposure tasks is to recreate the challenging situation as closely as possible and to help the lead member practice his/her TRAP and TRAC skills to navigate the problem in a more approach-oriented way. Exposure tasks can focus on specific situations and fears, such as giving a speech, asserting oneself in interpersonal conflicts, socializing at a party, asking a teacher for help, or negotiating demands with a parent. However, exposure tasks can also be designed to target more diffuse problems that are commonly associated with anhedonia (lack of interest in activities) and other general worries (e.g., "What happens if I don't get into college?"). In the case of anhedonia, the key is to simply practice getting active even when one's emotions and physiology are convincing one to act otherwise. Addis and Martell (2004) suggest that when one is feeling down or lost in unproductive rumination, this should be a "cue to action." For example, if a youth tends to "crash" in his bedroom after a hard day of school, the group practices helping the youth *do anything but* isolate himself in his bedroom and sleep. In this case, the group members can practice alternative, active coping the youth will enact at home (e.g., call a friend, take a walk) instead of his typical avoidant response (e.g., take a nap, isolating in room). In a school setting, many exposure tasks may be confined to the group room (typically a classroom or counselor's office); however, whenever possible, it is encouraged for exposures to take advantage of natural challenges and surroundings of the school. For example, there is no better exposure for a youth afraid of talking to new people, than to go to a crowded cafeteria and initiate a conversation. The group can serve as a place to prepare for the exposure and to process it afterwards, but the closer that exposures can come to real life challenge situations, the better. By the end of group, group leaders should endeavor to involve every member to be a lead member at least 2–3 times. While students are not serving as lead member, they can serve as role players, objective observers, or provide feedback.

Adaptation for Bullying-Related Anxiety and Mood Problems

The original GBAT protocol was adapted for use with bullied youth who experience anxiety and mood problems following a bullying incident (Chu, Hoffman, Johns, Reyes-Portillo, & Hansford, 2013). GBAT-Bullying (GBAT-B) teaches victims strategies to minimize the negative impact of bullying and builds social skills to minimize the risk of future bullying. GBAT-B contains four bullying-specific sessions to be completed prior to the traditional GBAT protocol (see Table 6.2). The first session ("Facts about School Life and Bullying") provides definitions and psychoeducation around bullying, endeavors to normalize the experience of being bullied, and challenges misperceptions of bullying perpetrators and victims. Different forms of bullying (physical, verbal, relational, cyberbullying) are discussed, and group members use a "Bullying Thermometer" to identify varying levels of distress associated with different kinds of bullying. It is stressed that different responses (e.g., official school action, interpersonal support, assertiveness) may be required depending on the type of bullying event experienced. Next, group members learn the skill "Build Your Social Network." This module was created in response to research suggesting that victims of bullying may be targeted because they are perceived as lacking social skills and have few reliable friends on which to depend (Fox & Boulton, 2006). To build their "Social Network," group members assess existing sources and gaps in their social network. For example, one group member may realize that she has many acquaintances on the bus and in the classroom but few close friends to sit with in the cafeteria. The group brainstorms possible ways for each member to increase their social connections, including joining groups, approaching new peers in the cafeteria, or choosing someone to invite to the movies. The group then problem solves potential barriers to these suggestions.

In the third session ("Standing Up For Yourself"), group members are taught three main communication styles: aggressive (impulsive reactive style), passive (avoidant style), and assertive (proactive style). Bullied youth often respond ineffectively to bullying events, making them more vulnerable targets in the future (Schwartz, Dodge, & Coie, 1993). Group members are taught verbal and physical ways to communicate assertiveness and use role-plays to practice assertiveness over passivity or aggressiveness. However, group leaders do stress that assertiveness may not be appropriate when physical harm is a realistic threat—in such cases, escape and help from an adult is recommended. In the last bullying-specific session, group members practice the skill "Mobilizing Your Forces," which help youth identify their preferred social supports in the event of bullying. Using the Social Network, group members select who they would contact in various situations. Peers and siblings may provide adequate support following mild forms of bullying (e.g., teasing in the classroom), but school personnel or parents might be preferred following more severe bullying incidents (e.g., being kicked in the hallway, cyberbullying). Upon completion of the bullying-specific sessions, the group resumes the traditional GBAT curriculum, where the focus shifts to preventing anxiety and mood symptoms following experiences with bullying.

Developmental Considerations

Awareness of the rapid developmental changes throughout childhood and adolescence should guide practitioners in their assessment, case conceptualization, and treatment of anxious and depressed youth. For example, biological factors such as gender and pubertal changes may impact the type of issues youth are exposed to at different periods of time. For instance, the peak of pubertal development occurs 2 years earlier in most females when compared to the average male (Holmbeck et al., 2006). Such changes can impact the quality of family relationships and certain indicators of psychosocial adaption and psychopathology. Early-maturing girls, for example, are at risk for a variety of adaptation difficulties, including depression, substance use, eating problems and disorders, and family conflicts (American Psychological Association, 2002; Holmbeck et al., 2006). Practitioners should keep these developmental norms in mind and shape program goals around relevant developmental issues.

Interpersonal contexts such as family, peers, and school should be considered. For example, the school environment is a key context for the development of one's personality, values, and social relationships (Holmbeck et al., 2006). It may be important to target issues unique to a particular school or its surrounding community, including recent bullying events, recovery from a natural disaster, high divorce rates in the community, unsafe neighborhoods, or poverty. Programs should be flexible to adapt to the school's individualized needs and make content changes as necessary. In one of our studies, we modified the TRAP acronym to stand for "Anger Pattern," in addition to Avoidant Pattern, which seemed to fit the response style and culture of the particular school (discussed more below).

Peer context is another critical variable, and it is important to understand the relative influence of peers and family members. In adolescence, the need for autonomy and personal choice commonly reaches a peak. School-based programs can help youth develop independence by teaching independent problem solving and decision-making while also identifying situations in which consultation from adults would be helpful.

Empirical Support for GBAT

The GBAT program has now been evaluated in a series of open trials and a small randomized controlled trial (Chu et al., 2009; Chu, Crocco et al., 2014), following recommended practice by the National Institute of Health. The intervention was developed in the schools where we ultimately hope it will be delivered. We actively consulted with school personnel and implemented early trials in schools, following recommendations of implementation and dissemination experts (e.g., Atkins, Frazier, & Cappella, 2006; Chorpita, 2002) who caution that the most important lessons do not emerge until the treatment itself is put into the community. Accordingly, treatment acceptability, therapist training, clinical supervision, and community beliefs were considered at each stage of development.

GBAT was first developed and piloted in a large public middle school (approximately 1,200 7th and 8th graders) representing a racially/ethnically (45 % African-American, 27 % non-Hispanic White, 15 % Asian, 13 % Hispanic) and socioeconomically (24 % of students qualified for free lunch and 8 % for reduced lunch) diverse student body (Chu et al., 2009). The initial open trial of five 7th and 8th grade students (ages 12–14) demonstrated positive diagnostic outcomes and significantly reliable change in anxiety/depression symptoms for three of the four (75 %) youth who stayed for the entire group (Chu et al., 2009). All treatment completers reported reduced avoidance on their top behavioral goal. Youth participants were initially referred by teachers and school counselors for anxiety or mood problems and then verified to have a clinical diagnosis by structured clinical interview, suggesting that school personnel can be a valuable source for student referrals. Attendance was generally good, with four members attending at least 10 sessions, and members rated group quality high, suggesting acceptability of the group in school settings. However, the small sample size and uncontrolled design limited conclusions.

Student feedback after the initial trial and after a second pilot group led to an important change in our GBAT model. Many had difficulty relating to the concept of avoidance as the primary factor maintaining their distress. Instead, feelings of anger characterized much of their distress and the students identified impulsive acts as getting them into trouble. For example, interpersonal conflict with a friend would trigger anger and result in lashing out verbally before ultimately ignoring the friend. Getting frustrated in class might result in acting dismissively to a teacher or refusing to do homework. Identifying the "avoidance" in these situations seemed counterintuitive even though one could point to the secondary avoidance of friends or homework as a key maintaining mechanism. To accommodate this experience, a third version was developed that included angry feelings as a target trigger (i.e., Trigger, Response, Anger Pattern). Conflict or frustration triggered anger which triggered the youth to choose the "easiest" solution. This solution typically included acting out in some aggressive way that ended the conflict quickly (e.g., yelling at one's friend in the hallway often led to both sides going their separate ways). However, neither the immediate solution nor the secondary avoidance ever solved the original problem (e.g., miscommunication). Thus, it was important to find Alternative Choices to get back on TRAC.

The third version of GBAT was evaluated in a small wait list-controlled RCT (Chu, Crocco et al., 2014). Double-gated screening with 895 7th grade students identified 35 youth (ages 12–14) who met criteria for either an anxiety or mood disorder and agreed to be randomly assigned to either GBAT ($n=21$) or a 15-week wait list ($n=14$). Diagnostic profiles were complex where 82.9 % had a principal anxiety disorder (GAD, SOP, SAD), 17.1 % had a principal depression disorder, 60 % had at least one comorbid anxiety disorder, and 14.3 % had comorbid depression. Four had a comorbid externalizing disorder, and 37 % of the youth had some kind of across-class comorbid disorder (e.g., anxiety and depression). Results indicated encouraging posttreatment diagnostic outcomes. GBAT was associated with greater posttreatment remission rates than WL in principal diagnosis (at the trend level) and secondary diagnosis (statistically significant level) and demonstrated greater improvement in overall impairment. Anxiety and depressive symptoms and functional outcomes were not significantly different at posttreatment. These findings suggested that overall diagnostic complexity and impairment decreased in GBAT relative to WL but that symptom severity did not differentially change—likely due to the small sample size. By 4-month follow-up, most outcomes showed linear improvement from pretreatment to follow-up in the combined sample of GBAT and WL (after they received the intervention). Thus, youth who participated in the original GBAT groups and those who received GBAT following the WL phase reported significant gains on diagnostic, symptom, and functional impairment measures 4 months after treatment.

Behavioral activation and automatic thoughts were assessed to evaluate potential mediator effects of GBAT. Increased behavioral activation and avoidance was seen in GBAT compared to WL at posttreatment at the trend level (large effect size), but no differences were found between treatment conditions on negative thoughts. Formal mediator analysis was not conducted given the small sample size, but these findings provided support that GBAT might have specific effects on behavioral activation compared to general effects on cognition.

Development and Evaluation of GBAT-Bullying

GBAT-B is currently being developed to address anxiety and mood problems secondary to peer victimization (Chu, Hoffman et al., 2013). Five 7th grade students (four boys, ages 12–13) participated in a 14-week GBAT-B group after being recruited by the school's harassment, intimidation, and bullying (HIB) officer, a position designated to address complaints of bullying. Most youth experienced improvements in anxiety and mood symptoms from pre- to posttreatment and reported less interference related specifically to bullying. Importantly, attendance records ($M = 13.2$ sessions attended) and satisfaction ratings suggested that the group was both feasible and acceptable in this setting. Overall, four of the five youth reported that they were at least "mostly satisfied" with the group and several noted that the group "did not stop bullying, but it helped me deal with it better." Satisfaction and attendance were key outcomes because we were concerned that bullied youth would be reluctant to participate in a group where bullying was a core topic. Group leaders and school personnel were careful to maintain confidentiality, but there was a concern that targeted youth would be taking a special risk by participating in the group.

We were gratified to learn that no group members experienced any additional stigma or targeting by virtue of attending the groups. The small sample and uncontrolled design dictate that further investigation is needed, but initial results are promising.

Implementation Potential

Early trials have shown encouraging support for the efficacy of GBAT, but we remain conscientious of its ultimate potential for dissemination and implementation. Even well-supported treatment protocols can go unused if they do not fit the needs of the intended setting or do not match the skill level of the intended end user (e.g., therapist, school counselor, teacher; Fixsen, Blase, Duda, Naoom, & Van Dyke, 2010). To assess the implementation potential of GBAT, we conducted a survey of potential GBAT users to determine opinions of the protocol's usability, feasibility, and acceptability (Areizaga, 2014). Eleven professionals with a doctoral degree in either clinical or school psychology and seven graduate students enrolled in either a clinical or school psychology doctoral program completed a survey after reading each session of the therapist manual and workbook. Participant ratings indicated highly positive impressions of the therapist manual and workbook. Items assessing clarity, consistency with theory, appropriateness for anxiety/mood, and usefulness received close to maximum ratings on acceptability. However, feasibility ratings were routinely lower, averaging slightly above the "somewhat feasible" range. Respondents found that the time allotted for tasks may have been less than desirable and that some of the assigned tasks may have been challenging to accomplish in school settings. Future development of the protocol will make sure to prioritize session activities to inform providers which skills to emphasize in the event of shortened time. It is also important to continue to involve school personnel in the development of GBAT to ensure that its structure and content is feasible and appropriate for schools. Despite potential challenges, individual professionals felt positive about the implementation potential of GBAT. On a specific measure of implementation potential (Forman, Fagley, Chu & Walkup, 2012), GBAT received high ratings on acceptability/efficacy (perceptions that the program is acceptable and efficacious), organizational support (perceptions that the school setting would support implementation of the group), and administrator support (perceptions that school principals and district administrators would support the group).

Case Examples

Several brief examples are offered to highlight the GBAT model in schools. Monique (names changed to protect confidentiality) was a 12-year-old, African-American 7th grade girl, living with both parents and a younger sister, and met DSM-IV-TR diagnostic criteria for social phobia (SOP), major depressive disorder (MDD), and subclinical generalized anxiety disorder (GAD). Monique was referred to GBAT by her guidance counselor for social anxiety, shyness, and noticeable isolation from other kids. Upon interview, she appeared shy (e.g., poor eye contact) and did not maintain her appearance optimally (e.g., slightly disheveled clothes, some poor hygiene habits). She complained of not fitting in with any "clique" at school. Monique identified three primary goals: "Get better grades," "Get along with my brother," and "To meet new people." Focusing on social situations, the group leaders used TRAP to identify her typical pattern of social avoidance, including T (finding herself at a party where she did not know anyone), R (feeling nervous and embarrassed) and AP (staying by herself in the corner, leaving early). Exposures then targeted socializing in novel settings where she practiced initiating and sustaining conversations, gaining comfort in self-disclosure, and increasing comfort with awkward situations (e.g., conversation lulls, disinterested conversation partners). Monique was an active participant throughout and benefitted from interacting with two older girls in the group. Behaviorally, she became significantly more socially skilled and became more interested in self-care and hygiene by the group's end. At posttreatment, Monique no longer met the criteria for any diagnoses and demonstrated a significant decrease in child-reported depressive symptoms and parent-reported anxiety symptoms.

Ryan, a 12-year-old, Caucasian 7th grade boy, was referred to GBAT-B after experiencing increased sadness following the death of his mother and experiencing several bullying incidents that occurred inside and outside of school. Ryan had reportedly been punched by older kids in his neighborhood, excluded from lunch tables, and left out of games in the neighborhood. Ryan met criteria for SOP, GAD, and subclinical MDD and separation anxiety disorder (SAD). Ryan had few friends and reported being the target of homophobic slurs. He reported that bullying most strongly impacted his relationship with his family as he became easily annoyed by his father and sister, did not want to spend time with them, and felt he could not confide in his family. The structured role-plays and exposure exercises of GBAT-B engaged Ryan's creative side and prompted him to think about solutions to bullying in ways previously not considered. For example, during a role-play practicing making new friends, he was especially persistent in asking a confederate peer to "hang out." He later reported that the skills practiced in the group helped him engage new friends. Ryan also utilized assertiveness skills learned in the group. Instead of responding passively when a friend returned a broken video game, he confronted his friend in a calm and descriptive (assertive) manner which avoided conflict but garnered an apology. On occasion, Ryan's sad mood was problematic in that he would present as moderately withdrawn from the group. The group leaders used this as an opportunity to model communication skills and to have Ryan practice appropriately communicating his expression of emotion to others. By the end of treatment, he no longer met criteria for any diagnoses. Ryan reported that he was still teased about once a week, but he was better equipped to deal with the bullying. He reported that being teased "messed up (his) mood," but only for a short period of time as he was now able to "let it go" more easily.

Other Practice Considerations

Initiating a psychosocial therapy program requires active, collaborative relationships with key stakeholders in the school, particularly if the program is initiated by consultants outside of the school. Support of school administration is essential to ensure smooth recruitment and scheduling of the group (e.g., Chu et al., 2009). For example, having school counselors cosign recruitment letters and call families can help connect group leaders to known school personnel. Teacher, counselor, and staff training may also be important to help educate school staff about the impact of internalizing problems which are often overlooked (Masia, Klein, Storch, & Corda, 2001; Weissman et al., 2008). Familiarity with state and district laws, as well as individualized school policies, may be critical. Therapists working in schools should become familiar with the school's local policy on confidentiality. Students, families, and school personnel should be clear on the kinds of information that might be shared with administrators, teachers, and guidance counselors (Fisher et al., 2004). Local and state laws may be particularly important in cases of bullying. For example, many states have adopted a zero-tolerance policy when it comes to bullying and have mandated that school staff report any type of bullying behavior to the school's anti-bullying specialist (US Department of Education, 2011). Such issues require good communication and collaboration among the therapist/group leader, school administration, and broader school community (teachers, parents, students). The need for good collaboration is amplified when the therapist is considered an "outsider" at the school, such as a district-level school psychologist or consulting psychologist.

These challenges should not discourage implementation of such programs. Schools provide unique advantages over typical outpatient settings. For example, conducting in vivo exposures in the naturalistic school setting provides unique opportunities to enhance ecological validity and generalization of skills. If making friends was an identified problem, we would first use TRAP to conduct a functional assessment: T (eating alone in the cafeteria), R (feeling nervous and embarrassed), and AP (skipping lunch, going to the library). We would then design exposures that made use of the group setting (e.g., initiating and maintaining conversation with group members) but then send the youth out to school grounds (e.g., approaching peers in the hallway, asking a classmate to sit with him or her at lunch).

Taking advantage of such opportunities helps a youth gain a more realistic sense of competence that helps expedite mastery of skills. While challenges may exist in implementing school-based psychosocial skills programs, the advantages encourage continued persistence. The emerging support for BA's efficacy, both in adults and youth, make it a promising candidate for further development. The GBAT program is unique in its transdiagnostic focus and its incorporation of in vivo exposure exercises. It has shown promising results as a school-based intervention that has been implemented by school counselors under some conditions. Given the paucity of resources currently available for depressed and anxious youth in schools, it is critical that promising interventions, like GBAT and BA, continue to be developed.

References

Addis, M. E., & Martell, C. R. (2004). *Overcoming depression one step at a time*. New Harbinger: Oakland, CA.

American Psychological Association. (2002). *Developing adolescents: A reference for professionals*. Washington, DC: American Psychological Association.

Angold, A., Costello, E. J., & Erkanli, A. (1999). Comorbidity. *Journal of Child Psychology and Psychiatry, 40*, 57–87.

Areizaga, M. (2014). *Feasibility and acceptability of implementing the SKILLS program, a group behavioral activation treatment for schools*. Unpublished doctoral dissertation. Rutgers University, Piscataway, NJ.

Atkins, M. D., Frazier, S. L., & Cappella, E. (2006). Hybrid research models: Natural opportunities for examining mental health in context. *Clinical Psychology: Science and Practice, 13*, 105–108.

Barlow, D. H., Allen, L. B., & Choate, M. L. (2004). Toward a unified treatment for emotional disorders. *Behavior Therapy, 35*, 205–230.

Chen, J., Lui, X., Rapee, R. M., & Pillay, P. (2013). Behavioural activation: A pilot trial of transdiagnostic treatment for excessive worry. *Behaviour Research and Therapy, 51*, 533–539.

Chorpita, B. F. (2002). Treatment manuals for the real world: Where do we build them? *Clinical Psychology: Science and Practice, 9*, 431–433.

Chu, B. C. (2008). Child and adolescent research methods in clinical psychology. In D. McKay (Ed.), *Handbook of research methods in abnormal and clinical psychology*. Thousand Oaks, CA: Sage.

Chu, B. C. (2012). Introduction to special series: Translating transdiagnostic approaches to children and adolescents. *Cognitive and Behavioral Practice, 19*, 1–4.

Chu, B. C., Colognori, D., Weissman, A. S., & Bannon, K. (2009). An initial description and pilot of group behavioral activation therapy for anxious and depressed youth. *Cognitive and Behavioral Practice, 16*, 408–416.

Chu, B. C., Crocco, S. T., Esseling, P., Areizaga, M. J., Staples, A. M., & Skriner, L. C. (2014). Transdiagnostic group behavioral activation therapy for youth anxiety and depression: Initial randomized controlled trial. Manuscript submitted for publication.

Chu, B. C., Hoffman, L. J., Johns, A. M., Reyes-Portillo, J., & Hansford, A. (2013). Transdiagnostic behavior therapy for bullying-related anxiety and depression: Initial development and pilot study. Manuscript submitted for publication.

Chu, B. C., Skriner, L. C., & Staples, A. M. (2014). Behavioral avoidance across child and adolescent psychopathology. In J. Ehrenreich-May & B. Chu (Eds.), *Transdiagnostic treatments for children and adolescents: Principles and practice*. New York: Guilford Press.

Coffman, S. J., Martell, C. R., Dimidjian, S., Gallop, R., & Hollon, S. D. (2007). Extreme nonresponse in cognitive therapy: Can behavioral activation succeed where cognitive therapy fails? *Journal of Consulting and Clinical Psychology, 75*(4), 531–541.

Costello, E. J., Egger, H. L., & Angold, A. (2005). Prevalence and comorbidity. *Child and Adolescent Psychiatric Clinics of North America, 14*, 631–648.

Craske, M. G., & Mystkowski, J. L. (2006). Exposure therapy and extinction: Clinical studies. In M. G. Craske, D. Hermans, & D. Vansteenwegen (Eds.), *Fear and Learning: Basic Science to Clinical Application* (pp. 217–233). Washington, DC: APA Books.

David-Ferdon, C., & Kaslow, N. J. (2008). Evidence-based psychosocial treatments for child and adolescent depression. *Journal of Clinical Child and Adolescent Psychology, 37*, 62–104.

Dimidjian, S., Barrera, M., Martell, C., Jr., Munoz, R. F., & Lewinsohn, P. M. (2011). The origins and current status of behavioral activation treatments for depression. *Annual Review of Clinical Psychology, 7*, 1–38.

Dimidjian, S., Hollon, S. D., Dobson, K. S., Schmaling, K. B., Kohlenberg, R. J., Addis, M. E., et al. (2006). Randomized trial of behavioral activation, cognitive therapy, and antidepressant medication in the acute treatment of adults with major depression. *Journal of Consulting and Clinical Psychology, 74*, 658–670.

Ehrenreich, J. T., Goldstein, C. R., Wright, L. R., & Barlow, D. H. (2009). Development of a unified protocol for the treatment of emotional disorders in youth. *Child and Family Behavior Therapy, 31*(1), 20–37.

Ehrenreich-May, J., & Chu, B. C. (2013). Overview of transdiagnostic mechanisms and treatments for youth psychopathology. In J. Ehrenreich-May & B. C. Chu (Eds.), *Transdiagnostic treatments for children and adolescents: Principles and practice*. New York: Guilford Press.

Feehan, M., McGee, R., & Williams, S. M. (1993). Mental health disorders from age 15 to age 18 years. *Journal of the American Academy of Child and Adolescent Psychiatry, 32*, 1118–1126.

Ferster, C. B. (1973). A functional analysis of depression. *American Psychologist, 28*, 857–870.

Fisher, P. H., Masia-Warner, C., & Klein, R. G. (2004). Skills for social and academic success: A school-based intervention for social anxiety disorder in adolescents. *Clinical Child and Family Psychology Review, 7*, 241–249.

Fixsen, D. L., Blase, K. A., Duda, M. A., Naoom, S. F., & Van Dyke, M. (2010). Implementation of evidence-based treatments for children and adolescents. In J. R. Weisz & A. E. Kazdin (Eds.), *Evidence-based psychotherapies for children and adolescents* (2nd ed., pp. 435–450). New York: Guilford.

Foa, E. B., & McNally, R. J. (1996). Mechanisms of change in exposure therapy. In R. M. Rapee (Ed.), *Current controversies in the anxiety disorders* (pp. 329–343). New York: Guilford.

Forman, S. G., Fagley, N. S., Chu, B. C., & Walkup, J. T. (2012). Factors influencing school psychologists' "Willingness to Implement" evidence-based interventions. *School Mental Health, 4*, 207–218.

Fox, C. L., & Boulton, M. J. (2006). Friendship as a moderator of the relationship between social skills problems and peer victimization. *Aggressive Behavior, 32*, 110–121.

Holmbeck, G. N., Friedman, D., Abad, M., & Jandasek, B. (2006). Development and psychopathology in adolescence. In D. A. Wolfe & E. J. Marsh (Eds.), *Behavioral and emotional disorders in adolescents* (pp. 21–55). New York: The Guilford Press.

Jacobson, N. S., Martell, C. R., & Dimidjian, S. (2001). Behavioral activation treatment for depression: Returning to contextual roots. *Clinical Psychology: Science and Practice, 8*, 255–270.

Kendall, P. C., Brady, E. U., & Verduin, T. L. (2001). Comorbidity in childhood anxiety disorders and treatment outcome. *Journal of the American Academy of Child and Adolescent Psychiatry, 40*, 787–794.

Langley, A. K., Bergman, R. L., McCracken, J., & Piacentini, J. C. (2004). Impairment in childhood anxiety disorders: Preliminary examination of the child anxiety impact scale-parent version. *Journal of Child and Adolescent Psychopharmacology, 14*, 105–114.

Lewinsohn, P. M., Clarke, G. N., Seeley, J. R., & Rohde, P. (1994). Major depression in community adolescents: Age at onset, episode duration, and time recurrence. *Journal of the American Academy of Child and Adolescent Psychiatry, 3*, 809–819.

Lewinsohn, P. M., & Graf, M. (1973). Pleasant activities and depression. *Journal of Consulting and Clinical Psychology, 41*, 261–268.

Lewinsohn, P. M., Hops, H., Roberts, R. E., Seeley, J. R., & Andrews, J. A. (1993). Adolescent psychopathology: I. Prevalence and incidence of depression and other DSM-III-R disorders in high school students. *Journal of Abnormal Psychology, 102*, 133–144.

Manassis, K., Wilansky-Traynor, P., Farzan, N., Kleiman, V., Parker, K., & Sanford, M. (2010). The feelings club: Randomized controlled evaluation of school-based CBT for anxious or depressive symptoms. *Depression and Anxiety, 27*(10), 945–952.

Masia, C. L., Klein, R. G., Storch, E. A., & Corda, B. (2001). School-based behavioral treatment for social anxiety in adolescents: Results of a pilot study. *Journal of the American Academy of Child and Adolescent Psychiatry, 40*, 780–786.

McCauley, E., Schloredt, K., Gudmundsen, G., Martell, C., & Dimidjian, S. (2011). Expanding behavioral activation to depressed adolescents: Lessons learning in treatment development. *Cognitive and Behavioral Practice, 18*, 371–383.

Merikangas, K. R., He, M. J., Burstein, M., Swanson, M. S. A., Avenevoli, S., Cui, M. L., et al. (2010). Lifetime prevalence of mental disorders in US adolescents: Results from the national comorbidity study-adolescent supplement (NCS-A). *Journal of the American Academy of Child and Adolescent Psychiatry, 49*(10), 980.

Mineka, S., & Zinbarg, R. (2006). A contemporary learning theory perspective on the etiology of anxiety disorders—It's not what you thought it was. *American Psychologist, 61*, 10–26.

O'Neil, K. A., & Kendall, P. C. (2012). Role of comorbid depression and co-occurring depressive symptoms in outcomes for anxiety-disordered youth treated with cognitive-behavioral therapy. *Child and Family Behavior Therapy, 34*, 197–209.

O'Neil, K. A., Podell, J. L., Benjamin, C. L., & Kendall, P. C. (2010). Comorbid depressive disorders in anxiety-disordered youth: Demographic, clinical, and family characteristics. *Child Psychiatry and Human Development, 41*, 330–341.

Rapee, R. M., Lyneham, H. J., Hudson, J. L., Kangas, M., Wuthrich, V. M., & Schniering, C. A. (2013). Effect of comorbidity on treatment of anxious children and adolescents: Results from a large, combined sample. *Journal of the American Academy of Child and Adolescent Psychiatry, 52*, 47–56.

Rhode, P., Clarke, G. N., Lewinsohn, P. M., Seeley, J. R., & Kaufman, N. K. (2001). Impact of comorbidity on a cognitive-behavioral group treatment for adolescent depression. *Journal of the American Academy of Child and Adolescent Psychiatry, 40*, 795–802.

Ritschel, L. A., Ramirez, C. L., Jones, M., & Craighead, W. E. (2011). Behavioral activation for depressed teens: A pilot study. *Cognitive and Behavioral Practice, 18*, 281–299.

Roblek, T., & Piacentini, J. (2005). Cognitive-behavior therapy for childhood anxiety disorders. *Child and Adolescent Psychiatric Clinics of North America, 14*, 863–876.

Schwartz, D., Dodge, K. A., & Coie, J. D. (1993). The emergence of chronic victimization in boys' peer groups. *Child Development, 64*, 1755–1772.

Silverman, W. K., & Ollendick, T. H. (2005). Evidence-based assessment of anxiety and its disorders in children and adolescents. *Journal of Clinical Child and Adolescent Psychology, 34*, 380–411.

Silverman, W. K., Pina, A. A., & Viswesvaran, C. (2008). Evidence-based psychosocial treatments for phobic and anxiety disorders in children and adolescents. *Journal of Clinical Child and Adolescent Psychology, 37*, 105–130.

Taylor, S., & Clark, D. A. (2009). Transdiagnostic cognitive-behavioral treatments for mood and anxiety disorders: Introduction to the special issue. *Journal of Cognitive Psychotherapy, 23*, 3–5.

U.S. Department of Education, Office of Planning, Evaluation and Policy Development Policy and Program Studies Service. (2011). *Analysis of State Bullying Laws and Policies*. Retrieved from http://www.ed.gov/about/offices/list/opepd/ppss/index.html

Weersing, V. R., Gonzalez, A., Campo, J. V., & Lucas, A. N. (2008). Brief behavioral therapy for pediatric anxiety and depression: Piloting an integrated treatment approach. *Cognitive and Behavioral Practice, 15*, 126–139.

Weersing, V. R., Rozenman, M. S., Maher-Bridge, M., & Campo, J. V. (2012). Anxiety, depression, and somatic distress: Developing a transdiagnostic internalizing toolbox for pediatric practice. *Cognitive Behavioral Practice, 19*(1), 68–82.

Weissman, A. S., Antinoro, D., & Chu, B. C. (2008). Cognitive behavioral therapy for anxiety in school settings: Advances and challenges. In M. Mayer, R. VanAcker, J. E. Lochman, & F. M. Gresham (Eds.), *Cognitive behavioral interventions for students with emotional/behavioral disorders* (pp. 173–203). New York: The Guilford Press.

Woodward, L. J., & Fergusson, D. M. (2001). Life course outcomes of young people with anxiety disorders in adolescence. *Journal of the American Academy of Child and Adolescent Psychiatry, 4*(9), 1086–1094.

Chapter 7
Obsessive-Compulsive Disorder

Carlos E. Rivera Villegas, Marie-Christine André, Jose Arauz, and Lisa W. Coyne

Obsessive-compulsive disorder (OCD) is characterized by persistent and intrusive thoughts, ideas, impulses, or images (obsessions) resulting in significant anxiety or distress, coupled with compulsions or rituals used to reduce this distress. According to the *Diagnostic and Statistical Manual of Mental Disorders* (DSM-V; American Psychiatric Association, 2013), common obsessions feature fears of contamination, self-doubts, desires to have things in a specific order, aggressive/horrific images of harming loved ones, and religiosity, or disturbing sexual imagery. Compulsions consist of repetitive behaviors and mental acts (i.e., mental compulsions) and commonly involve, but are not limited to, checking, repetition, and washing. They may also include repetitive motor movements that can appear tic-like, such as walking down the steps in a particular way or avoiding stepping on cracks or particular colors on the floor. According to Swedo and colleagues (1989), washing rituals constitute the most common symptom of childhood OCD, affecting more than 85 % of children diagnosed.

Clinically significant OCD symptoms resulting in significant distress are often associated with major functional impairment across social, occupational, and academic domains. Engagement in compulsions offers only momentary relief of these symptoms, usually leading to greater symptom severity. Childhood OCD is described as a chronic, enduring condition and, for about 60 % of subthreshold or

C.E. Rivera Villegas, B.S. (✉) • M.-C. André, M.A. • J. Arauz, M.A.
Clinical Psychology Department, Suffolk University, Boston, MA, USA
e-mail: cerivera@suffolk.edu; mandre@suffolk.edu; jlarauz@suffolk.edu

L.W. Coyne, Ph.D.
Clinical Psychology Department, Suffolk University,
Harvard Medical School/McLean Hospital, Boston, MA, USA
e-mail: lcoyne@suffolk.edu

© Springer Science+Business Media New York 2015
R. Flanagan et al. (eds.), *Cognitive and Behavioral Interventions in the Schools*, DOI 10.1007/978-1-4939-1972-7_7

threshold cases, is unlikely to remit on its own if left untreated, even though symptoms may shift and change over time (Stewart et al., 2004). Although there are important differences in phenomenology and prevalence of OCD across childhood, adolescence, and adulthood, OCD is generally considered to have a "childhood onset" if it occurs before puberty (Kalra & Swedo, 2009).

Community studies suggest that OCD affects 1–3 % of children over their lifetime and at the rate 0.7 % of children in a given year (American Psychiatric Association, 2000; Leckman et al., 1997; Zohar, 1999). In childhood, more boys than girls are affected (2:3.1; Leonard et al., 1994), although the gender disparity reverses by adolescence (Castle, Deale & Marks, 1995). More than half (56.5 %) of children with OCD begin experiencing significant, symptom-related impairments before 10 years of age (Chabane et al., 2005).

The essential features of OCD present in children and adolescents are mostly consistent with those found in adults (Bloch et al., 2008), with the exception of important differences in symptom presentation, patterns of comorbidity, and gender distribution. In addition, there appear to be differences in degree of insight and etiology (Kalra & Swedo, 2009). Firstly, children diagnosed with OCD are less likely than adults with OCD to recognize their thoughts as irrational (Storch et al., 2008). Secondly, about 40 % of children (compared with one-third of adults) deny that their compulsions are driven by obsessive thoughts (Karno et al., 1988; Swedo et al., 1989). It is notable that lack of insight is often a predictor of treatment resistance and poorer treatment outcome (Storch et al., 2008).

Etiology

Given the complex nature of the disorder, OCD is likely multiply determined. Biological models suggest that OCD may result from a dysfunction of the basal ganglia and, more specifically, with cortico-striato-thalamo-cortical circuitry (Saxena & Rauch, 2000). Neurotransmitter theories of OCD suggest that the disorder results from dysregulation of serotonin in the brain; however, this conjecture is based largely on pharmacotherapy studies noting symptom reduction when selective serotonin reuptake inhibitors (SSRIs) are used (Insel et al., 1985; Kalra & Swedo, 2009). To date, there has been little research into the role of serotonin in the pathophysiology of OCD. A recent review of the behavioral genetics literature suggested that OCD is, at least in part, heritable, with 45–65 % of variability accounted for by additive genetic influence (van Grootheest et al., 2005).

Learning theory has been more useful in terms of designing psychosocial treatments for OCD symptoms, since the theory focuses on describing and influencing maintaining factors. Behavioral models of OCD were developed from Mowrer's seminal work on a two-factor theory of fear and avoidance (Mowrer, 1939, 1960). Specifically, typical thoughts become associated with fear cues via classical conditioning. Individuals subsequently learn that engagement in rituals reduces fear by allowing escape from or avoidance of obsessional thoughts. Thus, OCD symptoms are maintained by negative reinforcement (Shafran, 2005). The momentary reduction in anxiety reinforces continued engagement in rituals (Albano, March, & Piacentini, 1999).

Cognitive-behavioral perspectives suggest that OCD results from either a dysfunction in cognitive processing or that obsessional thinking results from cognitive distortions (Salkovskis, Shafran, Rachman, & Freeston, 1999; Taylor, Abramowitz & McKay, 2007). Some studies suggest that compared to non-sufferers, individuals with OCD show deficits in varied cognitive tasks, with those deficits remaining after successful treatment (Nielen & Den Boer, 2003). With respect to cognitive distortion models, Salkovis posits that individuals with OCD experience intrusive thoughts and appraise them as dangerous, resulting in persistent attempts to suppress them via rituals (Salkovskis, 1996). A cognitive distortion hypothesized to underlie almost every manifestation of OCD is intolerance of uncertainty, or the need to be 100 % certain (Grayson, 2010). For example, a child might spend excessive amounts of time constantly rechecking that all his or hers school supplies are in his or hers backpack before leaving home and making him or her miss the bus. Studies evaluating cognitive-behavioral interventions have provided mostly positive support, with the majority of participants experiencing clinically meaningful reductions in OCD symptoms (Clark, 2004).

Functional Impairment

Roughly 90 % of children with OCD report significant functional impairment in at least one domain, and nearly half of them report experiencing difficulties in school, at home, and in social relationships. Parents tend to report more dysfunction in home and school than their children do, with the most common complaints being difficulty focusing on schoolwork and doing homework (Piacentini 2008). Level of functional impairment is related to symptom severity and comorbid depression; youngsters with good insight typically show less impairment. Rituals involving contamination or cleaning, aggression, or checking have been associated with greater functional impairment (Storch et al., 2010).

Classroom tasks may prove increasingly difficult as symptoms prevent the child from completing assignments in a timely manner. Ritualistic behaviors may also cause the child to withdraw from social activities due to embarrassment. Among adolescents, rituals may prevent engagement in typical teenage activities, such as dating, work, or driving (Albano, Chorpita, & Barlow, 2003). Teachers may inadvertently reinforce or accommodate rituals, such as providing extra time for tests to relieve the child's anxiety. While this can be a useful short-term strategy to reduce a child's distress, it may maintain or exacerbate symptoms over time.

OCD significantly impacts family members and disrupts family routines. Research suggests that family distress appears to be positively correlated with the degree to which family members accommodate a child's OCD symptoms (Storch et al., 2007). Although parents may perceive the accommodation of rituals as beneficial, the process serves to promote and maintain symptoms. Additionally, accommodation is counterproductive to the treatment process since it presents the child with opportunities to avoid participation in feared activities, thereby validating the child's fears and apprehension (Merlo, Lehmkuhl, Geffken, & Storch, 2009).

Functional impairment in OCD can be so profound that youngsters who suffer from OCD may need added supports. According to the International OCD Foundation, students may be eligible to receive special education services and accommodations under the Individuals with Disabilities Education Act (IDEA) if symptoms significantly impair functioning within school settings. Psychoeducational assessment and substantiation that previous academic and/or behavioral interventions were ineffective are typically required. It is important to clarify that accommodations provided in academic settings differ from the parent or teacher accommodations discussed earlier as playing a role in maintaining OCD symptoms. For example, an accommodation plan might include an aide helping the child decrease their rituals by coaching them through feared activities or situations.

OCD or Normal Fear?

Obsessions and compulsions differ from normative developmental fears and rituals. A study of 511 children and adolescents indicated a variety of fears are experienced, including worry about daily events and worry about their family's safety at night (Gordon, King, Gullone, Muris, & Ollendick, 2007). Distinguishing between normal developmental behaviors and maladaptive rituals can be challenging, as ritualistic behaviors among young children are common, particularly around bedtime and mealtime (Evans, Gray, & Leckman, 1999). This may include nighttime rituals with parents, such as being kissed on each cheek in a particular way.

A primary factor that distinguishes OCD behaviors from transient rituals or behavioral preferences is the level of the child's anxiety if a ritual is interrupted or prevented (Albano, Chorpita, & Barlow, 2003). Further, developmentally normal rituals are typically not as time consuming or impairing and usually end by age 8 or 9 (Geffken, Sajid, & MacNaughton, 2005). For example, an 11-year-old boy who insists on engaging in protracted rituals (e.g., rereading and rewriting homework assignments until everything feels "just right") is displaying developmentally inappropriate behavior.

Comorbid Conditions

OCD often does not occur alone. High rates of comorbidity in childhood OCD are common, and patterns of comorbidity change throughout development. Attention Deficit/Hyperactivity Disorder and tic disorders are commonly comorbid with childhood onset, and depression and anxiety are more frequently comorbid with adolescent onset (Mancebo et al., 2008). There are gender differences, with boys more likely to present with comorbid tic disorders than girls (Swedo et al., 1989), with almost 70 % of children with OCD presenting with tics (Leckman et al., 1997). Lebowitz and colleagues (2012) found that children with comorbid tic disorders and OCD displayed more severe tics than children with tic disorders alone. Additionally, the former group scored higher on measures of psychopathology, including depression, anxiety, and psychosocial stress. Distinguishing complex motor tics (e.g., repeating a particular action until it feels right) from compulsions can be challenging (Lewin, Chang, McCracken, McQueen, & Piacentini, 2010), particularly when rituals are simple, repetitive movements like tapping or stepping in specific ways (Kalra & Swedo, 2009). One difference is that tics typically occur with a premonitory urge, while rituals do not. Other comorbid conditions include other anxiety disorders and oppositional defiant disorder (Ale & Krackow, 2011).

Assessment

The assessment of OCD is complex. Grados and Riddle (1999) indicate that children with OCD may present to a variety of professionals not adequately trained to recognize the disorder, including pediatricians and dentists (e.g., bleeding gums from excessive toothbrushing). Moreover, high comorbidity with other disorders poses significant challenges given the numerous "OCD-like" symptoms that may be present. Therefore, it is important for clinicians to determine the *purpose* of presenting behaviors as opposed to simply assessing their form (Berman & Abramowitz, 2010). The progression of OCD may be intensified if symptoms are not recognized and treated promptly.

Clinicians should use a multi-method, multi-informant approach to assessment involving the use of structured and unstructured diagnostic interviews, self-report measures, clinician-administered inventories, and parent and teacher report measures. This approach offers qualitative and quantitative information regarding the onset, frequency, intensity, and duration of associated rituals. Sloman and colleagues (2007) argue that it is important to obtain a social developmental history from the child's parents to provide information regarding the child's psychological development and medical history. Behavioral observations across multiple time periods and settings to gain an understanding of the factors that maintain symptoms within the child's environment are indicated.

Standardized measures: Given that most children struggling with anxiety and obsessive compulsive spectrum disorders tend to underreport symptoms, it is critical to interview both parent(s) and child. Common diagnostic interviews include the Anxiety Disorders Interview Schedule for DSM-IV (ADIS-IV-C/P; Silverman & Albano, 1996) for children and adolescents and the Kiddie Schedule for Affective

Disorders and Schizophrenia (K-SADS) for younger children (Kaufman et al., 1997). The ADIS-IV-C/P was developed for children and adolescents aged 6–18 years and features questions to establish the history of the problem along with separate clinician rating scales that assess for degree of associated impairment (Silverman & Ollendick, 2008). These interviews offer the opportunity to differentiate OCD from other psychiatric disorders. The administration of diagnostic interviews may require extensive training and be time consuming, limiting their use (Merlo, Storch, Murphy, Goodman, & Geffken, 2005).

Thus, it is important to use self-report and other report measures to obtain additional information on symptoms, their severity, and functional impairment. The current gold standard is the Children's Yale-Brown Obsessive-Compulsive Scale (CY-BOCS). The CY-BOCS is a 10-item semi-structured questionnaire that measures OCD severity in children over the past week and includes a symptom checklist featuring a summary of commonly endorsed related symptoms (Freeman, Flessner, & Garcia, 2011). A downward extension of the Leyton Obsessional Inventory (LOI) features a 20-item child version designed for children aged 8–17 years that explores obsessive thoughts and accompanying rituals (Grados & Riddle, 1999), taking about 5 min to complete.

In addition to measures of OCD symptomatology, Calvoressi and colleagues (1999) developed the Family Accommodation Scale. This 9-item measure assesses the level of familial accommodation of a child's obsessive-compulsive behavior during the past month, including helping the child avoid objects/places and modifying family routines (Merlo et al., 2005). This scale has good psychometric properties and can be completed by parents or other family members in approximately 5 min. Items include "How often did you provide items for the patient's compulsions" and "Has the patient become distressed/anxious when you have not provided assistance? To what degree?"

Intervention/Treatment

Cognitive-behavioral therapy (CBT), specifically exposure and response prevention (ERP), and pharmacological treatment with SSRIs, or a combination of CBT and medication, are considered current evidence-based treatments for OCD in children and teens (Freeman et al., 2014; Pediatric OCD Treatment Study (POTS) Team, 2004). Recent studies also suggest the efficacy of family-based CBT and acceptance and commitment therapy (ACT). Since OCD is a chronic condition, people suffering from it often go back periodically for booster sessions (March & Mulle, 1998).

Although manualized treatments are available, treatment should be individualized for each child based on several factors, including symptom severity and comorbidity with other disorders. Given the amount of time children spend at school, educators and other school staff play an important role on the initial identification of OCD in children and assist in the development of a sound individualized treatment plan that helps the child achieve educational goals without making accommodations that may worsen symptoms.

Cognitive-Behavioral Treatment: Exposure and Response Prevention

March and Mulle (1998) developed a CBT treatment manual for children with OCD aged 7–17, composed of four steps: psychoeducation, cognitive training, mapping OCD, and graded exposure and response prevention. During the psychoeducation stage, OCD is described as a medical condition related to brain function. To help families understand the importance of treatment, OCD is presented as analogous to diabetes or asthma (CBT for OCD as exercise for diabetes). For younger children, OCD is described as "a worry monster" or "hiccups of the brain." By differentiating the child from the OCD, the child and family learn to externalize OCD and begin seeing it as something they can have control over by "bossing back" OCD.

Cognitive training involves teaching youngsters cognitive tools utilize to "boss back" OCD. ERP is identified as the main strategy for the child's battle against OCD, and the therapist, family members, and often educators are identified as allies of the child (March & Mulle, 1998). Child-friendly concrete examples are used to explain the rationale for ERP, for example, "bossing back the worry monster" who tries to tell you to do things it wants you to do (Freeman et al., 2008).

Mapping OCD focuses on assessing the child's symptom intensity, topography, triggers, and consequences. This assists the therapeutic team—the child, parents, and therapist—to learn situations in which the child is and is not successful in resisting compulsions. This "map" helps strengthen the externalization of OCD from the child and the belief that child and team are on the same side.

Graded Exposure and Response Prevention (ERP) is the core of CBT for OCD and is used with children as well as adults. Graded exposure consists of exposure to situations that produce unwanted feelings (anxiety, fear) in the child, such as touching a toilet seat when the child has contamination fears. Understandably, children may hesitate to engage in graded exposure. Clinicians should remind the child that each time a feared situation is practiced, the easier it will become. Response prevention consists of blocking or minimizing ritualistic and/or avoidance behavior, such as washing the hands after touching the toilet seat. The therapist and child review progress during every session in order to ensure the implementation of ERP exercises is appropriate and help the child learn to make these evaluations on his or her own. In the school setting, teachers should work with the child to help them respond obsessive thoughts in positive ways as opposed to providing excessive reassurance.

Other Cognitive-Behavioral Interventions

Intensive CBT (I-CBT)

Research suggests that more intensive CBT interventions may be beneficial for children and adolescents with severe symptoms and experiencing significant functional impairment. I-CBT uses similar tools that CBT treatments utilize; however, the protocol is condensed into a 3- to 4-week time frame, meaning there are multiple sessions per week. The main benefit of ICBT is rapid symptom relief (Storch et al., 2007).

Group Therapy

Several of the individual interventions for OCD have been adapted for group therapy settings. Group therapy has shown to be advantageous in several ways. When people share similar symptoms, they may feel motivated by hearing others in similar situations talk about their struggles and successes. Knowing that there are others going through similar situations might lessen stigmas and self-judgments associated with the disorder and provide validation. Delivering intervention to a group also tends to be cost and time effective compared to individual therapy (Muroff et al., 2009; Van Noppen, Steketee, McCorkle, & Pato, 1997).

However, group therapy also presents some drawbacks. OCD is private; obsessions can seem very strange to people who are not experiencing them. Thus, children with the disorder might feel more anxious and stigmatized when they open up and others do not relate to their experiences. It is also difficult to conduct ERP in group settings due to patients being at different stages of treatment. Lastly, therapeutic relationships are not as strong as in individual treatment; therefore, patients' rates of walking out of the group are more frequent. Studies have suggested difficulties in group settings when clients have different comorbid conditions, which might divert the course of therapy; in these instances, it is suggested that people receive additional individual therapy (Muroff et al., 2009).

Acceptance and Commitment Therapy

Acceptance and commitment therapy (ACT; Hayes, Strosahl, & Wilson, 1999) is a fairly recent empirically based intervention useful across many mental health problems and shows promise in the treatment of adolescent OCD (Armstrong, Morrison, & Twohig, 2013). Instead of changing the focus from a person's distorted thoughts to healthier ones (one of the main goals of CBT), ACT focuses on changing the relation a person has with his or her own thoughts by targeting the function of these thoughts and promoting behavior change in services of the person's values.

By practicing acceptance and mindfulness and exploring a person's values, ACT fosters willingness to experience obsessions and anxieties while encouraging one to act in ways consistent with the person's own values (Hannan & Tolin, 2005). For example, an adolescent with OCD may gradually realize that a thought is just a thought rather than a literal truth. Thus, the adolescent may attain the flexibility to engage in valued actions despite the occurrence of obsessions and anxieties. Lastly, given that ACT is an intervention that uses metaphors, it may be a better fit for adolescents, who tend to be in a stage of value exploration and are more capable of abstract thinking than younger children (Armstrong, Morrison, & Twohig, 2013; Greco, Blackledge, Coyne, & Ehrenreich, 2005). For example, the "chocolate cake" exercise instructs the individual *not* to think about a chocolate cake, thus illustrating the futility of attempting to control one's thoughts.

Pharmacotherapy

Research suggests that selective serotonin reuptake inhibitors (SSRIs) are the first options for psychopharmacological treatment for OCD in children and adolescents. However, medication for the treatment of OCD in children and adolescents should only be considered when symptoms are moderate or severe and in concert with CBT. Current US Food and Drug Administration (FDA)-approved medications for the treatment of OCD include the antidepressant clomipramine and the SSRIs Prozac, Zoloft, Paxil (in adults), and Luvox. As compared with clomipramine, SSRIs present fewer side effects, but some studies suggest clomipramine is superior to the SSRIs (Coyne, Freeman, Garcia, & Leonard, 2007). The "Expert Consensus Guidelines" suggests clomipramine be used after two or three trials of SSRIs and failed CBT (March et al., 1997). Side effects of clomipramine include drowsiness, dry mouth, and racing heart, among others. Side effects of SSRIs include nausea, inability to sit still, sleepiness or insomnia, and a heightened sense of energy. Antidepressants for children and teens might also lead to suicidal thoughts and urges, especially when starting a new medicine or increasing its dose. Therefore, it is of critical importance to assess for depression in the child at the outset of treatment. The FDA has issued "black box warnings" about suicidal thoughts and urges for all antidepressants in children and teenagers.

Although existing drugs help control and decrease symptoms, they do not "cure" the disorder. Therefore, it is recommended that children with OCD taking medication also undergo some kind of behavioral therapy (such as CBT). Since different drugs produce different results in people, it is not uncommon that a child would try several different medications before finding one that fits well. OCD medications work slowly and might take 10–12 weeks for them to start working properly. Once an appropriate drug and its dose have been identified, it might control symptoms of OCD well; however, these symptoms often return after medication is discontinued.

Developmental Considerations

When treating children and adolescents, it is essential to have a clear understanding of their developmental stage. Careful evaluation of a youngster's cognitive (not taken to mean cognitive ability) and emotional functioning will help guide the selection of therapeutic techniques. For example, children who are 8 years old and younger may have great difficulty with the more abstract, cognitive components of CBT, whereas older children might benefit greatly from these exercises. Similarly, younger children may have greater difficulty describing nuances in their level of anxiety compared with older children, thus complicating the development of exposure hierarchies. Thus, it is important to adjust what is said to the child so that it fits with their developmental level.

Similarly, parents may be helpful as guides of their younger children's attempts at behavior change, given that younger children are far more dependent on parents for structure and guidance. Engaging parents in treatment is important in two ways: first, they can report whether behavioral changes are occurring at home and homework is appropriately completed within a reasonable time frame; moreover, the clinician can intervene to address any parent behaviors that may inadvertently maintain or exacerbate their child's problems. In contrast, adolescents may benefit more if given greater autonomy to effect behavioral changes at their own pace rather than as stipulated by parents. Teachers may be used in an analogous manner if the target behaviors are manifesting in the classroom.

It is also crucial to consider the contextual factors that may impact a child or adolescent's behavioral presentation—namely, the home, school, and peer environments. Depending on a child's age and interests, their relative importance may vary over time. For instance, with adolescents, peer relationships may stand out as a critical treatment issue. Young children, on the other hand, may be more influenced by their parents. Additionally, youngsters' functioning may vary across each of these environments; thus, using multiple informants (e.g., self, teacher, parent) to describe behavior in each of these domains is encouraged.

K-6th Grades

In general, it is more difficult for younger children to understand questions about their own thoughts, as well as understanding concepts such as average, time, and estimates (Freeman et al., 2012). It is important to remember the difficulty for young children to assess hierarchies needed to utilize response prevention. When reporting the intensity of their feelings, children tend to describe their behavior dichotomously, rather than in increments. When this is the case, it would be beneficial to teach the child how to use a hierarchical rating scale. Using simple and concrete descriptions with younger children may help children understand concepts related to OCD (Coyne, Burke, & Freeman, 2008; Freeman et al., 2003). Since children in grades K-6 might find more difficulty monitoring their thoughts or engaging in rational disputation, it is easier to use functional disputation with them, for example, by asking them, "Did this help you stay less scared?"

Younger children may also rely more on adults for guidance. Thus, working with parents, caregivers, and teachers may be beneficial for youngsters. Hence, adults play an essential role in the treatment process for young children with OCD. There should be clear communication between teachers and caregivers, and a common way in which they will deal with situations, so that the child will find consistency in both home and school.

7th–12th Grades

As children develop and gain control over their own lives, they become less dependent on their caregivers and start placing greater value on peer relationships and their autonomy. Consequently, it is important to include caregivers and educators in ways in which the youth do not feel impotent, embarrassed, or infantilized. Teens can be, and often are, oppositional and more difficult to engage in treatment as compared with younger children. Therefore, striving toward strengthening a therapeutic alliance with them and motivating them to participate in therapy without making them feel coerced are a significant piece of the therapeutic process. It is important to keep in mind that adolescents tend to struggle more with self-esteem and social relationships, issues that could be easily exacerbated by the presence of OCD and that might lead to additional mental health problems such as depression, anger, disruptive behavior, and isolation, among others.

Teenagers' cognitive development makes it easier for them to monitor their cognitive processes because they are attaining formal operational thought and are able to express their own thoughts and emotions. Additionally, they are able to engage in rational disputation and utilize the concept of hierarchies, all of which are tools employed in the treatment of OCD. Adolescents tend to appreciate and understand more detailed and technical explanations of OCD and the treatment process and need more opportunity for discussion (March & Mulle, 1998).

Case Example

Individual features of client: Dimitri was a 15-year-old Caucasian male who presented to an outpatient child anxiety treatment center. He exhibited flat affect throughout the interview and demonstrated little excitement when discussing pleasurable activities. He also exhibited moderate understanding of his OCD and associated impairment. During the initial interview, Dimitri appeared motivated to received treatment for his OCD concerns. However, once treatment began, he resisted completing schoolwork, homework, and exposure exercises.

Presenting complaints: Dimitri's mother reported that he was often noncompliant, rigid about his routines, and anxious about bathroom incontinence. She also stated that he experienced a great deal of anxiety when starting new activities or visiting unfamiliar locations where he did not know where the bathroom was located. Additionally, his mother reported that Dimitri spent a long time in the bathroom and often used all of the toilet paper located in the household. Dimitri also reported forcing his bowel movements to ensure that he would not feel the urge to go again while on the school bus.

During school, Dimitri reported using the bathroom or at least sitting on the toilet about 8–10 times daily. Dimitri reported that he often became upset at his teachers if they did not allow him to use the bathroom. He specifically stated that he used the bathroom right before giving a presentation in front of the class for fear that he may need to use the bathroom while presenting. Dimitri's teachers also reported that Dimitri was not able to answer questions in class due to fear that he may not have the right answer.

Developmental factors: During the adaptation of the cognitive-behavioral treatment for Dimitri, several factors were considered. Firstly, a thorough assessment of Dimitri's bathroom rituals was conducted to differentiate between developmentally appropriate rituals and clinically significant rituals. Secondly, given Dimitri's age, it was crucial to determine his ability to recognize and express his anxiety in order to ensure his ability to create an accurate fear hierarchy during treatment.

Contextual factors: At home, Dimitri's family reported engaging in a significant amount of accommodation around his rituals. His mother reported that she almost always accommodated Dimitri's behavior in order to avoid upsetting him. Other familial factors became apparent during the assessment and became critical in implementing a course of CBT effectively. In particular, Dimitri's mother blamed herself for his symptoms because she used to give him reminders to clean and organize items in his room when he was younger. She had hoped he would outgrow these behaviors as he became older, especially given how suddenly they had emerged.

At school, Dimitri's teacher struggled with setting limits around his bathroom "breaks," and if she did not allow him to use the bathroom at will, he became extremely oppositional and disruptive in class. This contributed to his teacher feeling out of control of her classroom. In addition, Dimitri's teacher was concerned about the impact of Dimitri's behavior on his peer relationships. She reported increasing social isolation and deepening negative mood.

Assessment: Dimitri and his mother were interviewed separately using the Anxiety Disorders Interview Schedule for Children and Parent (ADIS-C/P) for DSM-IV. The Children's Yale-Brown Obsessive-Compulsive Scale (CY-BOCS) was also administered to assess symptoms and severity throughout the course of treatment (baseline, mid-treatment, and termination). Dimitri's mother and teacher completed the Child Behavior Checklist (CBCL) Parent and Teacher Forms, which provided a more general index of Dimitri's psychological functioning at home and school. Dimitri completed the Youth Self-Report (YSR), which is the self-report version of the CBCL. The data obtained by the CBCL and the YSR were consistent with the information provided during the ADIS-C/P interview and the CY-BOCS, suggesting that Dimitri experienced a great deal of symptoms which were interfering with his life.

Dimitri completed two additional self-report questionnaires: the Children's Depression Inventory (CDI; Kovacs, 1992) and the Penn State Worry Questionnaire (PSWQ; Meyer et al., 1990). These questionnaire scores were consistent with the information obtained during the interview, suggesting that Dimitri was not experiencing symptoms of depression but experienced a great deal of persistent worries.

Course of treatment and progress: Dimitri and his mother agreed to a course of CBT to target his symptoms. Dimitri attended most sessions individually, with his mother joining for the final 10 min of each session. One session was conducted with Dimitri's mother alone in order to allow her to express her thoughts and fears about the nature of Dimitri's symptoms and to discuss ways of coping with these fears on her own. At first, psychoeducation about the nature and course of anxiety was addressed followed by an overview of the three-component model of anxiety (thoughts, feelings, and behaviors). In the next sessions, psychoeducation about cognitive distortions and the use of cognitive restructuring techniques was covered, followed by multiple sessions on graduated exposure and ritual prevention. Cognitive restructuring strategies targeted Dimitri's catastrophic thinking about needing to use the bathroom and the possibility of having an accident in public, among other obsessions. The majority of treatment focused on ERP to help Dimitri resist his rituals and engage in behaviors that he would typically avoid. This part started with developing a fear hierarchy, which consisted of obtaining subjective units of distress (i.e., fear ratings) for each anxiety-provoking situation that Dimitri encountered. He was gradually exposed to these situations based on the order of his fear hierarchy.

In addition to the exposures completed in session and at home, consultation sessions were conducted with a school psychologist and Dimitri's teacher to help implement exposure exercises at school. Dimitri's teacher was provided with psychoeducation about OCD and was informed of the exposure exercises that Dimitri's was supposed to complete at school. The school psychologist assisted her in understanding that although disruptive in the short run, resisting accommodation of Dimitri's rituals was critical to his treatment. Thus, with the assistance of the school psychologist, his teacher stopped reassuring him, set limits around bathroom breaks, and helped reduce the number of rituals at school. Dimitri saw the school psychologist, who offered support and encouragement to remain engaged in treatment. She also provided help around peer issues that arose for Dimitri and helped build his social skills, which had suffered due to his engagement in rituals. Gradually, he was able to turn in assignments on time and significantly reduced the time spent checking for the "right" answers. Toward the end of the treatment, Dimitri was able to attend social outings that he previously avoided.

Other Practice Considerations

In addition to the developmental considerations discussed previously, it is important to understand cultural differences that may explain certain behaviors that are perceived as obsessive or ritualistic. For example, certain cultures or religions may have common practices that include a routine such as food restrictions or a specific pattern of activities shared by that community. It is crucial to consider these factors before starting treatment in order to avoid misdiagnosing behaviors that actually reflect cultural differences. Nevertheless, a differentiation between cultural practices and diagnosable compulsions can be made. For example, a child with OCD may feel like they need to pray a certain amount of time before they can feel "just right." In this example, even though the prayer ritual may be an activity shared by the whole community and the family, the clinician must assess whether the rigidity in the schedule or in the timing of the practice is prescribed by that culture or if the child is imposing those rules on himself or herself. The clinician can also solicit the assistance of a member of that community or that religion in order to get a more accurate picture of the practices and the expectations of that cultural/religious group.

Diagnostic issues should also be considered during the course of treatment, given the higher rates of comorbidity in youth. Thus, a child may meet criteria for an autism spectrum disorder (ASD) and also meet criteria for OCD. It is important to understand the symptom overlap. For example, children with both OCD and ASD may exhibit similar stereotypical and obsessive behaviors (e.g., repeating actions)—the underlying nature of these behaviors may be different—and the treatment differs accordingly. Children with OCD engage in ritualistic behaviors in an attempt to reduce their anxiety and control their obsessive thoughts; they tend to be distressed by their obsessive thoughts and try to avoid thinking about these thoughts by engaging in rituals. In contrast, children with ASD are not bothered by their thoughts and do not feel like they need to get rid of these thoughts. Worth noting is that the rigidity and hypersensitivity observed in ASD are similar to the "feel right" obsession present in OCD, yet it does not serve the same purpose. Children with ASD are not usually able to explain why they are sensitive to certain noises or why they like their routine, whereas children with OCD usually report that the specific behavior has to "feel right" and they fear that negative consequences will happen if the ritual is not completed. Regardless of this differentiation, ASD and OCD can co-occur in a small number of children. A thorough assessment for the presence of comorbid disorders is important because it guides the clinician to adapt the treatment protocol in order to maximize the gains for the patient. Diagnostic issues should also be considered because sometimes a diagnosis secondary to OCD may be slowing or impeding the course of treatment. Teenagers suffering from comorbid depression may have a difficult time engaging in exposure exercises, not necessarily because they are overly anxious but because they feel unmotivated to complete the exercises given their depressive symptomatology. Similarly, children with comorbid social anxiety may be reluctant to engage in exposure exercises in front of their peers, despite the focus of the exposure may be unrelated to their social anxiety. Clinicians must remain mindful of these nuances as they emerge in treatment.

In summary, OCD presents unique challenges across home and school settings. For parents and teachers, it is important to recognize the diversity of the disorder, including its varied presentations across individuals and the difficulty in differentiating between OCD and normal fears. Clinicians are encouraged to utilize a multi-method, multi-informant approach when assessing for OCD. Although several treatment options exist, treatment should be individualized for each child to maximize treatment efficacy. Although treatment may not completely eliminate symptoms, it offers the opportunity to learn new skills that may reduce the anxiety and impairment associated with OCD, thus permitting a more meaningful and enjoyable life.

References

Albano, A., Chorpita, B. F., & Barlow, D. H. (2003). Childhood anxiety disorders. In E. J. Mash & R. A. Barkley (Eds.), *Child psychopathology* (pp. 279–371). New York, NY: The Guilford Press.

Albano, A., March, J., & Piacentini, J. (1999). Cognitive-behavioral treatment of obsessive-compulsive disorder. In R. Ammerman, M. Hersen, & C. Lasts (Eds.), *Handbook of prescriptive treatments for children and adolescents* (pp. 193–215). Boston: Allyn & Bacon.

Ale, C. M., & Krackow, E. (2011). Concurrent treatment of early childhood OCD and ODD: A case illustration. *Clinical Case Studies, 10*, 312–323.

American Psychiatric Association. (2000). *Diagnostic and statistical manual of mental disorders (4th ed., text rev.).* Washington, DC: American Psychiatric Association.

American Psychiatric Association. (2013). *Diagnostic and statistical manual of mental disorders* (5th ed.). Washington, DC: American Psychiatric Association.

Armstrong, A. B., Morrison, K. L., & Twohig, M. P. (2013). A preliminary investigation of acceptance and commitment therapy for adolescent obsessive-compulsive disorder. *Journal of Cognitive Psychotherapy, 27*(2), 175–190.

Berman, N. C., & Abramowitz, J. S. (2010). Recent developments in the assessment and treatment of pediatric obsessive-compulsive disorder. *Child & Youth Care Forum, 39*(2), 125–127.

Bloch, M., Landeros-Weisenberger, A., Rosario, M., Pittenger, C., & Leckman, J. (2008). Meta-analysis of the symptom structure of obsessive-compulsive disorder. *American Journal of Psychiatry, 165*, 1532–1542.

Calvocoressi, L., Mazure, C. M., Kasl, S. V., Skolnick, J., Fisk, D., Vegso, S. J., et al. (1999). Family accommodation of obsessive-compulsive symptoms: Instrument development and assessment of family behavior. *Journal of Nervous and Mental Disease, 187*, 636–642.

Castle, D. J., Deale, A., & Marks, I. M. (1995). Gender differences in obsessive compulsive disorder. *Australian and New Zealand Journal of Psychiatry, 29*, 114–117.

Chabane, N., Delorme, R., Millet, B., Mouren, M., Leboyer, M., & Pauls, D. (2005). Early-onset obsessive compulsive disorder: A subgroup with a specific clinical and familial pattern? *Journal of Child Psychology and Psychiatry, 46*, 881–887.

Clark, D. A. (2004). Cognitive-behavioral therapy for OCD. Guilford Publication, New York, NY.

Coyne, L. W., Burke, A. M., & Freemen, J. B. (2008). Cognitive behavioral treatment. *Handbook of clinical psychology, children and adolescents*. Hoboken, NJ: John Wiley & Sons, Inc.

Coyne, L. W., Freeman, J. B., Garcia, A. M., & Leonard, H. L. (2007). Obsessive-compulsive disorder in children and adolescents. In G. O. Gabbard (Ed.), *Treatments of psychiatric disorders* (4th ed., pp. 39–46). Washington: American Psychiatric Publishing, Inc.

Evans, D. W., Gray, F., & Leckman, J. F. (1999). The rituals, fears and phobias of young children: Insights from development, psychopathology and neurobiology. *Child Psychiatry and Human Development, 29*, 261–276.

Freeman, J., Flessner, C. A., & Garcia, A. (2011). The Children's Yale-Brown Obsessive Compulsive Scale: Reliability and validity for use among 5 to 8 year olds with obsessive-compulsive disorder. *Journal of Abnormal Child Psychology, 39*, 877–883.

Freeman, J. B., Garcia, A. M., Benito, K., Conelea, C., Sapyta, J., Khanna, M., Franklin, M. (2012). The Pediatric Obsessive Compulsive Disorder Treatment Study for Young Children (POTS Jr): Developmental considerations in the rationale, design, and methods. *Journal of Obsessive-Compulsive and Related Disorders, 1*, 294–300.

Freeman, J. B., Garcia, A. M., Coyne, L. W., Ale, C., Przeworski, A., Himle, M., Leonard, H. L. (2008). Early childhood OCD: Preliminary findings from a family-based cognitive-behavioral approach. *Journal of the American Academy of Child and Adolescent Psychiatry, 47*, 593–602.

Freeman, J., Garcia, A., Frank, H., Benito, K., Conelea, C., Walther, M., & Edmunds, J. (2014) Evidence base update for psychosocial treatments for pediatric obsessive-compulsive disorder. *Journal of Clinical Child and Adolescent Psychology, 43*, 7–26.

Freeman, J. B., Garcia, A. M., Fucci, C., Karitani, M., Miller, L., & Leonard, H. L. (2003). Family-based treatment of early-onset obsessive-compulsive disorder. *Journal of Child and Adolescent Psychopharmacology, 13*, 71–80.

Geffken, G., Sajid, M., & MacNaughton, K. (2005). The course of childhood OCD, its antecedents, onset, comorbidities, remission, and reemergence: A 12-year case report. *Clinical Case Studies, 4*, 380–394.

Gordon, J., King, N., Gullone, E., Muris, P., & Ollendick, T. H. (2007). Nighttime fears of children and adolescents: Frequency, content, severity, harm expectations, disclosure, and coping behaviours. *Behaviour Research and Therapy, 45*, 2464–2472.

Grados, M. A., & Riddle, M. A. (1999). Obsessive-compulsive disorder in children and adolescents: Treatment guidelines. *CNS Drugs, 12*, 257–277.

Grayson, J. B. (2010). OCD and intolerance of uncertainty: Treatment issues. *Journal of Cognitive Psychotherapy, 24*(1), 3–15.

Greco, L. A., Blackledge, J. T., Coyne, L. W., & Ehrenreich, J. (2005). Integrating acceptance and mindfulness into treatments for child and adolescent anxiety disorders: Acceptance and commitment therapy as an example. In S. M. Orsillo & L. Roemer (Eds.), *Acceptance and mindfulness-based approaches to anxiety: Conceptualization and treatment*. New York: Kluwer/Plenum.

Hannan, S. E., & Tolin, D. F. (2005). Mindfulness and acceptance based behavior therapy for obsessive-compulsive disorder. In S. M. Orsillo & L. Roemer (Eds.), *Acceptance and mindfulness-based approaches to anxiety: Conceptualization and treatment* (pp. 271–299). New York: Springer.

Hayes, S. C., Strosahl, K. D., & Wilson, K. G. (1999). *Acceptance and commitment therapy: An experiential approach to behavior change*. New York: Guilford Press.

Insel, T. R., Mueller, E. A., Alterman, I., Linnoila, M., & Murphy, D. L. (1985). Obsessive-compulsive disorder and serotonin: Is there a connection? *Biological Psychiatry, 20*, 1174–1188.

Kalra, S. K., & Swedo, S. E. (2009). Children with obsessive-compulsive disorder: Are they just little adults? *The Journal of Clinical Investigation, 119*, 737–746.

Karno, M., Golding, J. M., Sorenson, S. B., & Burnam, M. A. (1988). The epidemiology of obsessive-compulsive disorder in five US communities. *Archives of General Psychiatry, 45*, 1094.

Kaufman, J., Birmaher, B., Brent, D., Rao, U., Flynn, C., Moreci, P., et al. (1997). Schedule for affective disorders and schizophrenia for school-age children—Present and lifetime version (KSADS-PL): Initial reliability and validity data. *Journal of the American Academy of Child and Adolescent Psychiatry, 36*, 980–988.

Kovacs, M. (1992). *Children's Depression Inventory*. New York, NY: Multi-Health Systems.

Lebowitz, E. R., Motlagh, M. G., Katsovich, L., King, R. A., Lombroso, P. J., Grantz, H., et al. (2012). Tourette syndrome in youth with and without obsessive compulsive disorder and attention deficit hyperactivity disorder. *European Child & Adolescent Psychiatry, 21*, 451–457.

Leckman, J. F., Grice, D. E., Boardman, J., Zhang, H., Vitale, A., Bondi, C., et al. (1997). Symptoms of obsessive-compulsive disorder. *American Journal of Psychiatry, 154*, 911–917.

Leonard, H. L., Topol, D., Bukstein, O., Hindmarsh, D., Allen, A. J., & Swedo, S. E. (1994). Clonazepam as an augmenting agent in the treatment of childhood-onset obsessive-compulsive disorder. *Journal of the American Academy of Child and Adolescent Psychiatry, 33*, 792–794.

Lewin, A. B., Chang, S., McCracken, J., McQueen, M., & Piacentini, J. (2010). Comparison of clinical features among youth with tic disorders, obsessive–compulsive disorder (OCD), and both conditions. *Psychiatry Research, 178*, 317–322.

Mancebo, M. C., Garcia, A. M., Pinto, A., Freeman, J. B., Przeworski, A., Stout, R., et al. (2008). Juvenile-onset OCD: Clinical features in children, adolescents and adults. *Acta Psychiatrica Scandinavica, 118*, 149–159.

March, J. S., Frances, A., Carpenter, D., & Kahn, D. A. (1997). The expert consensus guideline series: Treatment of obsessive-compulsive disorder. *Journal of Clinical Psychiatry, 58*, 1–72.

March, J. S., & Mulle, K. (1998). *OCD in children and adolescents: A cognitive-behavioral treatment manual*. New York: Guilford Press.

Merlo, L. J., Lehmkuhl, H. D., Geffken, G. R., & Storch, E. A. (2009). Decreased family accommodation associated with improved therapy outcome in pediatric obsessive–compulsive disorder. *Journal of Consulting and Clinical Psychology, 77*, 355–360.

Merlo, L. J., Storch, E. A., Murphy, T. K., Goodman, W. K., & Geffken, G. R. (2005). Assessment of pediatric obsessive-compulsive disorder: A critical review of current methodology. *Child Psychiatry and Human Development, 36*, 195–214.

Meyer, T. J., Miller, M. L., Metzger, R. L., & Borkovec, T. D. (1990). Development and validation of the Penn State Worry Questionnaire. *Behavior Research and Therapy, 28*, 487–495.

Mowrer, O. H. (1939). A stimulus-response analysis of anxiety and its role as a reinforcing agent. *Psychological Review, 46*, 553–565.

Mowrer, O. H. (1960). *Learning theory and behavior (Vol. 960)* (960). New York: Wiley.

Muroff, J., Steketee, G., Rasmussen, J., Gibson, A., Bratiotis, C., & Sorrentino, C. (2009). Group cognitive and behavioral treatment for compulsive hoarding: A preliminary trial. *Depression and Anxiety, 26*, 634–640.

Nielen, M. M. A., & Den Boer, J. A. (2003). Neuropsychological performance of OCD patients before and after treatment with fluoxetine: Evidence for persistent cognitive deficits. *Psychological Medicine, 33*(05), 917–925.

Pediatric OCD Treatment Study (POTS) Team. (2004). Cognitive behavior therapy, sertraline, and their combination for children and adolescents with obsessive-compulsive disorder. *Journal of the American Medical Association, 292*, 1969–1976.

Piacentini, J. (2008). Optimizing cognitive-behavioral therapy for childhood psychiatric disorders. *Journal of the American Academy of Child and Adolescent Psychiatry, 47*(5), 481–482.

Salkovskis, P. M. (1996). Cognitive-behavioral approaches to the understanding of obsessional problems. In R. M. Rapee (Ed.), *Current controversies in the anxiety disorders* (pp. 103–133). New York: Guilford.

Salkovskis, P., Shafran, R., Rachman, S., & Freeston, M. H. (1999). Multiple pathways to inflated responsibility beliefs in obsessional problems: Possible origins and implications for therapy and research. *Behaviour Research and Therapy, 37*, 1055–1072.

Saxena, S., & Rauch, S. L. (2000). Functional neuroimaging and the neuroanatomy of obsessive-compulsive disorder. *Psychiatric Clinics of North America, 23*(3), 563–586.

Shafran, R. (2005). Cognitive-behavioral models of OCD. In *Concepts and controversies in obsessive-compulsive disorder* (pp. 229–260). United States, New York, NY: Springer.

Silverman, W. K., & Albano, A. M. (1996). *The anxiety disorders interview schedule for DSM-IV-child and parent versions*. London: Oxford University Press.

Silverman, W. K., & Ollendick, T. H. (2008). Child and adolescent anxiety disorders. In J. Hunsley & E. Mash (Eds.), *Assessments that work* (pp. 181–206). Oxford, NY: Oxford University Press, Inc.

Sloman, G. M., Gallant, J., & Storch, E. A. (2007). A school-based treatment model for pediatric obsessive-compulsive disorder. *Child Psychiatry and Human Development, 38*, 303–319.

Stewart, S. E., Geller, D. A., Jenike, M. M., Pauls, D. D., Shaw, D. D., Mullin, B. B., et al. (2004). Long-term outcome of pediatric obsessive-compulsive disorder: A meta-analysis and qualitative review of the literature. *Acta Psychiatrica Scandinavica, 110*, 4–13.

Storch, E. A., Geffken, G. R., Merlo, L. J., Jacob, M. L., Murphy, T. K., Goodman, W. K., et al. (2007). Family accommodation in pediatric obsessive–compulsive disorder. *Journal of Clinical Child and Adolescent Psychology, 36*(2), 207–216.

Storch, E. A., Larson, M. J., Muroff, J., Caporino, N., Geller, D., Reid, J. M., et al. (2010). Predictors of functional impairment in pediatric obsessive-compulsive disorder. *Journal of Anxiety Disorders, 24*, 275–283.

Storch, E. A., Merlo, L. J., Larson, M. J., Marien, W. E., Geffken, G. R., Jacob, M. L., et al. (2008). Clinical features associated with treatment-resistant pediatric obsessive-compulsive disorder. *Comprehensive Psychiatry, 49*, 35–42.

Swedo, S. E., Rapoport, J. L., Leonard, H., Lenane, M., & Cheslow, D. (1989). Obsessive-compulsive disorder in children and adolescents: Clinical phenomenology of 70 consecutive cases. *Archives of General Psychiatry, 46*, 335–341.

Taylor, S., Abramowitz, J. S., & McKay, D. (2007). Cognitive-behavioral models of obsessive-compulsive disorder. In M. M. Antony, C. Purdon, & L. J. Summerfeldt (Eds.), *Psychological treatment of obsessive-compulsive disorder: Fundamentals and beyond* (pp. 9–29). Washington, DC: American Psychological Association.

van Grootheest, D. S., Cath, D. C., Beekman, A. T., & Boomsma, D. I. (2005). Twin studies on obsessive–compulsive disorder: A review. *Twin Research and Human Genetics, 8*, 450–458.

Van Noppen, B., Steketee, G., McCorkle, B. H., & Pato, M. (1997). Group and multifamily behavioral treatment for obsessive compulsive disorder: A pilot study. *Journal of Anxiety Disorders, 11*, 431–446.

Zohar, A. H. (1999). The epidemiology of obsessive-compulsive disorder in children and adolescents. *Child and Adolescent Psychiatric Clinics of North America, 12*, 33–36.

Chapter 8
Attention Deficit Hyperactivity Disorder: Use of Evidence-Based Assessments and Interventions

Linda Reddy, Erik Newman, and Arielle Verdesco

Attention deficit hyperactivity disorder (ADHD) is a complex chronic neurocognitive disorder that impairs students' academic, social, and behavioral functioning in school and home (e.g., Kent et al., 2011; Kessler et al., 2005). ADHD-related symptoms and high rates of comorbidity impact the teaching and learning process for children and pose unique challenges for practitioners, educators, and parents for assessment and intervention planning.

This chapter presents (1) an overview of ADHD as a heterogeneous neurocognitive disorder, highlighting common comorbid disorders and the symptom overlap with other conditions; (2) assessment and intervention frameworks; and (3) a case study using a multimodal intervention that employs teacher and student progress-monitoring methods.

ADHD as a Heterogeneous Disorder

The fundamental features that define ADHD include persistent patterns of inattention and/or hyperactivity-impulsivity, which are greater (in frequency or severity) than the patterns typically observed in individuals at a comparable level of

L. Reddy, Ph.D. (✉) • A. Verdesco, B.S.
Department of Applied Psychology, Graduate School of Applied
and Professional Psychology, Rutgers University,
152 Frelinghuysen Road, Piscataway, NJ 08854, USA
e-mail: LReddy@scarletmail.rutgers.edu; verdescoa2@gmail.com

E. Newman, Ph.D.
University of California, San Diego, 9500 Gilman Drive, La Jolla, CA 92093, USA

Integrative Psychotherapy Services of San Diego, Inc., 2333 State Street, Suite 102,
Carlsbad, CA 92008, USA
e-mail: newmanerik@gmail.com; enewman@ucsd.edu

© Springer Science+Business Media New York 2015
R. Flanagan et al. (eds.), *Cognitive and Behavioral Interventions
in the Schools*, DOI 10.1007/978-1-4939-1972-7_8

development (American Psychiatric Association Fifth Edition, 2013). The symptoms of ADHD typically fall into three categories: inattention, hyperactivity, and impulsivity. These symptoms relate to impairments in social and/or academic functioning and must be persistent across settings (home and school) (e.g., American Psychiatric Association, 2013). The three symptom categories help practitioners with differentiating the three ADHD subtypes: predominantly inattentive, predominantly hyperactive/impulsive, and combined. Typically, children with ADHD inattentive type appear distracted and withdrawn, while children with ADHD hyperactive/impulsive or combined type display high levels of motor activity (impulsive acts), including frequent moving and talking out of turn (see Reddy and Hale (2007) for a detailed discussion of ADHD subtypes).

ADHD affects approximately 4 % of all school-aged children, essentially at least one student in every classroom (National Health Interview Survey, 2009; Polanczyk, Silva de Lima, Horta, Biederman, & Rhode, 2007). Often misconstrued as a behavior disorder, ADHD is a complex neurocognitive disorder including both neuropsychological and behavior difficulties across settings such as impairments in attention, hyperactivity, impulsivity, planning, organization, evaluation skills, and mood stability (e.g., Douglas, 2005; Skirrow, McLoughlin, Kuntsi, & Asherson, 2009). These difficulties may stem from deficits in the cognitive abilities (i.e., executive functioning) necessary for implementing goal-directed behavior and adapting that behavior to social and environmental demands and changes (e.g., Castellanos & Tannock, 2002; DeShazo, Lyman, & Klinger, 2002). Children with executive functioning deficits typically experience difficulties in planning, self-monitoring, and social problem-solving skills, as well as low frustration tolerance and poor vigilance in the face of difficult tasks (Reddy, Weissman, & Hale, 2013).

Comorbidity and Common Symptom Dimensions

The assessment and intervention process for ADHD is complicated by high rates of comorbidity and symptom overlap with other conditions (Reddy & Hale, 2007). For example, children are sometimes misdiagnosed with ADHD when they have a related childhood disorder (e.g., learning disabilities, language-based disorders, disruptive behavior disorders, anxiety, and depression) or condition (e.g., medical, family, environmental). Approximately 66 % of children with ADHD have at least one additional psychiatric diagnosis, with oppositional defiant disorder being the most common (Elia, Ambrosini, & Berrettini, 2008). However, the comorbidity rate for this population varies across disorder, gender, and age.

Between 25 and 70 % of youth with ADHD have been identified as having a specific learning disability (Kellner, Houghton, & Douglas, 2003; Reddy, Weissman, & Hale, 2013), reading disabilities appearing in 25–40 % of youth with ADHD inattentive or combined type (Reddy & Hale, 2007; Willcutt & Pennington, 2000). Comorbid symptoms of inattention appear more often with reading disabilities (Willcutt, Pennington, Olson, & DeFries, 2007). Children with concurrent ADHD and reading disabilities may appear confused because they struggle with basic oral comprehension skills and tend to have difficulties following verbal and/or written directions (Muir-Broaddus, Rosenstein, Medina, & Soderberg, 2002; Tannock & Brown, 2000). ADHD can be distinguished from reading disabilities by way of phonological awareness, verbal memory, automatic processing skills, and other areas of functioning (O'Connor & Jenkins, 1999; Tannock & Brown, 2000).

Approximately 65 % of children with ADHD also have written expression disorder, suggesting that writing is an even greater challenge for these children than reading (Kellner, Houghton, & Douglas, 2003; Mayes, Calhoun, & Crowell, 2000). Executive functions are necessary to plan, organize, monitor, evaluate, and revise written expression. Therefore, the deficits in executive functioning that might underlie ADHD could also contribute to a comorbid learning disability in written language. Evidence suggests that children with ADHD have poorer handwriting, spelling, vocabulary, lexical-semantic knowledge, grammar, and syntax than children without ADHD. Students with ADHD tend to produce short, disorganized writing samples with many errors (e.g., Mayes, Calhoun, & Crowell, 2000; Re, Pedron, & Cornoldi, 2007).

Auditory processing disorder is a language-based disorder found in 5–10 % of school-aged children, with 45–75 % of these children having comorbid ADHD (Riccio, Hynd, Cohen, Hall, & Molt, 1994; Tannock & Brown, 2000). ADHD and auditory processing disorder have many shared symptoms including inattentiveness, distractibility, listening problems, and difficulties following oral instructions (Katz & Tillery, 2004; Moore, Ferguson, Edmonson-Jones, Ratib, & Riley, 2010). Also, ADHD-related symptoms may resemble the symptoms of sensory processing disorder, including difficulty processing sensory input (e.g., visual, auditory, tactile, smell, textures, taste) in the classroom (Yochman, Shula, & Ornoy, 2004). Children with ADHD also display some parallel symptoms with autism spectrum disorders, such as clinical levels of inattention and response inhibition (e.g., Happe, Booth, Charlton, & Hughes, 2006; Holtmann, Bolte, & Poustka, 2005).

Comorbid disruptive behavior disorders (i.e., oppositional defiant, conduct disorders) occur in 30–60 % of children with ADHD hyperactive/impulsive or combined type (Kadesjö, Hägglöf, Kadesjö, & Gillberg, 2003). Youth with coexisting ADHD and oppositional defiant disorder experience higher rates of teacher conflict, school refusal, anxiety, and depression than youth with either ADHD or oppositional defiant disorder alone (Johnston & Mash, 2001).

Comorbid anxiety and/or depression is common in youth with ADHD. Anxiety is one of the most common mental health problems in all children and is found in 25–50 % of youth with ADHD (e.g., Bowen, Chavira, Bailey, Stein, & Stein, 2008). Surprisingly, research suggests that children presenting with ADHD and anxiety may experience lowered rates of school failure, attention problems, and social impairments. Children with comorbid ADHD and anxiety might also benefit more from psychosocial interventions than children presenting with only ADHD (National Alliance on Mental Illness, 2013). Approximately 21 % of children and adolescents living with ADHD also have depression (Elia, Ambrosini, & Berrettini, 2008). Symptoms typical of both ADHD and depression include irritability, low self-esteem, and poor concentration. However, depression has distinct symptoms including fatigue, feelings of hopelessness, diminished interest in activities, and recurrent thoughts of death or dying (American Psychiatric Association, 2013).

Biological factors, medical conditions, and familial and environmental factors frequently resemble common symptoms of ADHD (Cushman & Johnson, 2001). For example, clinical levels of inattention can manifest from at least 38 different sources including family genetics history, low birth weight, prenatal exposure to alcohol, smoking, drugs, lead poisoning, asthma, and/or allergies (Goodman & Poillion, 1992; Reddy & Hale, 2007). The extent of inattention or impulsivity has been linked to the complexity of social or academic task demands, inconsistent use of home and/or classroom behavioral techniques, maternal overuse of control strategies (e.g., harsh comments, vague directives, physical restraints, lack of affection and praise), low family cohesion, and poor interpersonal relationships (e.g., Johnston, Murray, Hinshaw, Pelham, & Hoza, 2002; Samudra & Cantwell, 1999).

Framework for Assessment

We recommend that practitioners use comprehensive assessments that include both neuropsychological and behavioral/emotional assessments for two purposes. First, a diagnosis should be confirmed or disconfirmed by carefully assessing ADHD symptoms, ruling out other possible causes for those symptoms, and assessing for any comorbid disorders and conditions. Second, assessment should assess neurocognitive and behavioral strengths and impairments to inform interventions within and across contexts. Because ADHD is, by definition, a neurocognitive disorder that is present across multiple domains of functioning, assessment data should be collected from multiple informants (e.g., parent, teacher) whenever possible. A thorough clinical interview should include reports from the child's most informed parent regarding medical, developmental, social and academic histories, as well as descriptions of the child's behavior, symptoms, and interests. Symptom dimensions of ADHD (i.e., inattention, hyperactivity, impulsivity) should be addressed, as should common comorbid disorders and conditions previously described. For an older child, the practitioner may also want to probe the child for any additional behavioral reports (e.g., anxiety, depression, relationships with adults, siblings, and/or peers). Generally, parent and teacher reports tend to be most accurate for externalizing behaviors, but the child may be able to provide the most accurate information regarding any internalizing problems that are not readily apparent to observers.

While interviews are useful for describing the behaviors exhibited by the child, it is imperative that concerns are assessed directly using classroom/school observations and indirectly by using behavioral rating scales. We recommend school observation be conducted during both structured learning (e.g., math, language, and gym) and unstructured learning periods (e.g., transitions between classes, lunch, recess) at school. Practitioners should collect data on the teachers' classroom instructional and behavioral management practices (Reddy, Fabiano, Barbarasch, & Dudek, 2012). Likewise, data should be collected on the child's ability to follow and complete teacher instructions *during learning opportunities* (individual and small group) and *across learning opportunities* in the classroom. Indirect behavioral assessments (i.e., broadband and narrowband rating scales) are available for parents, teachers, and children. Examples of broadband behavior measures are available for parents, teachers, and children (e.g., Behavior Assessment System for Children-2, Behavior Youth Inventory-II,) that can screen for overall levels of inattention, hyperactivity, impulsivity, oppositional/defiant behavior, anxiety, and depression. Additionally, narrowband behavior measures should be used to further assess specific symptoms across contexts (e.g., Behavior Rating Inventory of Executive Functioning Scale; Conners 3, Children's Depression Inventory 2, Revised Children's Manifest Anxiety Scale-2).

Interviews, behavioral samples, and rating scales are helpful for confirming ADHD criteria and screening for comorbid disorders. However, a comprehensive (reliable) ADHD assessment should examine the severity of neurocognitive deficits (working memory, sustained or divided attention, planning, academic skills) through the use of neuropsychological and achievement assessments. The assessment process should begin with tests of cognitive functioning (e.g., WISC-IV) to include verbal, nonverbal, perceptual, working memory, and processing speed. In relation to cognitive functioning, tests of academic achievement (e.g., WIAT-III, WJ III ACH, WRAT4) are warranted to assess the child's abilities (consistency and inconsistency) across cognitive and achievement dimensions. Since oral language skills can significantly influence all academic achievement, testing of oral language functioning is strongly warranted. Also, tests of written language (e.g., TOWL-4) that assess child's organization of thoughts into writing as well as his/her graphomotor abilities are needed.

Depending on the age of the child, a number of tests can be used to measure attention and executive functioning. Sustained attention is frequently measured using a continuous performance task (e.g., Conners' Continuous Performance Test-III, Pediatric Attention Disorders Diagnostic Screener for Children), and other measures assess for selective and divided attention as well as cognitive flexibility and inhibitory control (e.g., TEA-Ch, NEPSY-II, D-KEFS). In cases where neurocognitive impairment seems more severe, practitioners may wish to assess deleterious effects on other processes such as memory and learning (e.g., CVLT-C, WRAML-2), language (e.g., CELF-4), and/or phonological processing (e.g., CTOPP). Assessment approaches that inform diagnosis and individualize interventions are warranted.

Framework for Intervention

According to the National Institute of Mental Health (2013), promising interventions for ADHD focus on reducing symptoms and improving functioning. A multimodal intervention approach which individualizes medical, educational, behavioral, and psychological interventions/services is recommended by the National Alliance on Mental Illness (2013). For a comprehensive review of recommended interventions by child age, see American Academy of Pediatrics ADHD Clinical Practice Guideline (2011).

To build upon these recommendations, we conducted a comprehensive literature review (PsycINFO, ProQuest, Google Scholar) and hand searched for meta-analyses/reviews on ADHD interventions. Keywords used were ADHD interventions, treatments for ADHD, meta-analysis ADHD interventions or treatments, and attention deficit hyperactivity disorder interventions. Articles included were (1) published in a peer-reviewed journal and (2) reviewed cognitive or behavioral interventions for youth with ADHD. A total of 14 meta-analyses/reviews (published 1998–2012) from 12 journals (see references denoted with *) were found. Table 8.1 provides a synthesis of the promising intervention approaches from this literature.

Based on the extensive literature, a multimodal cognitive-behavioral intervention framework is warranted that addresses the varied and individualized needs of children with ADHD in school and home. Our intervention approach is broadly conceptualized in six areas: assessment, behavior modification, parent training, teacher assessment and training, skill building, and accommodations. A case example is provided to illustrate the implementation of these methods in schools.

Assessment Implications

A comprehensive assessment will provide a wealth of information that can inform diagnostic decisions and intervention plans tailored to the child's specific needs. Once an ADHD diagnosis is confirmed, an assessment can help practitioners identify specific behavioral targets for intervention within and across settings (e.g., following directions, hyperactivity, tasks engagement, academic skills). Behavioral targets should be assessed for intensity (frequency), severity, and delivery process. Attention to specific contextual factors such as setting (morning routine, structure class time, mealtime), task (cognitive) demands required of the child, adult behaviors, peer behaviors, and temporal influences are warranted. Assessment information can inform the need for psychiatric consultation in addition to cognitive-behavioral interventions. Second, the neuropsychological assessment will provide information about the breadth and severity of related neurocognitive dysfunctions. This information is often helpful in informing skill building strategies and necessary accommodations. Comorbid disorders and conditions may require additional targets (e.g., reading or writing fluency, oral language skills) and interventions (e.g., academic, medical, occupational therapy, speech/language therapy). Additionally, youth with more severe cognitive impairment may limit the choice for interventions.

Behavior Modification

Although specific implementation of behavior modification strategies differs across settings, the basic principles are the same. Adaptive and prosocial behaviors are reinforced, and maladaptive behaviors are ignored, redirected, or, in limited

Table 8.1 Promising treatment approaches for children and adolescents with ADHD[a]

Approach	Description	Results
Multimodal approach	Any combination of parent and teacher interventions/training including pharmacological treatment	Interventions are most successful when combined with stimulant medication, especially for school-aged children with severe impairments. Multimodal treatment has the greatest effect on social outcomes and as good an effect on behavioral outcomes as pharmacological treatment. In addition, parent and teacher acceptance is enhanced and necessary drug dose may be lowered. Multimodal treatment has little or no effect on academic functioning.
Contingency management/ behavioral interventions	Includes contingency management (reinforcement and punishment/antecedent and consequence based), clinical behavior therapy, self-management approaches, and intensive behavioral interventions	There is strong and consistent evidence that behavioral treatments are effective for reducing ADHD symptoms, including disruptive and off-task behaviors. Empirical studies have supported the efficacy of behavioral interventions. Behavioral interventions tend not to be as effective as medical treatment.
Academic interventions	School-based interventions including behavioral classroom management, psychoeducation, organizational skills intervention, strategy training, teacher-based behavioral training, task and instructional modification, and computer-assisted instruction	Findings indicate that academic interventions may be weaker than behavioral interventions but are potentially effective. Behavioral classroom management is a well-established, evidence-based treatment for ADHD. A variety of school-based interventions were associated with moderate to large improvements in academic and behavioral functioning. Behavioral effect sizes were similar and academic effect sizes were superior to those found for pharmacotherapy. The effects on educational and cognitive outcomes were greatest for educational interventions. Strategies that directly address the academic difficulties experienced by students with ADHD (e.g., task and instructional modification, strategy training) should be incorporated into a multimodal treatment approach to achieve educational success. For school-aged children with moderate impairments, there is some evidence to suggest that classroom behavioral interventions and group parent training may suffice as first-line treatment.
	Academic interventions may incorporate other types of approaches if school-based (e.g., behavioral, self-regulation)	

(continued)

Table 8.1 (continued)

Approach	Description	Results
Parent training	Includes parent-based behavioral intervention training, behavioral management strategies, contingency training, and parent tutoring Parent training may incorporate other types of approaches that parents were trained to provide (e.g., behavioral)	Parent training is the most appropriate intervention for preschoolers. For school-aged children with moderate impairments, there is some evidence that group parent training and classroom behavioral interventions may suffice as first-line treatment. Behavioral parent training is supported as a well-established, evidence-based treatment for children with ADHD.
Peer interventions	Includes peer-focused behavioral interventions, social skills building, peer mediation, peer tutoring, assistance, instruction, and feedback Peer interventions may incorporate other types of approaches, but the main focus is on utilizing peers to create improvements	Behavioral peer interventions are supported as evidence-based treatments for children with ADHD. Intensive, peer-focused behavioral interventions implemented within recreational settings are well established. Some promising interventions for addressing social relationship difficulties among students have been developed. Peer tutoring is effective in enhancing academic engagement and scholastic performance, especially in combination with other treatments.
Self-regulation interventions	The regulation of cognitions or behaviors through strategies such as self-monitoring and self-management These results are examined independently of other approaches that may incorporate self-regulation components (e.g., contingency management, CBT)	Effect sizes for on-task behavior, inappropriate behavior, and academic accuracy and productivity were large, with similar results across different types of self-regulation interventions. Self-regulation interventions are effective for children with ADHD.
Cognitive-behavioral techniques	Includes cognitive-behavioral techniques such as self-reinforcement and cognitive rehearsal to develop self-control, problem solving skills, social skills, and metacognitive thinking	School-based cognitive-behavioral therapy was associated with improvements in the academic and behavioral functioning of students with ADHD. It is more effective to utilize cognitive-behavioral treatment along with medicine. Moderate mean weighted effect sizes were shown to improve social and behavioral outcomes, but multimodal and pharmacological treatment was more effective. Significant effects have been reported and some promise is shown for cognitive-behavioral treatment of ADHD.

Working memory training	The use of computerized programs to train working memory skills	Memory training programs appear to produce reliable short-term improvements in working memory skills that are not generalizable. For verbal working memory, limited evidence suggests that these effects might be maintained. In the absence of more general effects on cognitive performance or measures of scholastic attainment, working memory procedures should not be recommended as suitable for treating ADHD, although they may show promise in the future.
Cognitive training	Direct skills training of cognitive skills and remediation of deficiencies in thinking or cognitive processes	Studies have demonstrated significant effects for the cognitive treatment of ADHD, and some promise is shown across a larger age range.
Neural-based training	Including neurofeedback and maintaining effort and focus through metacognitive strategies	Studies have demonstrated significant effects, and promise is shown across a larger age range.

[a]Results are synthesized from 14 published reviews/meta-analyses from 1998 to 2012
Asterisk denotes review article in the reference section

circumstances, punished. Clear commands and cues are given to the child in order to form explicit expectations for appropriate behavior so she/he has an alternative option to the current behaviors that are deemed inappropriate. Research has indicated that children with ADHD should be given no more than one- or two-step clear directives (Reddy, Fabiano, Barbarasch, & Dudek, 2012; Reddy & Dudek, 2014). Contingencies are also managed in such a way that the child has many opportunities for success.

Several approaches are commonly used to accomplish the goals of behavior modification. One common strategy is to use praise (i.e., specific labeled immediate statements) as reinforcement for positive behaviors. Since teachers and parents often heavily rely on behavioral corrective feedback (pointing out what the child is doing wrong), it is imperative they are taught to (1) structure the environment to allow for frequent observation of the child and (2) "catch the child being good" followed by providing specific (labeled) praise immediately after appropriate behavior is observed. It is typically recommended that the child be praised 3–5 times for every one corrective command that is given in order to mitigate the adult and child frustration that occurs from constant corrective feedback. Reinforcement is also commonly given externally. Token economies are frequently used in which children earn points, stars, or stickers for meeting goals related to the performance of clearly specified target behaviors (e.g., homework completion, remaining quietly in seat for a specified period of time, doing specific chores). Children are typically given a menu of privileges that are associated with different point values and time periods, and they are allowed to choose a reward for which they earned enough points.

Reinforcement for positive behaviors is the primary approach that is recommended for behavior modification for ADHD. Punishment is generally not recommended because it does not usually produce long-lasting results, and may result in unintended consequences. However, there are situations in which punishment is warranted (e.g., child is actively engaged in inappropriate behavior, and it is necessary to stop it immediately). In these cases, time-out (focus on regaining positive self-control) may be needed. This strategy generally consists of the child spending a minimum specified amount of time in an isolated area where she/he is unable to interact with desired stimuli such as other people or objects (i.e., toys) until she/he has regained self-control.

The strategies outlined above are useful in many situations, but as noted, their implementation may look different across and within settings. For example, each parent may deal with different challenges during morning routines, homework, and bedtime routines. Similarly, different teachers may deal with varying challenges. Therefore, behavior modifications must be tailored to specific targets, contexts, and time periods. Furthermore, collaboration between key stakeholders (parents, teachers) within and between settings is urged for the child to fully benefit from a multimodal intervention.

Parent Training

A number of training programs have been developed over the past few decades for parents of children with ADHD. One such program is a cognitive-behavioral approach detailed by Anastopoulos and Farley (2003). In this approach, parent training typically begins with psychoeducation. This includes teaching parents about ADHD symptoms and associated behaviors, as well as a discussion about the implications of the diagnosis and the expectations that parents should have of their children. It can also include a discussion of child characteristics (e.g., demographics, temperament), parent characteristics (e.g., personality, parenting styles), fit between child and parent characteristics, and the impact of stress on the child and family. Psychoeducation is then followed by teaching of parent skills. Parents are taught how to give unambiguous 1- and 2-step directives and to avoid directives that invite compliance issues. They are also taught how to attend to and reinforce adaptive behaviors and to ignore maladaptive behaviors. Training is provided in the proper use of time-out when necessary.

Training may also focus on parents identifying their thoughts *and* behaviors during times when their child behavior is difficult or escalating. Anger and stress strategies can be identified and discussed for use in specific contexts. Finally, parents are taught how to engage their child in explicit problem-solving strategies.

Behavioral progress in the home is often assessed through the use of daily behavioral charts which require specific parent training on design, implementation, and monitoring. Parents of children with ADHD are often overwhelmed by a number of different behaviors that they consider problematic. However, they are encouraged to choose only a few (i.e., 2 to 3) targets for behavior modification. Behaviors should be as specific and concrete as possible so the child knows exactly what she/he needs to do to earn a point (e.g., brushed teeth by 7:15 am). A menu of rewards should also be constructed that involves a combination of short-term and longer-term goals. For example, daily rewards should consist of basic privileges that the child enjoys (e.g., 1 h of TV time after homework; 15 min of parent positive attention). Daily rewards can be further bridged with weekly rewards (relatively inexpensive bonus rewards) for obtaining a predetermined number of points for the week. Longer-term rewards can include special toys or trips to special places (e.g., Chuck E. Cheese, amusement park); however, it is strongly recommended that daily rewards be maintained to help the child to sustain efforts. Review of daily and weekly goal attainment through the use of behavior charts helps monitor progress, reevaluate targets, and revise reinforcements to sustain behavioral goals.

Teacher Assessment and Training

Teacher classroom instructional and behavioral management practices influence student learning and behavior. Students with ADHD often require changes in teacher's classroom-wide and student-specific practices/approaches. Teacher training with teacher formative assessment (visual performance feedback) can significantly improve educators' classroom practices related to student outcomes (Reddy, Fabiano, Barbarasch, & Dudek, 2012; Reddy & Dudek, 2014). The Classroom Strategies Scale (CSS) is a multisource, multi-method approach for identifying and monitoring teachers' usage of empirically supported instructional and behavioral management strategies (Reddy, Fabiano, Dudek, & Hsu, 2013a). The CSS was developed based on the effective teaching literature and principles from the response-to-intervention framework. The CSS generates scores that assess use of evidence-based practices, identify practice goals, and monitor progress toward practice goals following teacher training. The CSS Observer Form includes three parts centered on classroom observation: Part 1 Strategy Counts, Part 2 Instructional and Behavioral Management Strategies Scales, and Part 3 Classroom Checklist. The CSS Teacher Form includes two parts: Part 1 Instructional and Behavioral Management Strategies Scales and Part 2 Classroom Checklist. The Observer and Teacher Forms generate scores that can be used to enhance collaboration and communication among consultants (observers) and teacher to improve teacher practices and student learning and behavior (Reddy & Dudek, 2014). The CSS Strategy Counts include eight teacher strategies: (1) concept summaries, (2) academic response opportunities, (3) clear 1- to 2-step directives, (4) vague directives, (5) praise statements for academic performance, (6) praise for appropriate behavior, (7) academic corrective feedback, and (8) behavioral corrective feedback. The observer is to tally the number of times each behavior is observed in a specific lesson. For the Strategy Rating Scales, Instructional Scales (28 items) and Behavioral Management Scales (26 items), observers and teachers are asked to rate strategies/ items on a 7-point Likert scale on how often the teacher used each strategy (*Frequency Rating Scale*) and how often the teacher should have used each strategy (*Recommended Frequency Rating Scale*) in the lesson observed. The Classroom Checklist assesses the presence of specific classroom structures and resources and is completed by the observer and teacher after the completion of the Strategy Rating Scales. The CSS has evidence of content, construct, reliability, and validity (e.g., Reddy, Fabiano, Dudek, & Hsu, 2013a, 2013b, 2013c).

Using behavioral consultation, the CSS can be used to inform teacher practice targets and monitor progress toward targets and refine approaches for specific classroom-wide and ADHD student-specific needs. Likewise, teacher formative assessment and training guided by the CSS can be further enhanced with the use of a Daily Report Card (DRC) system employed by teachers and parents (Volpe & Fabiano, 2013; http://casgroup.fiu.edu/CCF/pages.php?id=1401. For a detailed case example using the CSS and DRC systems for students with ADHD, see Reddy, Fabiano, Barbarasch, & Dudek, 2012; Reddy & Dudek, 2014.)

Skill Building

While making clear and concise commands is an important way for children to understand what behaviors are expected of them, it is not sufficient in cases where the desired behaviors are skills that have not been developed as part of the child's repertoire. In these instances, skill building (self-regulated learning) strategies are an important component of intervention for ADHD (Reddy, Newman, & Verdesco, in press). Metacognitive skills can be taught and practiced in order to help the child "self-talk" his/her way through the steps to achieving a goal or solving a problem (see section "Stress-Inoculation Training (SIT) per Meichenbaum" in Chap. 12). This can help children with ADHD to slow down and think through a strategy before acting. Social skills may also be an important part of treatment for certain children with ADHD. Similar to other skill building exercises, social skills training groups help children to learn and practice effective steps toward getting along with others and forming and maintaining friendships. Peer and adult modeling during group training allow for repeated exposures to desired behaviors and are potentially effective ways of teaching these skills (Reddy, 2012). A specific type of peer modeling noted above that has shown some success is peer tutoring (see Table 8.1). Children with ADHD may be paired with other children of the same or slightly older age who have recently mastered academic skills with which the child is currently struggling. This provides the ADHD child with the opportunity for successful peer interactions as well as the opportunity to have problem-solving and learning strategies modeled by peers.

Accommodations

The flip side of skill building is that the child with ADHD may demonstrate certain limitations and/or delays that make it more difficult for him/her to learn skills than the typical child. Schools offer a variety of accommodations that have been shown to improve opportunities for success. Examples may include extra time (specified) on tests, fewer homework problems on page (specified), and/or modified test/homework instructions (e.g., simplified directives) or settings (e.g., a separate classroom to reduce distractions by other children). Next, a de-identified case study is presented using the proposed intervention framework.

Case Example

John is a 7-year-old Caucasian male in a 2nd grade general education classroom. His teacher is concerned because he is often disruptive in class. He frequently is out of his seat, talks to his peers, inconsistently completes his assignments, and appears to have difficulties understanding lessons. John's parents have observed that he is easily frustrated with his homework, distracted and inattentive when getting ready for school in the morning, struggling following directions, and tantruming on occasion when limits are set. His parents sought a comprehensive evaluation from a licensed psychologist. Based on the evaluation results, John was diagnosed with ADHD combined type exhibiting moderate deficits in attention, working memory, and executive functioning. It was recommended that John receive behavior therapy and be considered for an accommodation plan in school. A medication consult was noted if initial steps did not result in improvements.

John's parents sought behavior therapy from a licensed psychologist in the community. They reported that John is a sweet and loving boy, but that it is difficult to keep him on task and following directions. They often became frustrated and avoided dealing with his misbehavior because it became "too tiring to keep trying," eventually tending yell at him and saying things they regret. After reading John's assessment report and gathering information from his parents, it was determined that behavior modification through parent training would be appropriate. The goals were to help John's parents to understand their son's strengths and limitations, to clarify their expectations for themselves as parents and for John, and to implement a consistent behavior plan emphasizing particular target behaviors, reinforcement for performing those behaviors, and consequences for noncompliance and inappropriate behaviors.

The assessment report also went to John's school psychologist who evaluated him and arranged for an accommodation plan. The school psychologist also met with his teacher to discuss his needs. Although this teacher has had students with behavior problems in her classroom, she has never received formal training on effective behavioral strategies for these behaviors. To that end, she requested behavioral consultation with the school psychologist. The initial phase of consultation was focused on "fine-tuning" classroom instructional and behavioral management strategies (using the CSS).

Parent training consisted of 8 weekly 45-min sessions with John's parents in an out-of-school setting. Teacher consultation consisted of 30-min weekly meetings for 4 weeks. Both the licensed psychologist and school psychologist had John's parents sign authorizations to release information for the purpose of collaborative intervention, and they worked closely with the teacher and parents to ensure that they were working synergistically.

Teacher Training

Session 1

The consultant and teacher discussed her general classroom approaches to teaching and classroom management. The teacher and school psychologist/consultant reviewed and discussed the eight teacher strategies measured by the CSS. Initial plans for practice (strategy) goals were discussed. The teacher originally chose to work on corrective feedback for both academic performance and behavior (i.e., specific feedback on what was wrong with the child's academic response or what was inappropriate with the child's behavior). However, after further discussion, the consultant and teacher agreed to also work on increasing her use of academic and behavior praise statements. The teacher acknowledged that her use of praise for appropriate behavior and perhaps academic performance could be improved, especially for John. Thus, the identified strategy goals were (1) praise statements for academic performance (or effort), (2) corrective feedback for academic performance, (3) praise statements for appropriate behavior, and (4) corrective feedback for inappropriate behavior. The meeting concluded with the school psychologist arranging times to observe two different lessons in the classroom.

Session 2

The initial four strategy goals were confirmed. The consultant complimented the teacher on two lessons that were observed. The consultant and teacher first briefly reviewed the frequency in which she used the eight CSS strategies. Discussion then focused on the four identified strategy goals with particular emphasis on the two instructional goals. The objective was to establish a practical plan to build upon the teacher's current approaches, as well as define and operationalize the two target instructional strategies for improved implementation. For praise and corrective feedback for academic performance, it was observed that the teacher provided students with academic feedback (praise or corrective feedback) in about half of the opportunities she had to do so, which were numerous. It was noted that use of academic response opportunities was an area of strength for her.

The consultant/school psychologist suggested that the teacher increase the rate of praise and corrective feedback for academic performance (or effort) to approximate the number of times academic response opportunities were given. The teacher agreed with this goal. The consultant provided suggestions making corrective feedback a positive learning experience for students rather than a negative affirmation of poor performance. It was suggested that the teacher specifically explain what was incorrect about the students' responses. Because the teacher used concept summaries at the beginning of the lesson, it was suggested that the teacher try to increase summarizing concepts, facts, and instructional steps throughout the lesson to enhance student organization and recall of lesson content.

Session 3

The consultant and teacher briefly reviewed the frequency in which she used the CSS eight strategies (visual performance feedback). The four identified strategy goals were reviewed with particular emphasis on the two behavioral management goals. The teacher was praised for her efforts to improve her use of the two instructional goals. Similar to session 2, the goal for this session was to establish a plan to build upon the teacher's current approaches, as well as define and operationalize the two target behavioral management strategies for improved implementation. Although the teacher used behavioral corrective feedback, her feedback was somewhat vague and did not adequately specify (label) the inappropriate behavior. The consultant and teacher worked on how to deliver more specific corrective feedback and redirect John when behaving inappropriately. Of significant note, the teacher was observed using almost no behavioral praise during the lessons.

Further discussion revealed that the teacher struggled to separate academic and behavioral praise, as she saw behavioral praise as praising students for what they "should be doing." The consultant and the teacher discussed the differences between each type of praise and the benefits of each, especially for students with special needs like John. It pointed out that praising students for behaving appropriately increases their likelihood of engaging in more prosocial behavior while subsequently decreasing student inappropriate behavior and the need for corrective feedback. Implementation was strengthened by providing strategies to help remind the teacher to use behavioral praise (i.e., 10 pennies in a pocket, moving one penny from the left to right pocket after giving specific praise; taping a "p" on the front board and back windows). The teacher agreed to incorporate more praise strategies. While clear one- to two-step directives were not one of the teacher's goals, it was noted that she often made requests in the form of questions (i.e., favors; "Can you please clean up for me?") rather than directives (declarative statements). It was pointed out that the use of one- or two-step directives (declarative statements) will result in improved child follow-through.

Session 4

The teacher's progress on the eight teacher strategies and in particular the four practice goals was reviewed. She was commended for her improvements, noting strong efforts to use labeled praise statements during literacy and greater specificity in behavioral corrective feedback. Likewise, improvements in the teacher's use of praise statements and corrective feedback for academic performance were discussed.

While the teacher's use of academic response opportunities remained constant, the overall quality of her academic response opportunities improved as she asked students questions that fostered detailed answers and explanations on how they arrived at answers. Increases in the use of concept summaries were also observed. The teacher noted that the increased use of praise on her part appeared to improve the overall classroom climate and, consequently, she found herself using behavioral corrective feedback less often. She reported reprimanding John less and felt her relationship with John was beginning to improve. Overall, the teacher concluded that using the strategies increased student engagement.

Skills Training and Accommodations

John's assessment indicated a moderate level of executive dysfunction in comparison to his age peers that included difficulty finding his school supplies and being seemingly less able to attend to tasks at hand, especially when there are multiple things going on at once. The school psychologist met with John to help him organize his school supplies by making the organization explicit so he could understand it. However, she was concerned that his attentional difficulties were impacting his performance on assignments and tests during class, and so she worked with his teacher to make instructions simple, to provide extra time if needed, and to monitor his academic progress to determine whether he would benefit from shortened assignments. The school psychologist was hesitant to recommend removing him from the classroom to avoid distractions during assignments, as she did not want him to feel different from his classmates.

Parent Training

Session 1

The licensed psychologist discussed the general presentation of ADHD, its prevalence, and associated problems. He encouraged John's parents to depersonalize his symptoms by viewing them as separate from who he is, treating them as limitations that everyone has to take responsibility for rather than willful disobedience, and form an alliance with John in treating his symptoms. John's father acknowledged that he did tend to view John's misbehaviors as intentional, and both parents agreed to discuss this alternative conceptualization over the next week. Basic principles of behavior management were then discussed (as described above).

Session 2

John's parents expressed concern about several more instances of misbehavior throughout the past week; they worked to interpret John's actions as symptoms of a disorder. The psychologist underscored the importance of positive parent-child interactions. He recommended arranging 30-min play sessions with each parent (independently) twice a week. The parents were told not to instruct John on how to play but just to observe and participate in his play, to praise his efforts (catch him being good), and to ignore undesirable behaviors. Praise was described as being similar to depositing money in a bank account. That is, one earns frequent praise deposits—there is plenty to offset the inevitable withdrawals (corrective feedback) that occur.

Session 3

John's parents indicated they found it somewhat difficult to find the time to set aside 30-min play sessions, but they found that John responded positively to these sessions. The licensed psychologist recommended continuing the play sessions and that they also begin to use praise outside of these sessions whenever possible. They were also taught to issue simple directives that John is likely to comply with and to use praise immediately after compliance. The directives should be simple statements rather than questions, and adults should check for understanding by having John repeat the request. They chose to start with directives such as "John, please take off your shoes" and "please wash your hands and then sit down at the table."

Sessions 4–5

John's parents were beginning to feel comfortable making directives and praising John for his behaviors but continued to be concerned with compliance with basic routines. In session 4, the psychologist decided to help them implement a token economy. He encouraged them to make a list of the behaviors they would like him to perform as well as the problem behaviors they would like to extinguish. Their list initially consisted of ten items; they were asked them to prioritize their list and select the three most important behaviors to focus on. They chose brushing teeth in the morning, completing homework after school, and putting toys away after playing with them. They were encouraged to be as specific as is necessary to complete the task appropriately. They decided homework and cleaning up did not require a specific time frame, but that his teeth had to be brushed by a 7:45 am if he was going to make it to school on time. John was then to be awarded one sticker for meeting each of these target behaviors each day.

The parents were asked to make a tentative menu of rewards that John could choose from if he earned all his points in a day, as well as larger rewards for earning at least 12 stickers (out of a possible 15) over the course of a week, and even larger prizes for longer-term goals. Prior to completing this task, the psychologist explained the distinction between rights and privileges. Children take many things for granted (e.g., television time, play time, etc.) that are actually privileges that can be earned. His parents decided to offer one hour of TV time, or 30 min of video game or Internet time as daily rewards; trips to the mini-golf course, the arcade, or the movies as weekly rewards; and a trip to the nearest amusement or water park as long-term rewards.

In session 5, key elements were reviewed and progress discussed. John's parents brought their first week's behavior chart to session for review. John seemed to enjoy earning the stickers, and he was motivated to perform the tasks. He earned 13 out of

15 stickers for the week. Because he did not find the weekly rewards particularly motivating, other options were discussed with his parents. They indicated that John had recently become more interested in outdoor activities and that he enjoyed going on walks through nearby nature trails. They decided to substitute that activity for the movies. They also discussed ways of modifying target behaviors once he is consistently earning all his stickers.

Sessions 6–7

The next two sessions were dedicated to the incorporation of punishment into the behavioral plan. The psychologist explained that punishment should be used sparingly and tends to be as less effective than reinforcement. The removal of previously earned stickers as an option for dealing with noncompliance was discussed but warned the parents that frequent use of this strategy (response costs) could result in the child being in "debt," which would be highly unmotivating.

The use of time-out was described. The parents were told that when John throws a tantrum in response to a directive, he can be placed in time-out. They were taught that John should spend a minimum amount of time in time-out and that even after that time, John should not be approached unless he is quiet. The minimum duration for time-out should be determined by how long John can typically sit quietly. For example, if John has trouble sitting quietly for more than 5 min, time-out should be at least 3 min of silence, but not more, because he might eventually have difficulty meeting that target no matter how hard he tries. Finally, his parents were instructed to repeat the directive upon letting John out of time-out. The implementation of these strategies was practiced within session 6.

Session 7 consisted of a review of time-out. The parents were frustrated because the one time they attempted to implement time-out during the previous week, John kept screaming until they felt like they had to let him out. It was discussed with them that children often "up the ante" when they are not getting away with the same behavior did previously and that giving in just teaches the child that he or she can "win" by behaving worse. He attempted to reassure them that with practice, they would be able to implement time-out more effectively.

Session 8

The last session focused on anticipating problems and preparing for them. For example, the psychologist discussed the importance of anticipating when behavior problems are likely to arise in public when time-out is not an option. He suggested being very clear with John about expectations, positive reinforcement, and negative consequences for noncompliance. He discussed with them the importance of adherence to the behavioral program once parent training sessions are over. The parents were reassured they had the necessary skills to manage John's behavior effectively, the skills were reviewed and they were reminded that skills would improve with practice. Follow-up sessions were made available.

Conclusion

This chapter provides an overview of ADHD and frameworks for assessment and intervention planning. Effective interventions for ADHD typically involve implementing behavior management strategies in the home and school. Training in executive/metacognitive skills and/or social skills and developing school accommodations can be included. A medication consult may be indicated if symptoms are severe. Finally, parents *and* teachers are crucial to success intervention for this population. Strategies that effectively engage, train, and sustain stakeholders' implementation of evidence-based interventions are paramount for promoting social, behavioral, and academic success for youth with ADHD.

Acknowledgments The research reported here was supported by the Institute of Education Sciences, U.S. Department of Education, through Grant R305A080337 to Rutgers University. The opinions expressed are those of the authors and do not represent views of the Institute or the U.S. Department of Education.

References

American Psychiatric Association. (2013). *Diagnostic and statistical manual of mental disorders* (5th ed.). Washington, DC: American Psychiatric Association.

Anastopoulos, A. D., & Farley, S. E. (2003). *A cognitive-behavioral training program for parents of children with attention-deficit/ hyperactivity disorder. Evidence-based psychotherapies for children and adolescents*, 187–203. New York, NY: Guilford Press.

Bowen, R., Chavira, D., Bailey, K., Stein, M., & Stein, M. (2008). Nature of anxiety comorbid with attention deficit hyperactivity disorder in children from a pediatric primary care setting. *Psychiatry Research, 157*(1), 201–209. doi:10.1016/j.psychres.2004.12.015.

*Brown, R. T., Amler, R. W., Freeman, W. S., Perrin, J. M., Stein, M. T., Feldman, H. M., Pierce, K., & Wolraich, M. L. (2005). Treatment of attention-deficit/hyperactivity disorder: Overview of the evidence. *Pediatrics, 115*(6), e749–e757. Retrieved from http://pediatrics.aappublica-tions.org/content/115/6/e749.full

Castellanos, X., & Tannock, R. (2002). Neuroscience of attention-deficit/hyperactivity disorder: The search for endophenotypes. *Nature Reviews Neuroscience, 3*, 617–628. doi:10.1038/nrn896.

Center for Disease Control and Prevention. (2009). National Health Interview Survey. Retrieved from www.cdc.gov/nchs/nhis.htm

Cushman, T. P., & Johnson, T. B. (2001). Understanding 'inattention' in children and adolescents. *Ethical Human Sciences and Services, 3*(2), 107–125.

DeShazo, T., Lyman, R. D., & Klinger, L. G. (2002). Academic underachievement and attention-deficit/hyperactivity disorder: The negative impact of symptom severity on school performance. *Journal of School Psychology, 40*(3), 259–283. doi:10.1016/S0022-4405(02)00100-0.

Douglas, V. I. (2005). Cognitive deficits in children with attention deficit hyperactivity disorder: A long term follow-up. *Canadian Psychology, 46*(1), 23–31.

*DuPaul, G. J., & Eckert, T. L. (1998). Academic interventions for students with attention-deficit/hyperactivity disorder: A review of the literature. *Reading & writing quarterly: Overcoming learning difficulties, 14*(1). Retrieved from http://www.tandfonline.com/doi/pdf/10.1080/1057356980140104

*DuPaul, G. J., Eckert, T. L., & Vilardo, B. (2012). The effects of school-based interventions for attention deficit hyperactivity disorder: A meta-analysis. *School Psychology Review, 41*(4), 387–412.

*DuPaul, G. J., & Weyandt, L. L. (2006). School-based intervention for children with attention deficit hyperactivity disorder: Effects on academic, social, and behavioural functioning. *International Journal of Disability, Development, and Education, 53*(2). Retrieved from http://www.tandfonline.com. doi:10.1080/10349120600716141.

Elia, J., Ambrosini, P., & Berrettini, W. (2008). ADHD characteristics: I. Concurrent comorbidity patterns in children & adolescents. *Child and Adolescent Psychiatry and Mental Health, 2*(1), 2–15.

*Fabiano, G. A., Pelham, W. E., Coles, E. L., Gnagy, E. M., Chronis-Tuscano, A., & O'Connor, B. C. (2009). A meta-analysis for behavior treatments for attention-deficit/hyperactivity disorder. *Clinical Psychology Review, 29*(2), 129–140. doi:10.1016/j.cpr.2008.11.001.

Goodman, G., & Poillion, M. J. (1992). ADD: Acronym for any dysfunction or difficulty. *Journal of Special Education, 26*(1), 37–56. doi:10.1177/002246699202600103.

Happe, F., Booth, R., Charlton, R., & Huges, C. (2006). Executive function deficits in autism spectrum disorders and attention-deficit/hyperactivity disorder: Examining profiles across domains and ages. *Brain and Cognition, 61*(1), 25–39. doi:10.1016/j.bandc.2006.03.004.

Holtmann, M., Bolte, S., & Poustka, F. (2005). ADHD, Asperger syndrome, and high functioning autism. *Journal of the American Academy of Child and Adolescent Psychiatry, 44*(11), 1101. doi:10.1097/01.chi.0000177322.57931.2a.

Johnston, C., & Mash, E. J. (2001). Families of children with ADHD: Review and recommendations for future research. *Clinical Child and Family Psychology Review, 4*(3), 183–207. doi:10.1023/A:1017592030434.

Johnston, C., Murray, C., Hinshaw, S. P., Pelham, W. E., & Hoza, B. (2002). Responsiveness in interactions of mothers and sons with ADHD: Relations to maternal and child characteristics. *Journal of Abnormal Child Psychology, 30*(1), 77–88. doi:10.1023/A:1014235200174.

Kadesjö, C., Hägglöf, B., Kadesjö, B., & Gillberg, C. (2003) Attention-deficit-hyperactivity disorder with and without oppositional defiant disorder in 3- to 7-year-old children. *Child and Adolescent Psychiatry, 45*(10). doi:10.1017/S0012162203001282.

Katz, J., & Tillery, K. (2004). Central auditory processing. In L. Verhoeven & H. van Balkom (Eds.), *Classification of developmental language disorders: Theoretical issues and clinical implications* (pp. 191–208). Mahwah, NJ: Lawrence Erlbaum Associates.

Kellner, R., Houghton, S., & Douglas, G. (2003). Peer-related personal experiences of children with attention-deficit/hyperactivity with and without comorbid learning disabilities. *International Journal of Disability, Development and Education, 50*(2), 119–136. doi:10.1080/1034912032000089639.

Kent, K. M., Pelham, W. E., Molina, B. S. G., Sibley, M. H., Waschbusch, D. A., Yu, J., et al. (2011). The academic experience of male high school students with ADHD. *Journal of Abnormal Child Psychology, 39*, 451–462. doi:10.1007/s10802-010-9472-4.

Kessler, R. C., Adler, L. A., Barkley, R., Biederman, J., Conners, C. K., Faraone, S. V., et al. (2005). Patterns and predictors of attention-deficit/hyperactivity disorder persistence into adulthood: Results from the national comorbidity survey replication. *Biological Psychiatry, 57*(11), 1442–1451. doi:10.1016/j.biopsych.2005.04.001.

Mayes, S. D., Calhoun, S. L., & Crowell, E. W. (2000). Learning disabilities and ADHD: Overlapping spectrum disorders. *Journal of Learning Disabilities, 30*(5), 417–424. doi:10.1177/002221940003300502.

*Melby-Lervag, M., & Hulme, C. (2012). Is working memory training effective? A meta-analytic review. *Developmental Psychology*. Advance online publication. doi: 10.1037/a0028228.

Moore, D. R., Ferguson, M. A., Edmondson-Jones, A. M., Ratib, S., & Riley, A. (2010). Nature of auditory processing disorder in children. *Pediatrics, 126*(2), 382–390. doi:10.1542/peds.2009-2826.

Muir-Broaddus, J. E., Rosenstein, L. D., Medina, D. E., & Soderberg, C. (2002). Neuropsychological test performance of children with ADHD relative to test norms and parent behavioral ratings. *Archives of Clinical Neuropsychology, 17*(7), 671–689. doi:10.1093/arclin/17.7.671.

National Alliance on Mental Illness. (2013). About ADHD. Retrieved, from http://www.nami.org/Template.cfm?Section=ADHD&Template=/ContentManagement/ContentDisplay.cfm&ContentID=105610

O'Connor, R. E., & Jenkins, J. R. (1999). Prediction of reading disabilities in kindergarten and first grade. *Scientific Studies of Reading, 3*(2), 159–197. doi:10.1207/s1532799xssr0302_4.

*Pelham, W. E., & Fabiano, G. A. (2008). Evidence-based psychosocial treatments for attention-deficit/hyperactivity disorder. *Journal of Clinical Child and Adolescent Psychology, 37*(1). Retrieved from http://www.tandfonline.com, doi:10.1080/15374410701818681.

*Pelham, W. E., Wheeler, T., & Chronis, A. (1998). Empirically supported psychosocial treatments for attention deficit hyperactivity disorder. *Journal of Clinical Child Psychology, 27*(2), 190–205. doi:10.1207/s15374424jccp2702_6.

Polanczyk, G., Silva de Lima, M., Horta, B. L., Biederman, J., & Rohde, L. A. (2007). The worldwide prevalence of ADHD: A systematic review and metaregression analysis. *American Journal of Psychiatry, 164*(6), 942–948. doi:10.1176/appi.ajp.164.6.942.

*Purdie, N., Hattie, J., & Carroll, A. (2002). A review of the research on interventions for attention deficit hyperactivity disorder: What works best? *Review of Educational Research, 72*(61). Retrieved from http://rer.sagepub.com/content/72/1/61.full.pdf.html.

Re, A. M., Pedron, M., & Cornoldi, C. (2007). Expressive writing difficulties in children described as exhibiting ADHD symptoms. *Journal of Learning Disabilities, 40*(3), 244–255. doi:10.1177/00222194070400030501.

Reddy, L. A. (2012). *Group play interventions for children: Strategies for teaching prosocial skills*. Washington, DC: American Psychological Association Press. doi:10.1037/13093-001.

Reddy, L., Fabiano, G., Barbarasch, B., & Dudek, C. (2012). Behavior management of students with attention-deficit/hyperactivity disorders using teacher and student progress monitoring. In L. M. Crothers & J. B. Kolbert (Eds.), *Understanding and managing behaviors of children with psychological disorders: A reference for classroom teachers*. New York: Continuum International Publishing Group, Inc.

Reddy, L.A., & Dudek, C. (2014). Teacher progress monitoring of instructional and behavioral management practices: An evidence-based approach to improving classroom practices. *International Journal of School and Educational Psychology, 2*, 71–84.

Reddy, L.A., Fabiano, G. A., Dudek, C. M., & Hsu, L. (2013a). Development and construct validity of the classroom srategies scale. special series: Assessment of general education teachers' tier 1 classroom practices: Current science and practice. *School Psychology Quarterly. 28*, 317–341.

Reddy, L.A., Fabiano, G. A., Dudek, C. M., & Hsu, L. (2013b). Predictive validity of the Classroom Strategies Scale-Observer Form on statewide testing scores. *School Psychology Quarterly. 28*, 301–316.

Reddy, L.A., Fabiano, G. A., Dudek, C. M., & Hsu, L. (2013c). Instructional and behavioral management practices implemented by elementary general education teachers. *Journal of School Psychology. 51*(6), 683–700.

Reddy, L. A., & Hale, J. (2007). Inattentiveness. In A. R. Eisen (Ed.), *Treating childhood behavioral and emotional problems: A step-by-step evidence-based approach* (pp. 156–211). New York: Guilford Publications, Inc.

Reddy, L. A., Weissman, A., & Hale, J. B. (2013). Integration of neuropsychological assessment and clinical intervention for youth with ADHD. In L. A. Reddy, A. Weissman, & J. B. Hale (Eds.), Neuropsychological assessment and intervention for emotional and behavior disordered youth A step-by-step evidence-based approach. Washington DC: American Psychological Association Press.

Reddy, L. A., Newman, E., & Verdesco, A. (in press). Self-regulated learning interventions and students with ADHD. In T. Cleary (Ed.), *Self-regulated learning interventions with at-risk populations: Academic, mental health, and contextual considerations*. Washington, DC: American Psychological Association Press.

*Reid, R., Trout, A. L., & Schartz, M. (2005). Self-regulation interventions for children with attention deficit/hyperactivity disorder. *Exceptional Children, 71*(4), 361–377.

Riccio, C. A., Hynd, G. W., Cohen, M. J., Hall, J., & Molt, L. (1994). Comorbidity of central auditory processing disorder and attention-deficit hyperactivity disorder. *Journal of the American Academy of Child and Adolescent Psychiatry, 33*(6), 849–857. doi:10.1097/00004583-199407000-00011.

Samudra, K., & Cantwell, D. P. (1999). Risk factors for attention-deficit/hyperactivity disorder. In H. C. Quay & A. E. Hogan (Eds.), *Handbook of disruptive behavior disorders* (pp. 199–220). New York: Kluwer Academic/Plenum Publishers.

Skirrow, C., McLoughlin, G., Kuntsi, J., & Asherson, P. (2009). Behavioral, neurocognitive and treatment overlap between attention-deficit/hyperactivity disorder and mood instability. *Expert Review of Neurotherapeutics, 9*(4), 489–503.

Subcommittee on Attention-Deficit/Hyperactivity Disorder, Steering Committee on Quality Improvement and Management. (2011). ADHD: Clinical practice guideline for the diagnosis, evaluation, and treatment of attention-deficit/hyperactivity disorder in children and adolescents. *Pediatrics, 128*(5), 1–16. doi:10.1542/peds. 2011-2654.

Tannock, R., & Brown, T. E. (2000). Attention-deficit disorders with learning disorders in children and adolescents. In T. E. Brown (Ed.), *Attention-deficit disorders and comorbidities in children, adolescents and adults* (pp. 231–295). Washington, DC: American Psychiatric Publishing.

*Toplak, M. E., Connors, L., Shuster, J., Knezevic, B., & Parks, S. (2008). Review of cognitive, cognitive-behavioral, and neural-based interventions for attention-deficit/hyperactivity disorder(adhd). *Clinical Psychology Review, 28*, 801–823. Retrieved from http://www.sciencedirect.com/science/article/pii/S0272735807001870

*Trout, A. L., Lienemann, T. O., Reid, R., & Epstein, M. H. (2007). A review of non medication interventions to improve the academic performance of children and youth with ADHD. *Remedial and Special Education, 28*(207). Retrieved from rse.sagepub.com/content/28/4/207.full.pdf.

*Van der Oord, S., Prinsa, P. J. M., Oosterlaanb, J., & Emmelkampa, P. M. G. (2008). Efficacy of methylphenidate, psychosocial treatments and their combination in school-aged children with adhd: A meta-analysis. *Clinical Psychology Review, 28*(5), 783–800. Retrieved from http://www.sciencedirect.com/science/article/pii/S0272735807001869

Volpe, R. J., & Fabiano, G. A. (2013). *Daily behavior report cards: An evidence-based system of assessment and intervention*. New York, NY: Guilford Press.

Willcutt, E. G., & Pennington, B. F. (2000). Comorbidity of reading disability and attention-deficit/hyperactivity disorder: Differences by gender and subtype. *Journal of Learning Disabilities, 33*(2), 179–191. doi:10.1177/002221940003300206.

Willcutt, E. G., Pennington, B. F., Olson, R. K., & DeFries, J. C. (2007). Understanding comorbidity: A twin study of reading disability and attention-deficit/hyperactivity disorder. *American Journal Medical Genetics Part B: Neuropsychiatric Genetics, 144B*(6), 709–714. doi:10.1002/ajmg.b.30310.

Yochman, A., Shula, P., & Ornoy, A. (2004). Responses to preschool children with and without ADHD to sensory events in daily life. *American Journal of Occupational Therapy, 58*(3), 294–302. doi:10.5014/ajot.58.3.294.

*Young, S., & Amarasinghe, J. M. (2010). Practitioner review: Non-pharmacological treatments for ADHD: A lifespan approach. *Journal of Child Psychology and Psychiatry, 51*(2), 116–133. doi:10.1111/j.1469-7610.2009.02191

Chapter 9
Externalizing Disorders: Assessment, Treatment, and School-Based Interventions

Korrie Allen

Children with externalizing disorders (e.g., conduct disorder and oppositional defiant disorder) account for almost 25 % of all special services in schools and represent the most common reason for referral to pediatric and mental health clinics (Achenbach & Howell, 1993; Armbruster, Sukhodolsky, & Michalsen, 2004). Conduct problems often lead to increased use of psychiatric services and medication and are associated with significant emotional and physical distress in impacted children, families, and school personnel (Brosnan & Healy, 2011). The majority of children with an externalizing disorder receive few to no services, despite the high degree of impairment and poor prognosis (Lahey, Carlson, & Frick, 1997), and 70–80 % of those who do receive service use school-based services rather than services offered in the community (Burns et al., 1995). Schools represent the primary setting where children exhibit impairment and receive treatment (Ginsburg, Becker, Kingery, & Nichols, 2008). Providing evidence-based interventions in the school setting is therefore imperative to effectively prevent and treat externalizing disorders.

The purpose of this chapter is to review the developmental and environmental factors, assessment tools, and school-based interventions for children diagnosed with an externalizing disorder. The chapter focuses on conduct disorder and oppositional defiant disorder; the reader is referred to Chap. 8 to learn more about attention-deficit hyperactivity disorder. Conduct disorder (CD) is characterized by a long-standing pattern of rule violations and antisocial behavior. Approximately 6–16 % of boys and 2–9 % of girls meet the diagnostic criteria for conduct disorder (Esser, Schmidt, & Woerner, 1990; Kashani et al., 1987). Oppositional defiant disorder (ODD) is characterized by patterns of hostile and defiant behavior toward adults and other authority figures over a period of at least 6 months, and it occurs in

K. Allen, Psy.D. (✉)
Innovative Psychological Solutions, Fairfax, VA, USA
e-mail: korrie.allen@gmail.com

© Springer Science+Business Media New York 2015
R. Flanagan et al. (eds.), *Cognitive and Behavioral Interventions in the Schools*, DOI 10.1007/978-1-4939-1972-7_9

about 1–16 % of the general population (American Academy of Child and Adolescent Psychiatry, 2007; Loeber, Burke, Lahey, Winters, & Zera, 2000). Certain features may overlap between the two disorders; however, there are important distinctions. Children with ODD, although argumentative, do not display significant physical aggression and are less likely to have a history of problems with the law as is common with CD. If left untreated, child conduct problems (irrespective of extent) intensify following entry into school, putting children with emergent behavior problems at increased risk for peer rejection, academic difficulties, substance abuse, delinquency, school dropout, and depression (Campbell, 1995).

Impact of Externalizing Disorders on the School Environment

Administrators and teachers face enormous pressure to ensure the academic success of all students. When students exhibit disruptive behavior, teachers are challenged with the arduous task of maintaining high academic standards while simultaneously managing problem behaviors (e.g., hitting, talking out, noncompliance) that are disruptive to the learning environment. Research indicates that teachers report spending almost 50 % of their class time managing behavior problems rather than focusing on educational instruction (e.g., Clapp, 1989). The management of problem behaviors has been identified as the most persistent issue facing schools (Center & McKittrick, 1987; Elam, Rose, & Gallup, 1992; Cotton, 1990; Colvin, Kame'enui, & Sugai, 1993). Teacher behaviors and school characteristics, such as low emphasis on teaching social and emotional competence, low rates of praise, and high student-teacher ratio, are associated with classroom aggression, delinquency, and poor academic performance (Webster-Stratton & Reid, 2010). Furthermore, aggressive children frequently develop poor relationships with teachers and are often expelled from classrooms (Webster-Stratton & Reid, 2010). Taken together, inadequate teacher support and exclusion from the classroom exacerbate social problems and academic difficulties.

Empowering school personnel to effectively treat behavior problems improves the overall educational environment for all students. This particularly needs to occur with early childhood education teachers, as externalizing behavior problems often start preschool. As a result, an increasing number of prekindergarten students are being expelled from early childhood education classrooms (Perry, Dunne, McFadden, & Campbell, 2008). Nationally, 6.67 prekindergarteners were expelled per 1,000 enrolled in early childhood education classrooms (Gilliam, 2005). Results from a national study of 3,898 prekindergarten classrooms revealed that 10.4 % of prekindergarten teachers reported that they expelled at least one student in the past 12 months with 19.9 % of those students being expelled more than once (Gilliam, 2005). Unfortunately, one of the main consequences of expulsion at the prekindergarten level is that it shifts the focus of early intervention and education away from the students who need it the most (Gilliam, 2008).

Severe behavior problems manifesting in childhood have long been considered precursors to juvenile delinquency and adult criminality (e.g., Broidy et al., 2003). The period from infancy to preschool is one of the most critical periods in the development of learned aggressive patterns (Aguilar, Sroufe, Egeland, & Carlson, 2000; Bor, Duncan, & Owen, 2001; Farrington, 1994). For instance, longitudinal studies examining preschool children have shown that almost 50 % of children exhibiting aggressive behavior problems in the preschool years will continue to experience similar problems in middle childhood and into adolescence (Campbell, 1995; Cummings, Iannotti, & Zahn-Waxler, 1989). More specifically, empirical studies that track the development of behavior problems over time have found continuity between aggressive, noncompliant behaviors measured between 1 and 3 years of age and externalizing behavior problems measured at 5 years of age (e.g., Cummings et al., 1989). Additionally, preschool children identified as aggressive at 5 years of age are five times more likely to be aggressive at age 14 and that 86 % of children identified with conduct and oppositional defiant behaviors at age 7 tend to display these same behaviors at age 15 (e.g., Moffitt, 1993). Nagin and Tremblay (1999) found that physical aggression in early childhood is a distinct risk factor for later violent offending independent of other disruptive behavior problems. Broidy et al. (2003) indicated that chronic physical aggression during the elementary school years among boys markedly increased their risk of demonstrating physical violence during adolescence.

Contextual Social-Cognitive Model

Violent and aggressive behavior rarely occurs spontaneously. It usually has a long developmental pathway impacted by many environmental variables (Rappaport & Thomas, 2004). The child's environment tends to either promote or buffer conduct problems. Aggressive, impulsive, and violent behavior is often the end result of a complex interaction among many different types of causal mechanisms, including individual vulnerabilities (e.g., poor impulse control, low intelligence), problems in the rearing environment, and stressors in the larger social ecology (Frick, Bodin, & Barry, 2000). Lochman and colleagues (2012) developed the contextual social-cognitive model which is based on empirically identified risk factors associated with antisocial behavior. The model provides a framework to understand how conduct problems develop and worsen over time and includes malleable risk factors such as family, peer groups, community and neighborhood, and the child's social-cognitive processes and emotional regulation abilities that can guide intervention efforts (Lochman & Wells, 2002a, 2002b).

Family

Parental discord, criminality, antisocial family values, and unemployment are often associated with ODD and CD. Children with conduct problems tend to reflect the dysfunction, conflict, and maladaptive processes within the family (Kazdin, 1996). Parents of children with conduct problems often have limited skills to manage the child's behavior appropriately and often inadvertently end up reinforcing the child's negative behavior. They tend to engage in harsh and inconsistent discipline, poor monitoring and supervision, and low levels of warmth and involvement (e.g., Patterson, Reid, & Dishion, 1992). Children's behavior also influences parenting, as youth who present challenging behaviors may elicit less effective parenting (Fite, Colder, Lochman, & Wells, 2006). Though difficult and often resistant to change, parenting style is important to understand and assess as the family plays a primary role in the development and maintenance of conduct problems.

Social Cognition

The most common behavioral problem exhibited by children with externalizing disorder is aggression. Aggression is typically the reason for referral, suspension, and other negative outcomes. Aggressive behavior is complex and associated with social, emotional, and cognitive factors (Feindler & Engel, 2011). Aggressive children typically have underdeveloped social skills (Glick, 2003) due to cognitive distortions and deficiencies that often interfere with accurate encoding and appraisal of social information (Powell et al., 2012). Specifically, children with ODD and CD appear to excessively recall hostile cues and to inaccurately attribute hostile intent to other's motives (Lochman & Dodge, 1994). This "antisocial belief system" justifies their aggressive responses and perceived injustices (Glick, 2003) and, not surprisingly, delinquent youth function at lower levels of moral reasoning than their nondelinquent peers (Feindler & Engel, 2011; Glick, 2003; Kohlberg, 1981, 1984; Nelson, Smith & Dodd, 1990).

Biological Factors

Genetic factors account for about 50 % of the variance in aggressive/antisocial behavior (Nelson, Finch, & Ghee, 2012). Research demonstrates that aggression may be a function of the behavioral activation system, which stimulates behavior and responses to signals of reward or non-punishment, coupled with deficits in the behavioral inhibition system, which is responsible for anxiety and inhibiting behavior (Nelson et al., 2012). Recently, researchers have begun studying the association between aggression in youth and fluctuations in testosterone, cortisol, and neurotransmitters (Rappaport & Thomas, 2004); however, at this time no definite mechanisms have been identified. There is some evidence to suggest that there is a correlation between higher levels of testosterone and physical aggression in boys (Scerebo & Kolko, 1994). Additionally, other studies have found that the neurotransmitter serotonin may modulate aggressive behavior in youth (Conner, 2002; Clarke, Murphy, & Constantino, 1999).

Peers

Rejection from prosocial peers can lead aggressive youth to congregate, forming deviant peer groups (Miller-Johnson et al., 1999). In addition, research demonstrates that associating with deviant peers raises the likelihood of more serious conduct problems (Fite, Colder, Lochman, & Wells, 2007).

Complexity of Assessment and Diagnosis

The diagnostic criteria for oppositional defiant disorder and conduct disorder have largely remained the same in the *Diagnostic and Statistical Manual of Mental Disorders*, 5th ed. (DSM-5), as in the prior edition. In order to make the diagnosis of oppositional defiant disorder, the behavioral disturbances must cause significant impairment in the child's social, academic, or occupational functioning, and the behaviors must not occur exclusively during the course of a psychotic or mood disorder. Additionally, the child must not meet criteria for conduct disorder, which is a more serious behavioral disorder. If the youth is 18 years or older, he or she must not meet criteria for antisocial personality disorder. Conduct disorder is the repetitive and persistent pattern of behavior that violates societal norms or the basic rights of others, covering four symptom areas: (1) aggressive behavior that threatens or causes physical harm to other people or animals, (2) nonaggressive conduct that causes property loss or damage, (3) deceitfulness or theft, and (4) serious violation of rules (e.g., truancy).

The assessment and diagnostic process for ODD and CD is complicated by high rates of comorbidity and symptom overlap with other conditions. ODD and CD are associated with increased risk of other mental disorders during childhood (e.g., Burke, Loeber, Lahey, & Rathouz, 2005). For instance, Nock, Kazdin, Hiripi, and Kessler (2007) found that 42.3 % of children with ODD develop CD and 25 % develop attention-deficit hyperactivity disorder (ADHD). ADHD is found to influence the development, course, and severity of CD. Youth with comorbid ADHD have a much earlier age of onset of disruptive behavior than youths with CD alone (Moffit, 1990). Furthermore, studies have reported that ODD and CD are associated with elevated rates of mood and anxiety disorders (Nock, Kazdin, Hiripi, & Kessler, 2007; Burke et al., 2005). Biederman and colleagues (1996) found that a diagnosis of ODD doubles the risk of both severe major depression and bipolar disorder.

In addition, children with externalizing disorders tend to exhibit many anger outbursts. This is typically the primary reason for referral. Angry students tend to see themselves as victims of injustice and, consequently, often reject the goal of eliminating their anger. Once children with behavior problems enter school, negative academic and social experiences escalate the development of conduct problems (Webster-Stratton & Reid, 2010).

For many of these children, anger and aggression occur with high rates of noncompliant behavior. McMahon and Forehand (2003) describe noncompliance as refusing to follow instructions or established rules and arguing with adults during day-to-day activities. As described above, noncompliance is one of the core features of ODD and CD. Examples of noncompliance in the school setting include refusing to follow teacher commands or follow expected behaviors such as completing class-work, arguing, whining, and refusing to "take no" for an answer. Typically noncompliance and aggressive behavior occur simultaneously; however, they represent different types of disruptive behavior and may require separate treatments (Sukhodolsky, Cardona, & Martin, 2005). The complexity of ODD and CD makes diagnosis and determination of long-term outcomes difficult. The majority of children with internalizing and externalizing disorders exhibit disruptive behavior, aggression, and irritability.

Assessment Methods

School practitioners should use a battery of assessment tools when evaluating children for ODD and CD due to the heterogeneous nature of the disorders. Similar to all other psychosocial problems, it is important to use multimethod, multi-informant, multisetting approach and to use multiple data collection points (Nelson et al., 2012). Comprehensive assessment of the family characteristics, culture, and preferences helps the school psychologist understand the scope of the problem and implement effective interventions (Nelson et al., 2012). In the school setting, the depth of the assessment is often impacted by practical factors such as time and availability of measures. When assessing conduct problems, it is important to look at the context of observable behavior problems, interaction styles, and environmental factors (Lochman, Powell, Whidby, & FitzGerald, 2012).

Behavior Rating Scales

The use of a behavior checklist is a quickly and easy method to understand the breadth and severity of the problems (Lochman, Powell, Whidby & FitzGerald, 2012; McMahon & Forehand, 2005). A commonly used rating scale to assess for clinically significant externalizing behaviors (e.g., ODD and CD) is the Behavior Assessment System for Children-Second Edition (BASC-2; Reynolds & Kamphaus, 2004). The BASC-2 aids in the identification and differential diagnosis of emotional/behavioral disorders (in accordance with special education laws) among children and adolescents based on a 4-point Likert scale ranging from "never" to "always." Additional rating scales include the Achenbach Child Behavior Checklist (CBCL; Achenbach & Rescorla, 2001), Eyberg Child Behavior Inventory (Eyberg & Pincus, 1999), and Revised Behavior Problem Checklist (RBPC; Quay & Peterson, 1996).

Interviews and Behavioral Observations

Interviews with the child, parent, and teacher can be helpful in identifying variables related to the occurrence of disruptive behavior. In the school setting, it is important to determine the function of the behavior. The reader is referred to Chap. 2 for a detailed review of conducting functional behavior assessments. Overall, identifying the antecedents and consequence of the behavior will help the teachers effectively modify the behavior in classroom.

Impairment and Other Areas of Functioning

Longitudinal studies have demonstrated that persistent difficulty in adulthood is better predicted by functional impairment than by diagnostic symptoms (Pelham et al., 2005). Children's Impairment Rating Scale (CIRS; Fabiano et al., 2006) is a brief measure which assesses impairment in important areas. The scale has parent and teacher versions which ask about the degree to which the child has problems that warrant treatment, intervention, or special services in specific areas of functioning. The measure assesses the following areas of functioning: peer, sibling, parent, teacher, academics, self-esteem, classroom/family, and global performance. In addition, peer ratings are often helpful in identifying a subgroup of aggressive, socially rejected children who exhibit a combination of risk factors that point to possible situational factors related to their experience of frustration and aggressive outbursts (Lochman, Powell, Boxmeyer, Andrade, Stromeyer & Jimenez-Camargo, 2012).

Interventions for Youth with Externalizing Behavior Disorders

The research indicates that school-based interventions for children with externalizing disorders have yielded mixed results. In some instances, especially in urban high-risk schools, some intervention programs were found to be ineffective or even iatrogenic (Farahmand, Grant, Polo, & Duffy, 2011; Franklin, Kim, & Tripodi, 2009). Children with ODD and CD exhibit disruptive behavior that negatively impacts classroom instruction, other students, and the child's ability to function. Due to the complex nature of ODD and CD, interventions require a multifaceted approach that includes school mental health providers working with teachers, parents, and the student. This section includes three intervention modalities: (1) manualized programs for school personnel and families, (2) individual skill building techniques, and (3) teacher consultation.

Evidence-Based Manualized Treatments

There are several evidence-based treatments already in use for the treatment of ODD and CD in the school setting. Due to the heterogeneity of the disorder and sensitivity to environmental variables, most programs include a school and parent training component, although implementing the parent component is not always feasible in school settings. Research indicates that of the two types of evidence-based treatments for youth with ODD—(1) individual approaches with a focus on problem-solving skills and (2) family interventions with a focus on parent management training—parent management programs have the greatest amount of empirical support (American Academy of Child and Adolescent Psychiatry, 2007).

Most parent management interventions adhere to four main principles: (1) reduce positive reinforcement for negative or disruptive behaviors, (2) increase positive reinforcement for appropriate behaviors, (3) establish consequences or punishment for negative or disruptive behaviors, and (4) provide consistent, predictable responses to behaviors (American Academy of Child and Adolescent Psychiatry, 2007). Brestan and Eyberg (1998) identified ten treatments for ODD that had sufficient research outcome reports to designate them as probably efficacious. Pardini and Lochman (2006) outlined several of these treatments, including Incredible Years Program and Dinosaur School, Montreal Delinquency Prevention Program, Anger Coping and Coping Power programs, and Problem-Solving Skills Training. The major components of these programs are presented briefly because they each contain a school component.

The Incredible Years Program (3–8 years) includes a teacher and parent training program. Though most of the research focuses on the teacher program which consists of six workshops focusing on building positive relationships with children and families, providing encouragement and incentives, teaching effective discipline, and supporting the development of children's emotion regulation, social skills, and problem-solving abilities (Webster-Stratton & Reid, 2010), research shows that children in the program demonstrate reduced behavior problems in the classroom and improved prosocial skills with peers and that teachers demonstrate improvements in classroom management skills (Webster-Stratton & Reid, 2010).

The Montreal Delinquency Prevention Program (Tremblay, Masse, Pagani, & Vitaro, 1996) is designed as a 2-year program for children in early elementary school and also involves both parent and child components. In the child component, small groups of children meet for 45-min weekly sessions, totaling to nine sessions during the first year and ten during the second year. The groups of children consist of equal numbers of target children with ODD and typical children, and these children work together to learn social skills and self-control techniques.

The Anger Coping program consists of both school-based and outpatient programs for children in fourth through sixth grade (see Larson & Lochman, 2013). There are 18 sessions lasting between 45 and 90 min, and the program employs both a point system for compliant behavior and a goal-setting aspect, in which the children identify areas of their behavior that need improvement; they monitor their progress through weekly progress reports. The program also involves segments for anger management, perspective-taking, social problem-solving skills, and role-playing. The Coping Power program is a more comprehensive, lengthier version of the Anger Coping program, extending it to 33 sessions, and includes additional topics such as emotional awareness, managing peer pressure, social and personal goals, relaxation techniques, and social skills enhancement (Lochman et al., 2008; Wells, Lochman, & Lenhart, 2008). The extension of this program is designed to improve long-term effects. Moreover, the Coping Power program includes a parent component of sixteen 2-h sessions extended over the same period of time as the child component. In these sessions, parents are taught to effectively manage problem behaviors, set house rules, and reinforce the skills and techniques learned in the child component.

The Problem-Solving Skills Training and Parent Management Training is a well-researched form of cognitive-behavioral therapy (CBT) designed for children aged 7–13 years and involves 25 weekly individual sessions, each lasting about 50 min (Kazdin, 2010). This program teaches children prosocial problem-solving skills and techniques for managing difficult interpersonal relationships. Therapists work with the children to practice these skills through role-playing, reinforcement, modeling, and feedback. Parents are taught and encouraged to help their children with these new skills at home. The Parent Management Training aspect consists of 16 individual 2-h sessions over the course of 6–8 months, during which parents are instructed on techniques to use when managing problematic behaviors at home. This parent training aspect also employs role-playing and modeling to reinforce techniques. Parents are also taught school-based reinforcement to improve their children's performance in school through goal-setting and positive reinforcement.

Skill Building Strategies

The above programs were selected because they include school-based components or individual/group techniques that are easily translated to the school setting. However, administering a comprehensive program may not be feasible in the school setting due to financial, environment, and time constraints. Please see Chap. 14 for additional methods to adjust programs to the school setting. Children with ODD and CD often lack the skills to effectively identify triggers or cope with perceived threats. There are additional skill building strategies that are beneficial for children with ODD and CD. The key goal of teaching new strategies is to help the students *develop* and *use* skills during a conflict. This review only covers a few of the several research-based interventions, primarily focusing on those that are amenable to the school setting. These include self-monitoring and problem-solving skills. For a more extensive review of common treatment components for children with conduct problems, see Eyberg, Nelson and Boggs (2008) and Lochman, Powell, Boxmeyer, and Jimenex-Camargo (2012).

Emotion Awareness and Self-Monitoring

Students with conduct disorder typically do not perceive their behavior as problematic. Often the first phase of change involves helping the child to identify their destructive behaviors and to understand the triggers for their behaviors (Lochman et al., 2012). Improving the child's ability to recognize negative emotions helps the child identify conditions where they are prone to engage in negative behavior. This involves teaching students to identify physiological sensations, behaviors, and cognitions. One technique to achieve this is the use of a "Hassle Log," a self-monitoring tool, designed to identify variables associated with both the antecedent and consequent conditions surrounding anger provocations and aggressive behavior (Feindler & Engel, 2011). The Hassle Log provides information that helps children determine the triggers for their behaviors and to create scripts for role-play and practice. It also teaches self-observation and self-evaluation and encourages self-reinforcement for instances of effectively managed anger (Feindler & Engel, 2011).

Another tool is the emotion "thermometer." Using a "thermometer" analogy, school practitioners teach students to identify the intensity of different emotions. Friedberg and McClure (2002) also suggest using an anger "gauge" or "speedometer" to help the student track feelings and behaviors. Specifically, speeds in the "danger" or "overload" zone would indicate high levels of negative emotions; the goal is to help keep the student's speed (e.g., anger, frustration) out of the danger zone. Christner, Friedberg, and Sharp (2006) recommend developing the metaphor further by asking "what happens if a car is driven constantly at high speeds…" (e.g., it is likely to lose control). This helps the child see the importance of "slowing down" the anger to control the speed.

Social Problem Solving

Teaching effective problem-solving skills to children with ODD and/or CD is instrumental to behavioral improvements. Interventions often focus on changing stressful situations that are within the child's control. The primary goal of problem solving is to teach the students to identify the problem, create multiple responses, and evaluate the consequences of the response before acting. Kazdin (1996) also developed the five self-instructions to promote effective problem solving: (1) What am I supposed to do, (2) I have to look at all my possibilities, (3) I had better concentrate and focus in, (4) I need to make a choice, and (5) I did a good job or I made a mistake. Overall, the goal is to teach the student to stop and reflect prior to reacting in key components of these interventions including education, modeling, coaching, rehearsal, and feedback.

In the Coping Power program, students are taught the PICC (problem identification, choices, and consequences) model which helps the student identify problem areas in objective and behavioral terms (Lochman et al., 2012). Students are encouraged to discuss several responses to the problems with both positive and negative outcomes.

They then evaluate the choice and decide which will have the most positive outcome. The students are encouraged to practice their problem-solving skills through activities such as rehearsal, role-plays, and story writing and effort to improve the likelihood they will engage in proactive behavior and reduce aggressive and disruptive behaviors.

Gaps in Behavior Management Training

The results of studies conducted on the effect of using evidenced-based classroom behavior management strategies demonstrate that teachers can significantly alter student behavior. Research demonstrates that teachers are not adequately trained to address negative behavior in the classroom (Hamre, Pianta, Downer, & Mashburn, 2008), particularly planned ignoring and time-out. This could be due to inadequate knowledge of the procedures and how one troubleshoots such procedures (see Witt, VanDerHeyden, and Gilbertson (2004) for a discussion) rather than a complete lack of preservice and professional development training, a condition often resulting from one-time in-service programs. Alternatively, this may be a function of personal preference for a strategy—*or* (emphasis added) the ease of carrying it out. While it is good practice to first utilize positive strategies that utilize positive reinforcement, there are behaviors, situations, or individuals that respond better to strategies that incorporate negative reinforcement or punishment. Unfortunately, this tends to occur far more with ODD and CD compared to other disorders. This is most likely related to the tenacity of the problem as well as the child's hope or expectation that the teacher will not force the issue. Moreover, adults applying behavior management strategies based on negative procedures can become frustrated because the behavior almost always becomes worse before it improves, as is common to extinction procedures (Kazdin, 2001).

School psychologists and mental health providers have the training that can be used to promote better understandings of behavioral intervention principles among teachers. In regard to in-service training, schools frequently offer teachers 1 or 2 h of what equates to foundational knowledge about a specific classroom strategy. Conditions do not often exist that allow for follow-up, in-depth understanding, practice, and supervision. Unfortunately, when a strategy that contains a negative component is misused, the incidence of the problematic behavior may increase rather than decrease. Teachers would benefit from guidance from school psychologists and with the theoretical knowledge to allow them to identify when an intervention strategy is progressing, as it should. For example, teachers may get frustrated if a child's behavior is not changing as rapidly as desirable. School personnel may reinforce a positive behavior and expect immediate change as they would expect with reading remediation. Change takes time, particularly when children are expected to change behavior that they have little intrinsic motivation to modify. Too often, behavior modification plans fail because there is the perception that conceptual underpinnings to an intervention are straightforward and obvious and that therefore the change in behavior will be easily and quickly achieved. Regular consultation and follow-up by the school psychologist is one possible solution in encouraging longer-term commitment to interventions and achieving optimal outcomes.

Teacher Consultation: Effective Classroom Behavior Management Strategies

School psychologists are often called upon to consult with teachers to modify problem behaviors among students. Though psychologists may not interact directly with the student, the guidance they provide teachers can prevent the emergence of problem behavior and/or reduce the severity. Teacher actions in the classroom have a significant impact on student achievement, with classroom management having the greatest effect on student achievement (Wang, Haertel, & Walberg, 1993). School administrators rely heavily on teachers to maintain appropriate student behavior in the classroom. Teachers with poor classroom management skills can unwittingly create classroom environments that maintain behavior problems (Shernoff & Kratochwill, 2007). Such teachers often use ineffective strategies that focus on controlling students rather than modifying behavior (Burke, Guck, & O'Neill Fichtner, 2006) and frequently create academic lesson plans that are geared toward decreasing problem behavior rather than encouraging learning (Martin, Shoho, Yin, Kaufman, & McLean, 2003). For example, a common behavior modification plan used in elementary school classrooms is the stoplight system. Students start the day on green, and if they are "good" all day, they remain on green; however, if they misbehave, they change their color to orange and then red. This system lacks opportunities to reinforce positive behavior and only draws attention to negative behavior. Moreover, once the child enters the orange zone, there is less incentive to behave appropriately because reinforcement will be less likely to be forthcoming. Although punishment temporally suppresses negative behavior, it fails to reinforce or teach positive behaviors. This type of classroom management and teaching often causes student learning to suffer and teacher self-efficacy to diminish, resulting in teacher burnout and academic underachievement for all students. Difficulty managing student behavior is often cited as a significant source of frustration for teachers and is the primary reason for leaving the profession (Morris-Rothschild & Brassard, 2006). A more encouraging whole class system would be to drop a marble in a jar in the front of the classroom when a student engages in a positive behavior such as raising their hand or saying something nice to another student. Another more individualized system frequently used is providing students with tickets or stickers to reinforce positive behaviors. Unfortunately, few teacher training programs offer sufficient education on basic classroom management skills or the implementation of prevention programs.

In aggregate, the research on classroom behavior management systems suggests that when teachers correctly employ strategies with proven effectiveness, disruptive classroom behaviors can be significantly reduced, and academic achievement for all students strengthened through better use of instructional time. Teachers that create a more supportive classroom environment reduce the adverse impact of behavioral problems on academic outcomes (Hester & Kaiser, 1997). Young students often rely on teachers to provide encouragement and a foundation that will allow them to maximize gains from their classroom interactions (Myers & Pianta, 2008). School psychologists can use their training in consultation, counseling, and the systematic delivery of interventions to help teachers with these tasks.

Effective teachers utilize multiple resources and avenues to maintain positive classroom management. There are several specific classroom behavior management strategies that foster good behavior. The strategies that have been reviewed extensively are (1) positive reinforcement and positive attending, (2) planned ignoring, and (3) effective rules and instructions. However, it is important to note that for these strategies to be successfully implemented, teachers must also devote resources to building relationship skills and to establishing a good rapport with students—as positive relationships with students have assisted teachers in facilitating management techniques and strategies (Cothran, Kulinna, & Garrahy, 2003). Negative teacher attitudes, perceptions, and comments on student conduct can affect problem behavior in the classroom resulting in an increase in problem behaviors (Cothran et al., 2003).

In the next section, the following case sample is used to describe specific interventions in the classroom:

> Jonathon's kindergarten teachers report that he is the "enemy of the 5-year-olds." He punches or bites children and pushes them off the swings in the playground without provocation. He pulled the fish out of the tank and smashed them between his fingers in front of the students despite being told how it hurts the animal. His parents report that he has been difficult to manage since he was a toddler due to his anger, aggression, and noncompliance.

Positive Reinforcement and Positive Attending

Positive reinforcement and positive attending include feedback encouraging a student to repeat a desired behavior. Research on positive teacher communication found that verbal praise from teachers is a powerful motivator and can increase behavioral compliance when used correctly. An extensive review (Beaman & Wheldall, 2000) reported that historically, teachers praised students' positive academic performance more often than they addressed positive social behavior. Moreover, inappropriate social behavior attracts teacher attention and is often addressed with punishment or negative verbal response. Sutherland et al. (2000) reported that only 5 % of teacher praise was directed toward behavior; they found that as the teacher's praise for behavior increased, the students appropriate classroom behavior increased. Conversely, during the short period that teacher praise ceased, appropriate student behavior decreased. These findings suggest that teacher praise directly impacts student behavior and can be used effectively in successful classroom management. Teachers' positive attentive behavior toward students such as responding in a timely manner and anticipating student needs and emotions encourages student scholastic and social competence in the early childhood classroom setting (Hamre & Pianta, 2001):

> In the case of Jonathon, the teacher needs to recognize and reinforce any positive behavior, striving to achieve a 5 to 1 ratio of positive to negative comments. It is typical for children with ODD and CD to increase their negative behavior when the teacher starts to praise positive behavior. They are accustomed to receiving negative attention. For example, the teacher may say, "I really like how carefully you are coloring and the student may scribble across

the paper and throw it away." In most situations, the automatic response is to say, "Why would you do that? I cannot believe it. I just told you how nicely you wrote on the paper." Often the adult shows much more emotion and attention when providing the second comment than the initial comment that would be positively reinforced. School personnel working with children should ignore those attention-seeking behaviors and focus on reinforcing any positive behavior even as simple as walking in line or holding hands in their lap. The child must be provided with a "to-do" behavior and immediately reinforced. The first behavior to address with Jonathon is positive use of his hands, which include keeping his hands on the desk, handing the teacher his paper, and giving a high five to children. When he engages in such behaviors, the teacher provides enthusiastic and specific positive reinforcement, "that is so great that you handed your paper in the first time I asked." Avoid providing backward compliments such as "thank you for handing in your paper, it is about time."

Planned Ignoring

Promoting appropriate classroom behavior can take several forms. While communicating praise as positive reinforcement for appropriate behavior is an effective tactic, ignoring students' inappropriate behavior can be another effective classroom management strategy (Sigler & Aamidor, 2005). Buck (1992) defines planned ignoring as "the planned and systematic use of ignoring inappropriate student behavior and reports that it works well with attention-getting behaviors" (p. 4). Ideally, once the student realizes that the behavior is not gaining attention, the behavior is extinguished, as its effectiveness is tied to a child's social learning that misbehavior gains adult attention. Ignoring the misbehavior and praising alternative good behavior redirects the student toward more appropriate classroom conduct.

> For example, Jonathon frequently crumples up his papers, slaps his desk, and calls out answers. The behaviors are annoying but do not endanger other students and can be ignored. To maximize the impact of ignoring, try to focus on one behavior at time and reward the opposite or to-do behavior frequently and immediately. Specifically, to begin, the teacher may focus on calling out answers. During group lessons, every time Jonathon is quiet or raises his hand, the behavior should be immediately reinforced: "I love how quietly you are sitting or thank you so much for raising your hand." At the same time, if he yells an answer out, ignore him and reinforce the students who raise their hand. It should be noted that planned ignoring should not be used to address violent behaviors such as hitting.

Effective Instructions and Rules

There are several steps teachers can use to set students up for success. Most importantly, use of clear instructions and identifying the "to-do" behavior (i.e., walking in a straight line with your hands at your sides) rather than the "what not to do" (i.e., do not touch others in line) provides a specific goal for the child to achieve success. Also when delivering instructions, obtain eye contact from the student, state request clearly, give one command/instruction at a time, and *only* make a request if it is feasible to follow-up and ensure the student complies. School psychologists and mental health providers often use the supervisor metaphor with teachers where they ask the teachers to identify the positive attributes of a good supervisor and the negative aspects of a bad supervisor. Essentially, teachers play the role of the supervisor in the lives of their students, and effectively explaining instructions and consequences will help children behave appropriately in class.

Striepling-Goldstein (2004) offers six "rules for making rules": (1) make few rules (between three and six), (2) negotiate rules with the children, (3) state them behaviorally and positively, (4) make a contract with the children to adhere to them, (5) post them on the classroom wall, and (6) send a copy to parents.

Responses from the teachers to children following or not following the rules should be consistent and immediate. Striepling-Goldstein (2004) indicates that rewards can be social (teacher praise, peer recognition, notes home to parents), material (stickers, certificates, tokens to exchange for food, etc.), or privileges (e.g. extra break time, games, parties, computer time).

Conclusions

Over the last 25 years, children 10–17 years of age, who constitute less than 12 % of the population, have been offenders in approximately 25 % of serious acts of violence (CDC, 2007). As a result, many school systems are implementing evidence-based programs designed to address significant behavioral disorders and to teach children skills such as anger management, problem solving, and the development of impulse control. School-based interventions typically involve teachers training children how to deal with anger in a prosocial manner through promoting empathic understanding, emotion management, impulse control, social problem solving, and a sense of self-efficacy and self-worth (e.g., Grossman et al., 1997). Research on school-based programs has revealed that there are over 150 different violence prevention programs currently available (McMahon & Washburn, 2003). Meta-analyses conducted to examine the intervention effects of school-based programs on aggressive behavior have found modest overall mean effect sizes, with programs that have teachers employ cognitive-behavioral and behavioral modification strategies demonstrating the largest beneficial effects (e.g., Wilson, Lipsey, & Derzon, 2003).

The field of school psychology has evolved focusing on prevention and building capacity within the schools. The response-to-intervention framework uses a multi-tiered model of intervention that involves universal, targeted, and intensive levels of intervention in an effort to address problems school-wide. This model applies to instructional as well as behavioral, emotional, and social problems. The research indicates that programs using cognitive-behavioral interventions demonstrate the largest beneficial effects across all levels of intervention (e.g., Mennuti, Freeman, & Christner, 2006). Teachers can markedly influence a child's behavior by modeling and reinforcing prosocial attitudes and behaviors within the classroom. Thus, schools can provide clear behavioral expectations and counter public and familial messages of disruptive behavior by providing prosocial alternatives (e.g., Walker, Colvin, & Ramsey, 1995).

References

Achenbach, T. M., & Howell, C. T. (1993). Are American children's problems getting worse? A 13-year comparison. *Journal of the American Academy of Child and Adolescent Psychiatry, 32*, 1145–1154.

Achenbach, T. M., & Rescorla, L. (2001). *ASEBA school-age forms & profiles*. Burlington: ASEBA.

Aguilar, B., Sroufe, L., Egeland, B., & Carlson, E. (2000). Distinguishing the early-onset/persistent and adolescence-onset antisocial behavior types: From birth to 16 years. *Development and Psychopathology, 12*(02), 109–132.

American Academy of Child and Adolescent Psychiatry. (2007). Practice parameter for the assessment and treatment of children and adolescents with oppositional defiant disorder. *Journal of the American Academy of Child and Adolescent Psychiatry, 46*, 126–141.

Armbruster, P., Sukhodolsky, D., & Michalsen, R. (2004). The impact of managed care on children's outpatient treatment: A comparison study of treatment outcome before and after managed care. *American Journal of Orthopsychiatry, 74*, 5–13. doi:10.1037/0002-9432.74.1.5.

Beaman, R., & Wheldall, K. (2000). Teachers' use of approval and disapproval in the classroom. *Educational Psychology, 20*(4), 431–446.

Biederman, J., Faraone, S., Mick, E., Wozniak, J., Chen, L., Ouellette, C., et al. (1996). Attention-deficit hyperactivity disorder and juvenile mania: an overlooked comorbidity? *Journal of the American Academy of Child and Adolescent Psychiatry, 35*(8), 997–1008.

Bor, J., Duncan, J., & Owen, A. M. (2001). The role of spatial configuration in tests of working memory explored with functional neuroimaging. *Scandinavian Journal of Psychology, 42*, 217–224.

Brestan, E. V., & Eyberg, S. M. (1998). Effective psychosocial treatments of conduct-disordered children and adolescents: 29 years, 82 studies, and 5,272 kids. *Journal of Clinical Child Psychology, 27*(2), 180–189.

Broidy, L. M., Nagin, D. S., Tremblay, R. E., Bates, J. E., Brame, B., Dodge, K. A., et al. (2003). Developmental trajectories of childhood disruptive behaviors and adolescent delinquency: a six-site, cross-national study. *Developmental Psychology, 39*(2), 222.

Brosnan, J., & Healy, O. (2011). A review of behavioral interventions for the treatment of aggression in individuals with developmental disabilities. *Research in Developmental Disabilities, 32*(2), 437–446.

Buck, G. H. (1992). Classroom management and the disruptive child. *Music Educators Journal, 79*(3), 36–42.

Burke, R. V., Guck, T. P., & O'Neill Fichtner, L. (2006). Overcoming resistance to implementing classroom management strategies: Use of the transtheoretical model to explain teacher behavior. *Research in the Schools, 13*(2).

Burke, J. D., Loeber, R., Lahey, B. B., & Rathouz, P. J. (2005). Developmental transitions among affective and behavioral disorders in adolescent boys. *Journal of Child Psychology and Psychiatry, 46*(11), 1200–1210.

Burns, B., Costello, E., Angold, A., Tweed, D., Stangl, D., Farmer, E., et al. (1995). Children's mental health service use across sectors. *Health Affairs, 14*(3), 147–159.

Campbell, S. B. (1995). Behavior problems in preschool children: A review of recent research. *Journal of Child Psychology and Psychiatry, 36*(1), 113–149.

Center, D., & McKittrick, S. (1987). Disciplinary removal of special education students. *Focus on Exceptional Children, 20*, 1–9.

Centers for Disease Control. (2007). Surveillance summaries prevalence of autism spectrum disorders – autism and developmental disorders monitoring network, six sites, United States 56 (S001). *CDC Morbidity and Mortality Weekly Report*, 1–11.

Christner, R. W., Friedberg, R. D., & Sharp, L. (2006). Working with angry and aggressive youth. In R. B. Menutti, A. Freeman, & R. W. Christner (Eds.), *Cognitive-behavioral interventions in educational settings: A practitioner's handbook* (pp. 203–220). New York, NY: Routledge.

Clapp, B. (1989). The discipline challenge. *Instructor, 99*, 32–34.

Clarke, R. A., Murphy, D. L., & Constantino, J. N. (1999). Serotonin and externalizing behavior in young children. *Psychiatry Research, 86*, 29–40.

Colvin, G., Kame'enui, E., & Sugai, G. (1993). Reconceptualizing behavior management and school wide discipline in general education. *Education and Treatment of Children, 16*, 361–381.

Conner, D. F. (2002). *Aggression and antisocial behavior in children and adolescents: Research and treatment*. New York, NY: Guilford Press.

Cothran, D. J., Kulinna, P. H., & Garrahy, D. A. (2003). "This is kind of giving a secret away…": Students' perspectives on effective class management. *Teaching and Teacher Education, 19*(4), 435–444.

Cotton, K. (1990). *School improvement series, close-up #9: School wide and classroom discipline*. Portland, OR: Northwest Regional Educational Laboratory.

Cummings, E. M., Iannotti, R. J., & Zahn-Waxler, C. (1989). Aggression between peers in early childhood: Individual continuity and developmental change. *Child Development, 60*, 887–895.

Elam, S., Rose, L., & Gallup, A. (1992). The 24th annual Gallup/Phi Delta Kappa poll of the public's attitudes toward public schools. *Phi Delta Kappan, 74*, 41–53.

Esser, G., Schmidt, M. H., & Woerner, W. (1990). Epidemiology and course of psychiatric disorders in school-age children—Results of a longitudinal study. *Journal of Child Psychology and Psychiatry, 31*, 243–263. doi:10.1111/j.1469-7610.1990.tb01565.

Eyberg, S. M., Nelson, M. M., & Boggs, S. R. (2008). Evidence-based psychosocial treatments for children and adolescents with disruptive behavior. *Journal of Clinical Child and Adolescent Psychology, 37*(1), 215–237.

Eyberg, S. M., & Pincus, D. (1999). Eyberg child behavior inventory and sutter- eyberg student behavior inventory-revised: Professional manual. *Psychological Assessment Resources*.

Fabiano, G. A., Pelham, W. E., Waschbusch, D. A., Gnagy, E. M., Lahey, B. B., Chronis, A. M., et al. (2006). A practical measure of impairment: Psychometric properties of the impairment rating scale in samples of children with attention deficit hyperactivity disorder and two school-based samples. *Journal of Clinical Child and Adolescent Psychology, 35*(3), 369–385.

Farahmand, F. K., Grant, K. E., Polo, A. J., & Duffy, S. N. (2011). School-based mental health and behavioral programs for low-income, urban youth: A systematic and meta-analytic review. *Clinical Psychology: Science and Practice, 18*(4), 372–390.

Farrington, D. (1994). Early developmental prevention of juvenile delinquency. *RSA Journal*, 22–34.

Feindler, E. L., & Engel, E. C. (2011). Assessment and intervention for adolescents with anger and aggression difficulties in school settings. *Psychology in the Schools, 48*(3), 243–253.

Fite, P. J., Colder, C. R., Lochman, J. E., & Wells, K. C. (2006). The mutual influence of parenting and boys' externalizing behavior problems. *Journal of Applied Developmental Psychology, 27*(2), 151–164.

Fite, P. J., Colder, C. R., Lochman, J. E., & Wells, K. C. (2007). Pathways from proactive and reactive aggression to substance use. *Psychology of Addictive Behaviors, 21*(3), 355.

Franklin, C., Kim, J. S., & Tripodi, S. J. (2009). A meta-analysis of published school social work practice studies 1980–2007. *Research on Social Work Practice, 19*(6), 667–677.

Frick, P. J., Bodin, S. D., & Barry, C. T. (2000). Psychopathic traits and conduct problems in community and clinic-referred samples of children: further development of the psychopathy screening device. *Psychological Assessment, 12*(4), 382.

Friedberg, R. D., & McClure, J. M. (2002). *Clinical practice of cognitive therapy with children and adolescents: The nuts and bolts*. New York, NY: Guilford Press.

Gilliam, W. (2005). *Prekindergarteners left behind: Expulsion rates in state prekindergarten systems*. New Haven, CT: Yale Child Studies Center.

Gilliam, W. (2008). *Implementing policies to reduce the likelihood of preschool expulsion*. Yale University Child Study Center.

Ginsburg, G. S., Becker, K. D., Kingery, J. N., & Nichols, T. (2008). Transporting CBT for childhood anxiety disorders into inner-city school-based mental health clinics. *Cognitive and Behavioral Practice, 15*(2), 148–158.

Glick, B. (2003). Cognitive programs: Coming of age in corrections. *Corrections Today, 65*(1), 78–80.

Grossman, D. C., Neckerman, H. J., Koepsell, T. D., Liu, P. Y., Asher, K. N., Beland, K., et al. (1997). Effectiveness of a violence prevention curriculum among children in elementary school: A randomized controlled trial. *Journal of the American Medical Association, 277*(20), 1605–1611.

Hamre, B. K., & Pianta, R. C. (2001). Early teacher–child relationships and the trajectory of children's school outcomes through eighth grade. *Child development, 72*(2), 625–638.

Hamre, B. K., Pianta, R. C., Downer, J. T., & Mashburn, A. J. (2008). Teachers' perceptions of conflict with young students: Looking beyond problem behaviors. *Social Development, 17*(1), 115–136.

Hester, P. P., & Kaiser, A. P. (1997). Prevention of conduct disorders through early intervention: A social-communicative perspective. Behavioral Disorders, 22(3), 117–130.

Kashani, J. H., Beck, N. C., Hoeper, E. W., Fallahi, C., Corcoran, C. M., McAllister, J. A., …, & Reid, J. C. (1987). Psychiatric disorders in a community sample of adolescents. *American Journal of Psychiatry, 144*(5), 584–589.

Kazdin, A. E. (1996). Problem solving and parent management in treating aggressive and antisocial behavior. In E. D. Hibbs & P. S. Jensen (Eds.), *Psychosocial treatments for child and adolescent disorders: Empirically based strategies for clinical practice* (pp. 377–408). Washington, DC: American Psychological Association. doi: 10.1037/10196-015.

Kazdin, A. E. (2001). Progression of therapy research and clinical application of treatment require better understanding of the change process. *Clinical Psychology: Science and Practice, 8*(2), 143–151.

Kazdin, A. E. (2010). Problem-solving skills training and parent management training for oppositional defiant disorder and conduct disorder. In J. R. Weisz & A. E. Kazdin (Eds.), *Evidence-based psychotherapies for children and adolescents* (2nd ed., pp. 211–226). New York, NY: Guilford.

Kohlberg, L. (1981). *The philosophy of moral development: Moral stages and the idea of justice (essays on moral development, volume 1)*. San Francisco, CA: Harper & Row.

Kohlberg, L. (1984). *Essays on moral development. Vol. 2, The psychology of moral development: the nature and validity of moral stages* (Vol. 2). New York City, NY: Harper & Row.

Lahey, B., Carlson, C., & Frick, J. (1997). Attention-deficit disorder without hyperactivity. In T. A. Widiger, A. J. Frances, H. A. Pincus, R. Ross, M. B. First, & W. Davis (Eds.), *DSM-IV Sourcebook 3* (pp. 163–188). Washington, DC: American Psychiatric Association.

Larson, J., & Lochman, J. E. (2013). *Helping school children cope with anger: A cognitive-behavioral intervention*. New York, NY: Guilford Press.

Lochman, J. E., & Dodge, K. A. (1994). Social-cognitive processes of severely violent, moderately aggressive, and nonaggressive boys. *Journal of Consulting and Clinical Psychology, 62*(2), 366.

Lochman, J. E., Wells, K. C., & Lenhart, L. A. (2008). *Coping Power program*. Oxford: Oxford University Press.

Lochman, J. E., Powell, N., Boxmeyer, C., Andrade, B., Stromeyer, S. L., & Jimenez-Camargo, L. A. (2012). Adaptations to the coping power program's structure, delivery settings, and clinician training. *Psychotherapy, 49*(2), 135.

Lochman, J. E., Powell, N., Whidby, J. M., & FitzGerald, D. P. (2012). Aggression in children. In P. C. Kendall (Ed.), *Child and adolescent therapy: Cognitive procedures* (4th ed., pp. 27–60). New York, NY: Guildford Press.

Lochman, J. E., & Wells, K. C. (2002a). Contextual social-cognitive mediators and child outcome: a test of the theoretical model in the Coping Power Program. *Development and Psychopathology, 14*, 945–967.

Lochman, J. E., & Wells, K. C. (2002b). The Coping Power Program at the middle school transition: Universal and indicated prevention effects. *Psychology of Addictive Behaviors, 16*, S40–S54.

Loeber, R., Burke, J. D., Lahey, B. B., Winters, A., & Zera, M. (2000). Oppositional defiant and conduct disorder: a review of the past 10 years, part I. *Journal of the American Academy of Child and Adolescent Psychiatry, 39*(12), 1468–1484.

Martin, N. K., Shoho, A. R., Yin, Z., Kaufman, A. S., & McLean, J. E. (2003). Attitudes and beliefs regarding classroom management styles: The impact of teacher preparation vs. experience. *Research in the Schools, 10*(2), 29–34.

McMahon, R. J., & Forehand, R. (2003). *Helping the noncompliant child: A clinician's guide to effective parent training*. New York, NY: Guilford.

McMahon, S. D., & Washburn, J. J. (2003). Violence prevention: An evaluation of program effects with urban African American students. *Journal of Primary Prevention, 24*(1), 43–62.

McMahon, R. J., & Forehand, R. L. (2005). *Helping the noncompliant child: Family-based treatment for oppositional behavior*. New York, NY: Guilford Press.

Mennuti, R., Freeman, A., & Christner, R. (2006). *Cognitive-behavioral interventions in educational settings*. New York, NY: Routledge.

Miller-Johnson, S. H., Coie, J., Maumary-Gremaud, A. N., Hyman, C., Terry, R., & Lochman, J. (1999). Motherhood during the teen years: A developmental perspective on risk factors for childbearing. *Development and Psychopathology, 11*(01), 85–100.

Moffitt, T. E. (1990). Juvenile delinquency and attention deficit disorder: Boys' developmental trajectories from age 3 to 15. *Child Development 61*, 893–910.

Moffitt, T. E. (1993). Adolescence-limited and life-course-persistent antisocial behavior: A developmental taxonomy. *Psychology Review, 100*, 674–701.

Morris-Rothschild, B. K., & Brassard, M. R. (2006). Teachers' conflict management styles: The role of attachment styles and classroom management efficacy. *Journal of School Psychology, 44*(2), 105–121.

Myers, S. S., & Pianta, R. C. (2008). Developmental commentary: Individual and contextual influences on student–teacher relationships and children's early problem behaviors. *Journal of Clinical Child & Adolescent Psychology, 37*(3), 600–608.

Nagin, D., & Tremblay, R. E. (1999). Trajectories of boys' physical aggression, opposition, and hyperactivity on the path to physically violent and nonviolent juvenile delinquency. *Child Development, 70*(5), 1181–1196.

Nelson, J. R., Smith, D. J., & Dodd, J. (1990). The moral reasoning of juvenile delinquents: A meta-analysis. *Journal of Abnormal Child Psychology, 18*(3), 231–239.

Nelson, W. M., Finch, A. J., & Ghee, A. C. (2012). Anger management with children and adolescents. In P. C. Kendall (Ed.), *Child and adolescent therapy: Cognitive procedures* (4th ed., pp. 92–139). New York, NY: Guilford.

Nock, M. K., Kazdin, A. E., Hiripi, E., & Kessler, R. C. (2007). Lifetime prevalence, correlates, and persistence of oppositional defiant disorder: results from the National Comorbidity Survey Replication. *Journal of Child Psychology and Psychiatry, 48*(7), 703–713.

Pardini, D. A., & Lochman, J. E. (2006). Treatments for oppositional defiant disorder. In M. A. Reinecke, F. M. Dattilio, & A. Freeman (Eds.), *Cognitive therapy with children and adolescents: A casebook for clinical practice* (pp. 43–69). New York, NY: Guilford Press.

Patterson, G. R., Reid, J. B., & Dishion, T. J. (1992). *Antisocial boys: A social interactional approach*. Eugene, OR: Castalia.

Pelham, W. E., Burrows-MacLean, L., Gnagy, E. M., Fabiano, G. A., Coles, E. K., Tresco, K. E., et al. (2005). Transdermal methylphenidate, behavioral, and combined treatment for children with ADHD. *Experimental and Clinical Psychopharmacology, 13*(2), 111.

Perry, D., Dunne, M., McFadden, L., & Campbell, D. (2008). Reducing the risk for preschool expulsion: Mental health consultation for young children with challenging behaviors. *Journal of Child and Family Studies, 17*, 44–54.

Powell, N. P., Boxmeyer, C. L., Baden, R., Stromeyer, S., Minney, J. A., Mushtaq, A., et al. (2012). Assesssing and treating aggression and conduct problems in schools: Implications from the Coping Power program. *Psychology in the Schools, 48*, 233–242.

Quay, H. C., & Peterson, D. R. (1996). Revised behavior problem checklist. *Psychological Assessment Resources.*

Rappaport, N., & Thomas, C. (2004). Recent research findings on aggressive and violent behavior in youth: Implications for clinical assessment and intervention. *Journal of Adolescent Health, 35*, 260–277.

Reynolds, C. R., & Kamphaus, R. W. (2004). *Behavior assessment system for children—2 (BASC-2).* Bloomington, MN: Pearson Assessments.

Scerebo, A., & Kolko, D. (1994). Salivary testosterone and cortisol in disruptive children: Relationship to aggressive, hyperactive, and internalizing behaviors. *Journal of the American Academy of Child and Adolescent Psychiatry, 33*, 1174–1184.

Shernoff, E. S., & Kratochwill, T. R. (2007). Transporting an evidence-based classroom management program for preschoolers with disruptive behavior problems to a school: An analysis of implementation, outcomes, and contextual variables. *School Psychology Quarterly, 22*(3), 449.

Sigler, E. A., & Aamidor, S. (2005). From positive reinforcement to positive behaviors: An everyday guide for the practitioner. *Early Childhood Education Journal, 32*(4), 249–253.

Striepling-Goldstein, S. H. (2004). The low aggression classroom: A teacher's view. In J. C. Conoley & A. P. Goldstein (Eds.), *School violence intervention: A practical handbook* (pp. 23–53). New York, NY: Guilford Press.

Sukhodolsky, D. G., Cardona, L., & Martin, A. (2005). Characterizing aggressive and noncompliant behaviors in a children's psychiatric inpatient setting. *Child Psychiatry and Human Development, 36*(2), 177–193.

Sutherland, K. S., Wehby, J. H., & Copeland, S. R. (2000). Effect of varying rates of behavior-specific praise on the on-task behavior of students with EBD. *Journal of Emotional and Behavioral Disorders, 8*(1), 2–8.

Tremblay, R. E., Masse, L., Pagani, L., & Vitaro, F. (1996). From childhood physical aggression to adolescent maladjustment: The Montreal Prevention Experiment. In R. D. Peters & R. J. McMahon (Eds.), *Preventing childhood disorders, substance abuse, and delinquency* (pp. 268–298). Thousand Oaks, CA: Sage Publications.

Walker, H. M., Colvin, G., & Ramsey, E. (1995). *Antisocial behavior in school: Strategies and best practices.* Pacific Grove, CA: Thomson Brooks/Cole Publishing Co.

Wang, M. C., Haertel, G. D., & Walberg, H. J. (1993). Toward a knowledge base for school learning. *Review of Educational Research, 63*(3), 249–294.

Webster-Stratton, C., & Reid, M. J. (2010). The incredible years parents, teachers, and children training series. In J. R. Weisz & A. E. Kazdin (Eds.), *Evidence-based psychotherapies for children and adolescents* (2nd ed., pp. 194–210). New York, NY: Guilford.

Wells, K., Lochman, J. E., & Lenhart, L. (2008). *Coping power: Parent group facilitator's guide.* Oxford, NY: Oxford University Press.

Wilson, S. J., Lipsey, M. W., & Derzon, J. H. (2003). The effects of school-based intervention programs on aggressive behavior: a meta-analysis. *Journal of Consulting and Clinical Psychology, 71*(1), 136.

Witt, J. C., VanDerHeyden, A. M., & Gilbertson, D. (2004). Troubleshooting behavioral interventions: A systematic process for finding and eliminating problems. *School Psychology Review, 33*(3).

Chapter 10
Using CBT to Assist Children with Autism Spectrum Disorders/Pervasive Developmental Disorders in the School Setting

Erin Rotheram-Fuller and Rachel Hodas

Autism Spectrum Disorders (ASD) encompasses a wide variety of behavior. While the descriptions of students across the spectrum can differ, it is most often students with mild or moderate ASD who are included in general education classrooms. It is also these same students who are more likely to benefit from CBT interventions. Thus, the majority of ASD-specific issues discussed in the text will highlight concerns more common to this higher functioning population.

ASD presents unique challenges within the school setting relative to working with other children with challenging behaviors. While many of the behaviors that are the focus of treatment with this population are externalizing behaviors that may look similar to other students, there are several underlying abilities that must be considered and addressed in the development of a treatment plan for students with ASD. Hallmarks of ASD are difficulties in social interaction, repetitive behaviors and a strong hold to routines (APA, 2013), all of which are directly challenged in the social and ever-changing worlds of schools. These difficulties can lead to tantrums or acting out, social isolation, or conflicts with peers, and often need additional intervention beyond the classroom. Cognitive Behavioral Therapy (CBT) offers an opportunity to not only directly address overt behavioral concerns, but also understand and alter the underlying cognitive assumptions of children with ASD, who may not interpret events in ways similar to their peers.

Children with ASD can exhibit a wide variety of behavioral challenges within the school setting. Behavioral concerns may include issues from hand flapping

E. Rotheram-Fuller, Ph.D. (✉)
Division of Educational Leadership and Innovation, Arizona State University,
Tempe, AZ, USA
e-mail: erf@asu.edu

R. Hodas, M.Ed.
Psychological, Organizational, and Leadership Studies in Education, Temple University,
Philadelphia, PA, USA
e-mail: tuc69986@temple.edu

© Springer Science+Business Media New York 2015
R. Flanagan et al. (eds.), *Cognitive and Behavioral Interventions in the Schools*, DOI 10.1007/978-1-4939-1972-7_10

(potentially distracting to peers near the child with ASD) to aggressive behaviors (e.g., throwing chairs during a tantrum and endangering peers). Given the spectrum nature of these disorders, it is extremely difficult to anticipate all of the challenges of students with ASD within the school setting to reduce the likelihood or severity of these difficult behaviors. Each individual student is unique, and their behaviors may be equally unique within the classroom. For example, some students with ASD are extremely quiet, and others have difficulty controlling verbalizations. In considering social interactions with peers, some students with ASD fit in well with classmates, share common interests, and understand and follow the rules of social interaction, while others can have very basic social misunderstandings based on an inability to read the social cues of their peers. It is critical to understand the unique needs of each child with ASD prior to considering intervention, and how an intervention like CBT might work best with that individual child.

As inclusion of children with ASD in general education classrooms is increasing (Simpson, de Boer-Ott, & Smith-Myles, 2003), schools are called upon to intervene and ensure that these students are both academically and socially progressing. Even when academics are intact (supporting placement in the general education classroom), socialization is often a larger challenge for children with ASD. Research demonstrates that in general education classrooms, children with ASD are more often neglected and rejected than their peers (Chamberlain, Kasari, & Rotheram-Fuller, 2007; Kasari, Locke, Gulsrud, & Rotheram-Fuller, 2011; Rotheram-Fuller, Kasari, Chamberlain, & Locke, 2010). These difficulties increase with age as well, as children in later grades have increasing problems with social inclusion relative to their younger counterparts (Rotheram-Fuller et al., 2010). These challenges can also be so intense as to make teachers less likely to accept children with ASD into their classroom (McGregor & Campbell, 2001).

Behavioral problems for children with ASD may appear similar to other children. These can include an inability to stay on-task for long periods of time, difficulty expressing wants or concerns to teachers or peers, feeling overwhelmed by academic or social demands, or an uncertainty about expectations within the school setting. What can be different about this population, however, are the underlying cognitions that accompany such behaviors in the classroom. Whereas a peer within the classroom may not understand class expectations on the first day or week of school, they may be able to infer expectations from the behavior of others, or recognize and follow expectations if explained once by an adult. For children with ASD, however, these expectations must be explained in far more detail, with concrete terminology, and with ongoing practice opportunities to ensure comprehension. Children with ASD have difficulty reading the non-verbal behavior of others (Baron-Cohen, Campbell, Karmiloff-Smith, Grant, & Walker, 1995), which extends into reading cues that are not explicit within the classroom or school setting.

Children with ASD can also be dealing with a variety of co-morbid conditions. The rates of anxiety among children with ASD range from 35 to 84 % (Gillott, Furniss, & Walter, 2001; Muris, Steerneman, Merckelbach, Holdrinet, & Meesters, 1998; Sze & Wood, 2007), making it a highly prevalent issue to deal with in interventions for this population. Within the school setting, anxiety related concerns (e.g., social anxiety and/or performance anxiety) can significantly impact a child's ability to perform academically and socially at school (Reaven et al., 2009). Ensuring that this anxiety is addressed along with any ASD specific social concerns is necessary to increase the likelihood of progress throughout the intervention. Given this likelihood of co-occurring issues, it is important to assess all psychological concerns prior to initiating treatment.

Existing Interventions for Children with ASD

There is an increasing need to develop appropriate interventions to assist school personnel in ensuring the appropriate inclusion of children with ASD within the school. Common interventions for children with ASD include behavioral techniques (e.g., discrete trial or pivotal response training; Koegel & Frea, 1993; Smith, 2001), or social skills interventions focused on training the child with ASD (Bellini, Peters, Benner, & Hopf, 2007; Rao, Beidel, & Murray, 2008; White, Keonig, & Scahill, 2007). Applied Behavioral Analysis (ABA) is currently the most empirically supported approach to treating individuals with ASD (Dawson & Burner, 2011; Kasari & Lawton, 2010; Vismara & Rogers, 2010). ABA focuses on the manipulation of variables that can be effective in improving socially relevant behaviors (Baer, Wold, & Risley, 1968). When working with children with ASD, behavioral techniques have been used to facilitate improvements in their cognitive abilities (Lovaas, 1987; McEachin, Smith, & Lovaas, 1993), communication and language skills (Mancil, 2006; Yoder & Stone, 2006), adaptive behaviors (Cohen, Amerine-Dickens, & Smith, 2006; McEachin et al., 1993), anger management (Brosnan & Healy, 2011), and social skills (DeRosier, Swick, Davis, McMillen, & Matthews, 2011; Frankel et al., 2010).

One of the most common ABA techniques used with children with ASD is Discrete Trial (DT) Training. DT interventions aim to increase positive behavioral responding using contingencies like a penny board (earning a penny for each positive behavior or correct response) until the child earns enough pennies to trade in for a larger desired reward. In this case, behavioral reinforcement is provided to support the acquisition of new positive behaviors or skills.

Within the classroom, teachers often use reward charts, stickers, tokens etc., to increase either correct academic or behavioral responding (e.g., get a token for every time you raise your hand instead of calling out, or get a token for each time you answer a question correctly). DT strategies can be used alone, or in combination with other interventions, but often form the basis of behavioral interventions within the classroom.

Another type of intervention for children with ASD that is typically used within the school setting is social skills interventions. Social skills interventions seek to improve social interactions and functioning of children with ASD. These social skills sessions often cover basic social interaction skills, such as verbal initiations to peers, responses, joining or maintaining an activity, and learning to read or understand social cues. These interventions are often conducted by adults directly working with the child with ASD, however, these social skills training sessions can also be implemented as group interventions that include other children within the classroom or school (Paul, 2003). Interventions such as these focus on providing direct instruction to the child with ASD, and can include didactic instructional sessions, or practice-based instruction (e.g., trying out learned skills on the playground as a part of sessions; Paul, 2003). Social skills interventions such as these have been shown to be effective in improving social initiations, responses, and overall interactions, as well as more structured teacher or parent ratings of social skills (Bellini et al., 2007; Rao et al., 2008; White et al., 2007).

Although CBT is commonly used to treat a variety of childhood problems such as anxiety or aggression, it has not been as widely used within the school setting for children with ASD. Thus, information from clinic-based studies of CBT with children with ASD is evaluated and shows how some of these studies have been applied to issues that arise within schools. These strategies are growing in popularity, however, and an increasing number of studies have utilized CBT, showing promise for its effectiveness with children with ASD.

CBT is composed of strategies that address changing behaviors, as well as underlying cognitions in treatment. Thus, it can incorporate behavioral techniques from the ABA research with this population in combination with direct instructional techniques such as those used in social skills trainings. We know that CBT has been effectively used in both single subject and group studies to improve social skills (Cardaciotto & Herbert, 2004) and daily living skills (Drahota, Wood, Sze, & Dyke, 2011), as well as to reduce anxiety (Chalfant, Rapee, & Carroll, 2007; Puleo & Kendall, 2011; Reaven, 2011; Reaven et al., 2009; Reaven & Hepburn, 2003; Sofronoff, Attwood, & Hinton, 2005; Storch et al., 2013; Sung et al., 2011; Sze & Wood, 2007; Wood et al., 2009), and depression (Hare, 1997).

Research Background

The most common use of CBT among children with ASD is in the management of anxiety symptoms. A number of single-subject studies conducted within clinical settings have looked at improving specific target symptoms within this population and have found CBT to be predictive of improvements in anxiety symptoms such as those related to OCD (e.g., compulsions/obsessions) social anxiety and self-injurious behavior (e.g., Cardaciotto & Herbert, 2004; Hare, 1997; Reaven & Hepburn, 2003; Sze & Wood, 2007; 2008). Larger studies have conducted randomized trials of CBT versus wait list control groups (e.g., Chalfant, Rapee, & Carroll, 2007; Drahota et al., 2011; Reaven et al., 2009; Reaven, Blakeley-Smith, Leuthe, Moody, & Hepburn, 2012; Storch et al., 2013; Wood et al., 2009), but few of these were conducted within the school setting. Many of these studies have, however, focused on skills relevant to schools and classrooms, such as social skills (e.g., Drahota et al., 2011; Sung et al., 2011; Sze & Wood, 2007; Wood et al., 2009) and some have even measured outcomes across settings, including schools (e.g., Chalfant, Rapee, & Carroll, 2007; Wood et al., 2009).

Bauminger (2007) and Wood and colleagues (2009) have conducted some of the few trials that have looked at CBT within school settings. While the Bauminger (2007) study was conducted completely within the school, using teachers as interventionists, Wood and colleagues (2009) conducted the CBT portion of the study within a clinical setting, and provided school consultation as a component of the intervention. These studies both targeted anxiety symptoms and social challenges among children with ASD, and were successful in improving targeted skills as a result of intervention. Bauminger (2007) found improvements in companionship, problem-solving, affective matching and Theory of Mind skills, while Wood and colleagues (2009) showed reductions in anxiety symptoms and improvements in friendship skills. These studies highlight the ability to use CBT within the school setting, and are helpful in suggesting necessary modifications to the CBT process for use with children with ASD (see the section below on suggested intervention modifications).

Currently, CBT treatment manuals have not been fully developed and published specifically for children with ASD. There were three programs mentioned in the literature that were specifically developed for children with ASD, however, they have not yet been fully evaluated and made publicly available. These programs included the Facing-Your Fears (FYF) curriculum (Reaven, Blakeley-Smith, Nichols, & Hepburn, 2011), the Multi-Component Integrated Treatment (MCIT) program (White et al., 2010), and the Behavioral Interventions for Anxiety in Children with Autism (BIACA) program (Wood & Drahota, 2005). Each of these manuals differed in terms of length (ranging from 12 to 16 sessions) and intensity of treatment (ranging from 60 to 90 min each). While each of these curriculums was used in multiple studies, the majority of publications are within the same research group. Thus, more studies are needed to fully evaluate these programs before fully recommending their use more broadly with children with ASD.

A number of studies in CBT for children with ASD have utilized existing models of CBT that were adapted to meet developmental needs of this population. The most commonly used programs included the Building Confidence CBT Program (Wood & McLeod, 2008), the Cool Kids Program (Lyneham, Abbott, Wignall, & Rapee, 2003), the Coping Cat Cognitive-Behavioral Therapy for Anxious Children (Kendall & Hedtke, 2006), and the Mind over Mood Workbook (Greenberger & Padesky, 1995; Padesky & Greenberger, 1995). Similar to the programs developed specifically for children with ASD, these programs also ranged from 12 to 16 sessions, and were simply modified from their original curriculum to adapt to the developmental needs of the child with ASD. The intensity of treatment (length of individual sessions) was not always provided in manuscripts.

Assessment and Intervention Planning

There are a wide variety of skills used in CBT interventions. Thus, it is important to identify the child's skills and skill deficits prior to starting any intervention, and to know what necessary adaptations may need to be made to CBT to work best with any individual child. A trained professional is needed who understands both common challenges for children with ASD, as well as a good understanding of the CBT process to best match a child's cognitive functioning level to the intervention techniques used within CBT. This strategy has most often been provided to this population using clinicians outside the school setting; however, it has also been shown to be effective using special education teachers as intervention agents (Bauminger, 2007). Thus, although we should consider the training and expertise of individuals within the school setting who might best understand the needs of these children and intervention itself (e.g., School Psychologists or School Counselors), other personnel within the school who might have similar expertise should also be considered.

A number of different cognitive skills are necessary for components in cognitive behavioral interventions. Therefore, in order to determine whether CBT is an appropriate treatment option for a specific child, different aspects of the child's functioning should be evaluated and specific modifications to the treatment plan should be developed based on the child's cognitive profile. First, it is important to gauge a student's overall cognitive abilities in order to determine the appropriateness of CBT for a child. CBT, and psychotherapy in general, has commonly been believed to be inappropriate for individuals with lower cognitive abilities, as they are considered to lack the abstraction skills required by many psychotherapeutic approaches (Rutter, 1983; Sturmey, 2005). However, there is a growing body of literature supporting the use of CBT with individuals with intellectual disability (ID) (Taylor, Lindsay, & Willner, 2008). For example, one study using a randomized controlled design found CBT to be effective in reducing levels of depression and automatic negative thoughts and increasing positive feelings about the self in a sample of adults with mild/moderate ID (McCabe, McGillivray, & Newton, 2006). Similarly, in Beail's (2003) review of studies using a variety of different treatment approaches for individuals with intellectual disabilities, the author concluded that CBT has promise in being an effective treatment for this population. While the existing literature on the use of CBT in adults with ID appears promising, there is not enough research on its use in school-age children.

Children with ASD are at increased risk for intellectual disability, with approximately 70 % of children diagnosed with ASD experiencing some degree of impairment, and 40 % of children with ASD experiencing severe to profound levels of impairment (Fombonne, 2003). Thus, it is important to note that cognitive abilities for this population can vary dramatically, from impairments that result in concrete and literal language skills to more global severe impairments, such as low IQ. Given the high rates of cognitive impairments in children with ASD, it is critical that a child's cognitive abilities are assessed in order to determine whether CBT could be suitable for that child as well as to develop appropriate modifications to treatment based on the child's abilities and needs. Although the assessment of a student's overall cognitive abilities can be an important indicator of the overall appropriateness of using CBT, there are other specific aspects of cognition and social functioning that should also be evaluated to aid in treatment planning once CBT has been selected. Because one of the defining features of an ASD diagnosis includes challenges in communication (APA, 2013), a child's verbal abilities should be assessed, as CBT typically requires high levels of verbal ability for establishing therapeutic relationships and being able to express thoughts and feelings. Other common features of ASD are likely to impact the effectiveness of CBT, such as difficulty with emotion recognition, self-reflection, perspective taking, and causal reasoning (Lickel, MacLean, Blakely-Smith, & Hepburn, 2012; Rutter, 1983). These areas should also be assessed to determine whether CBT is appropriate, to identify skills in need of remediation, and to guide adjustments to treatment. Table 10.1 includes a list of suggested areas to asses prior to the use of CBT, along with some possible measures to use in the assessment process.

Table 10.1 Assessment and intervention modifications relevant to children with ASD

Area of functioning	Importance in CBT	Examples of possible assessment tools	Possible modifications needed to CBT
Cognitive abilities	CBT requires abstract thinking, and the ability to recognize the difference between thoughts, feelings, and behaviors	Kaufman Assessment Battery for Children (KABC-II) Stanford-Binet Intelligence Scales (SB5) Woodcock-Johnson III Tests of Cognitive Abilities (WJ-III) Wechsler tests are not recommended due to high verbal demand	Use of concrete language and explicit explanation for each topic Some topics may need to be simplified or removed to ensure comprehension during sessions
Verbal abilities	Verbal abilities are important in establishing rapport with therapist and/or group members, as well as in expressing thoughts and feelings	Bracken Basic Concept Scale: Receptive and Expressive (BBCS-III) Receptive-Expressive Emergent Language Test (REEL-3)	Use of visual materials to support verbal explanations Modeling the use of specific language when practicing skills
Emotion recognition/ empathy	CBT typically requires children to recognize emotions and discriminate between different feelings	Select subtests from the NEPSY-II, including affect recognition Informal emotional vocabulary tests Pictures of Facial Affect system (Ekman & Friesen, 1976) Thought/Feeling/Behavior Discrimination Task (Oathamshaw & Haddock, 2006)	Discussion of emotions may be ongoing throughout sessions to ensure comprehension Practice and explain the process of empathy explicitly
Perspective taking/causal reasoning/ theory of mind	These skills are needed in social understanding	Select subtests from the NEPSY-II, including Theory of Mind	May need to assess for ToM ability prior to beginning treatment and focus on this skill during intervention if not established. Theory of Mind ability should never be assumed

Modifying CBT for Children with ASD

While CBT is a well-validated technique, it has not been used as widely with children with ASD. CBT can be a good match for children with ASD, however, as it is a structured and predictable therapeutic process (following the same session outline each week), and offers repetition, uses concrete evidence in problem solving, and offers opportunities to practice skills (Weiss & Lunsky, 2010). After a thorough assessment of the child with ASD, it would be clear what level of concrete language must be used, how much detail to go into in descriptions of behavioral expectations and how much practice may be needed to master skills. The child's assessment will also determine the specific skills to be targeted during intervention.

There is also some evidence that emotion comprehension can be taught to children with ASD, which can help them benefit from CBT activities. Golan and colleagues (2010) found that children with ASD who were repeatedly shown an animated video designed to teach different emotions or mental states performed better on tests of emotional vocabulary and emotion recognition. Even if a child is showing difficulties on initial assessments prior to intervention, it is important not to immediately eliminate those elements, but instead focus on them more intensely throughout the intervention. The assessment prior to intervention can highlight areas in which intervention will be most important, as well as some possible modifications to the therapeutic process. CBT overall appears to be a promising intervention for children with ASD, when conducted with appropriate modifications.

The most common modifications to CBT interventions for children with ASD are provided in Table 10.1, and will be described here in more detail. Given the core difficulty of children with ASD in social skills, it is important to teach explicit social skills during intervention (e.g., Cardaciotto & Herbert, 2004; Sofronoff et al., 2005; Sze & Wood, 2008). Additionally, it may be necessary to use visual aides to teach important skills (e.g. Chalfant, Rapee, & Carroll, 2007; Reaven et al., 2009; Sze & Wood, 2008), and not rely on the child's abstract thinking ability. Attwood (2004) suggests using social stories to help teach cognitive skills, having students create tangible objects, such as drawings or images to help them define emotions, and teaching students to use coping strategies that are not dependent on abstract language, such as deep breathing and other relaxation techniques. Lang, Regester, Lauderdale, Ashbaugh and Haring (2010) note that many common CBT modifications tend to focus on teaching practical skills, such as social and self-help skills, while reducing the emphasis on cognitive-based components of the treatment.

Other common methods used within interventions for children with ASD include using a child's perseverative interests in order to increase engagement (Bryson et al., 2007), and using systematic reinforcement for appropriate behavior (Smith, 2001). Children with ASD often have perseverative or restricted interests (APA, 2013), and using those interests to motivate the child to learn new skills can be an effective way to encourage them to try new activities or to reach out to others when their inclination may be to avoid those situations. In addition, using reinforcements for approaching behaviors that they may otherwise avoid can also be an effective tool in motivating students with ASD to try new behaviors. For example, if trying to increase a child's level of social interaction, the therapist may want to offer a tangible reward during the next session for initiating to peers as part of their homework. The child is then motivated to approach these peers and to try the behavior in order to get the tangible reward from the therapist. It is hoped that with repeated positive exposure to the peers (presumably achieved through appropriate approach behaviors), the child may be more willing to ultimately continue the behavior without needing a tangible reward in the future.

Given the differences in the spectrum of ASD, it is important to consider individualized modifications to the treatment that acknowledge the variability in how these children present for treatment. For example, as described in Table 10.1, children with limited vocabulary may need picture representations of information and materials to better understand core concepts. More universally, it is recommended to use concrete language (e.g., avoid the use of sarcasm or joking, as it is generally not as well understood by children with ASD), as well as to ensure probing for comprehension throughout sessions.

While it may appear that children with ASD understand core concepts, the application of these concepts across settings is often a core difficulty for these students (Bellini et al., 2007). While children may understand social rules in structured settings (e.g., classrooms—where rules are both explained and posted), unstructured settings can be much more challenging. For example, when walking into a cafeteria, it is not always readily apparent where to sit (even when tables are assigned to classes). Simultaneously, students also need to balance engagement with peers with the task of eating in a socially appropriate manner. Thus, it is important to be as concrete as possible about alternatives, and perhaps practice alternatives with the child, so that they are aware of the range of potential responding in ambiguous situations.

Practicing alternatives can be a large component of the CBT process, as children with ASD often hold strictly to the routine or script that they are taught. Thus, it is important not to suggest only one alternative, but to instead practice a range of alternatives that can occur in any particular situation. Practicing responding in these situations can be done with social stories or comic strip stories for students who need concrete representations about the situation, while other students may be able to role play or simply describe the situation more abstractly and discuss multiple potential outcomes. By prompting the child with different, but similar scenarios, the child can practice flexibility in responding to multiple situations that may occur within the same setting.

When using any intervention with children with ASD, it is also important to ensure that if a child has mastered a skill in one setting (e.g., initiating to peers in the cafeteria) that they are then able to understand when and how to adapt that skill to other settings (e.g., initiating to peers on the playground). Whereas typically developing peers may be able to learn a skill and apply that skill in all situations, this is far more difficult for the child with ASD (Rogers, 2000). Context specific learning is common, and children may have to be shown the direct linkages between how to behave in two similar, but different settings.

Another common challenge for children with ASD is a lack of understanding the thoughts or perspective of others (Theory of Mind). While this understanding is not critical in all skill development, it is a key concern in social situations (which are often of concern within schools). Focusing directly on this skill of understanding the view of other people may be a key to helping students socially adapt. Using these perspective taking strategies during CBT may also allow the opportunity to show how the child can deduce another's perspective in different situations. For example, for a child who is assessed to have poor perspective taking skills, it is important to review this skill repeatedly, asking about what another child might think or feel in each situation you discuss throughout each session (and generate multiple situations to practice this skill). Moving on to more complex social skills may be difficult when the child is unable to understand the perspectives of others.

Finally, a common modification to treatment when working with children with ASD, is to include parents in the treatment process (e.g., Reaven et al., 2009; Storch et al., 2013; White et al., 2010). Including parents in CBT interventions offers the best opportunity to help with the generalization of skills across settings, as well as to teach parents critical skills in working with their own child (Sofronoff et al., 2005). One study even compared family vs. individual CBT, and found greater effects from working with the family than the individual child alone (Puleo & Kendall, 2011). However, it can be challenging to get parental involvement for school-based services due to the timing of the sessions and/or some parents' reluctance to participate in school-based activities. Interventions with parents may be more successful in the evenings after school hours, when parents are less likely to have conflicts with work, and run groups concurrently with students and parents to ensure childcare needs are addressed.

Adapting CBT to the School Setting

Schools can be an ideal setting to provide students with evidence-based mental health services. As mental health problems can produce barriers to student learning, it can be considered a school's responsibility to provide struggling students with mental health services (Adelman & Taylor, 2003). Because many students, particularly those in urban settings, do not get the mental health services that they need, schools may increase rates of service delivery by removing some of the common barriers to services such as attendance difficulties and fear of stigma (Atkins, Frazier, Adil, & Talbott, 2003). Additionally, school-based clinicians often have information about students that a mental health worker in another setting might not have access to, such as students' academic and behavioral records. They are also able to observe students interact with their teachers and peers (Creed, Reisweber, & Beck, 2011).

CBT as an intervention itself may be particularly well suited to the school setting. Because CBT sessions are often highly structured, clinicians are able to work around school scheduling constraints and use shorter, more frequent sessions in an effective way (Creed et al., 2011). Additionally, because students are used to being assigned homework in school, they may feel more inclined to practice using the skills outside of the sessions than they would if they were working with a clinician in another setting. CBT has already been used in schools to prevent and/or treat a variety of disorders, including anxiety (Bernstein, Bernat, Victor, & Layne, 2008; Mifsud & Rapee, 2005) and depression (Gillham et al., 2007; Shirk, Kaplinksi, & Gudmundsen, 2009), which also suggests its potential use for more populations within schools.

Despite these benefits, there are some specific challenges to providing mental health services in a school setting. Mental health workers in schools typically have very large caseloads and may not have the time to provide one-on-one or small group therapy. Additionally, because of high stakes testing, students' academic days are usually very busy and it may be difficult to schedule times where teachers are comfortable with students being pulled out of class.

When considering modifications needed to make CBT more appropriate for children with ASD, other barriers arise. In order to fit CBT into students' schedules, they often need to be pulled out of class or other activities. Because children with ASD do not respond well to changes in routine, they may be more resistant to attending sessions. It is recommended that children be told about sessions prior to the first one to prepare them for changing their routine from what they expect. It is also recommended that sessions be held at the same time each week on a regular basis in order to help make this part of a new routine for the child with ASD.

Another challenge conducting CBT in the school setting relates to the length of CBT sessions. For example, in McNally, Keehn, Lincoln, Brown, and Chavira's (2013) study, a manualized CBT was adapted for the ASD population by extending the length of sessions to allow greater time for introducing and practicing concepts. However, due to the scheduling challenges during a school day, it may be unrealistic to adjust treatment in this way, even if it is recommended for a specific child with ASD. Instead, more frequent, shorter sessions may be a better way to increase practice opportunities. As stated above, this adjustment in session time (more frequent but shorter sessions) is also one of the advantages of using CBT within the school setting, where students are on site for intervention on a daily basis, instead of having to ask children and families to come to a clinical setting repeatedly during a week.

In explaining CBT to students with ASD, it may also be helpful to prepare them for the format of sessions, as well as what will be discussed ahead of time, as much as possible. Letting them know how much time you will spend together and some of the activities you might be doing together can help to ease any discomfort they may have from being pulled out of regular class routines for this new activity. Building a therapeutic relationship with the child (e.g., gaining trust or showing interest in the student's favorite activities or topics) is also critical to increase the likelihood of participation in sessions, and allowing time for adjustment to a practitioner can be important by first focusing on building rapport over several sessions before introducing "work" to be done by the student.

Within the school setting, there can also be flexibility in who takes the responsibility for implementing therapeutic interventions. School counselors, social workers, and school psychologists are typically relied on within the school setting to provide mental health services. However, as previously mentioned, one of the only school-based studies of CBT found that students' special education teachers were effective group leaders (Bauminger, 2007). Regardless of who provides the intervention, it is critical to maintain the same therapist once a therapeutic relationship has been established with a student. Changing therapists regularly can disorient the student to the purpose of sessions or meetings, and halt therapeutic progress.

Building the therapeutic relationship may take longer with children with ASD. Many of these children have often been exposed to numerous providers (e.g., doctors, therapeutic support staff, case workers, behavioral health professionals, etc.). With so many individuals involved in their care, it can mean that they are either more or less receptive to having new adults in their lives. It is important that the individual responsible for working with a child with ASD is both familiar with the child as well as general characteristics of ASD. Understanding common challenges for children with developmental delays can help the therapist to know what to look for, specifically, in assessments, and how to adapt interventions to meet these needs.

A big advantage to any intervention within the school setting is the opportunity to include peers in the practice component of the intervention. Having peers allows the possibility for group work, as well as practice opportunities during unstructured time. Peers can include those who are typically developing (perhaps serving as models), or those with different special needs within the school. Peers can be selected based on a common need for intervention or strength in a specific area (e.g., social skills). It is recommended, however, to have a heterogeneous group in terms of the type of problems and degree of impairment to provide opportunities for all students to be models as well as learn from others. Group work saves time for interventionists (who can work with multiple children at one time), as well as increasing the likelihood of generalization of skills for the child with ASD, as these group members can help each other during non-group times within the school. Practice opportunities (e.g., homework) are critical to the continued use of the skill within the school setting, and having peers who understand the assignment along with the child with ASD can potentially increase the likelihood that they will try the homework between sessions.

Conclusions

The research that has been done on CBT for children with ASD has shown promising results, especially around anxiety concerns. A comprehensive assessment should be conducted prior to intervention to best determine both concerns for intervention, as well as necessary modifications to the CBT process. Common modifications should be considered, and outcomes should be monitored to assess the efficacy of the intervention for specific children with ASD.

While the use of CBT has been increasing among children with ASD, it has not yet been fully developed with this population, especially within the school setting. More research is needed to identify an effective school-based model of CBT for children with ASD that can be widely disseminated within schools. What has been shown in the research thus far, however, is that CBT offers an opportunity to provide consistent and reliable intervention services in schools where students are more likely to attend sessions. In addition, because of the specific social deficits common to ASD, it is an ideal intervention for schools where peers can both be included in sessions, as well as helpers in ensuring the generalization of skills (providing practice during non-intervention situations). As more students with ASD are being included in general education settings, the need for interventions for this population are increasing. CBT offers a promising treatment option for this group.

References

Adelman, H. S., & Taylor, L. (2003). Toward a comprehensive policy vision for mental health in schools. In M. Weist, S. Evans, & N. Lever (Eds.), *Handbook of school mental health: Advancing practice and research*. New York, NY: Springer.

American Psychiatric Association. (2013). *Diagnostic and statistical manual of mental disorders* (5th ed.). Arlington, VA: American Psychiatric Publishing.

Atkins, M. S., Frazier, S. L., Adil, J. A., & Talbott, E. (2003). School-based mental health services in urban communities. In M. Weist, S. Evans, & N. Lever (Eds.), *Handbook of school mental health: Advancing practice and research*. New York, NY: Springer.

Attwood, T. (2004). Cognitive behavior therapy for children and adults with Asperger's syndrome. *Behaviour Change, 21*, 147–161.

Baer, D. M., Wold, M. M., & Risley, T. R. (1968). Some current dimensions of applied behavior analysis. *Journal of Applied Behavior Analysis, 1*, 91–97.

Baron-Cohen, S., Campbell, R., Karmiloff-Smith, A., Grant, J., & Walker, J. (1995). Are children with autism blind to the mentalistic significance of the eyes? *British Journal of Developmental Psychology, 13*(4), 379–398.

Bauminger, N. (2007). Brief report: Group social-multimodal intervention for HFASD. *Journal of Autism and Developmental Disorders, 37*, 1605–1615.

Beail, N. (2003). What works for people with mental retardation? Critical commentary on cognitive-behavioural and psychodynamic psychotherapy research. *Mental Retardation, 41*, 468–472.

Bellini, S., Peters, J. K., Benner, L., & Hopf, A. (2007). A meta-analysis of school-based social skills interventions for children with autism spectrum disorders. *Remedial and Special Education, 28*, 153–162.

Bernstein, G. A., Bernat, D. H., Victor, A. M., & Layne, A. E. (2008). School-based interventions for anxious children: 3-, 6-, and 12-month follow-ups. *Journal of the American Academy of Child and Adolescent Psychiatry, 47*, 1039–1047.

Brosnan, J., & Healy, O. (2011). A review of behavioral interventions for the treatment of aggression in individuals with developmental disabilities. *Research in Developmental Disabilities, 32*, 437–446.

Bryson, S. E., Koegel, L. K., Koegel, R. L., Openden, D., Smith, I. M., & Nefdt, N. (2007). Large scale dissemination and community implementation of pivotal response treatment: Program descriptionand preliminary data. *Research & Practice for Persons with Severe Disabilities, 32*, 142–153.

Cardaciotto, L., & Herbert, J. D. (2004). Cognitive behavior therapy for social anxiety disorder in the context of Asperger's syndrome: A single-subject report. *Cognitive and Behavioral Practice, 11*, 75–81.

Chalfant, A. M., Rapee, R., & Carroll, L. (2007). Treating anxiety disorders in children with high functioning autism spectrum disorders: A controlled trial. *Journal of Autism and Developmental Disorders, 37*, 1842–1857.

Chamberlain, B., Kasari, C., & Rotheram-Fuller, E. (2007). Involvement or isolation? The social networks of children with autism in regular classrooms. *Journal of Autism and Developmental Disorders, 37*, 230–242.

Cohen, H., Amerine-Dickens, M., & Smith, T. (2006). Early intensive behavioral treatment: Replication of the UCLA model in a community setting. *Journal of Developmental & Behavioral Pediatrics, 27*, 145–155.

Creed, T. A., Reisweber, J., & Beck, A. T. (2011). *Cognitive therapy for adolescents in school settings.* New York, NY: The Guilford Press.

Dawson, G., & Burner, K. (2011). Behavioral interventions in children and adolescents with autism spectrum disorder: A review of recent findings. *Current Opinion in Pediatrics, 23*, 616–620.

DeRosier, M. E., Swick, D. C., Davis, N., McMillen, J., & Matthews, R. (2011). The efficacy of a social skills group intervention for improving social behaviors in children with high functioning autism spectrum disorders. *Journal of Autism and Developmental Disorders, 41*, 1033–1043.

Drahota, A., Wood, J., Sze, K., & Dyke, M. (2011). Effects of cognitive behavioral therapy on daily living skills in children with high-functioning autism and concurrent anxiety disorders. *Journal of Autism and Developmental Disorders, 41*, 257–265.

Ekman, P., & Friesen, W. V. (1976). Measuring facial movement. *Journal of Environmental Psychology, 1*, 56–75.

Fombonne, E. (2003). Epidemiological surveys of autism and other pervasive developmental disorders: An update. *Journal of Autism and Developmental Disorders, 33*, 365–382.

Frankel, F., Myatt, R., Sugar, C., Whitham, C., Gorospe, C. M., & Laugeson, E. (2010). A randomized controlled study of parent-assisted children's friendship training with children having autism spectrum disorders. *Journal of Autism and Developmental Disorders, 40*, 827–842.

Gillham, J. E., Reivich, K. J., Freres, D. R., Chaplin, T. M., Shatte, A. J., Samuels, B., et al. (2007). School-based prevention of depressive symptoms: A randomized controlled study of the effectiveness and specificity of the Penn Resiliency Program. *Journal of Consulting and Clinical Psychology, 75*, 9–19.

Gillott, A., Furniss, F., & Walter, A. (2001). Anxiety in high-functioning children with autism. *Autism, 5*, 277–286.

Golan, O., Ashwin, E., Granader, Y., McClintock, S., Day, K., Leggett, V., et al. (2010). Enhancing emotion recognition in children with autism spectrum conditions: An intervention using animated vehicles with real emotional faces. *Journal of Autism and Developmental Disorders, 40*, 269–27.

Greenberger, D., & Padesky, C. A. (1995). *Mind over mood: Change how you feel by changing the way you think.* New York, NY: Guilford Press.

Hare, D. J. (1997). The use of cognitive behavioral therapy with people with Asperger syndrome. *Autism, 1*, 213–225.

Kasari, C., & Lawton, K. (2010). New directions in behavioral treatment of autism spectrum disorders. *Current Opinion in Neurology, 23*, 137–143.

Kasari, C., Locke, J., Gulsrud, A., & Rotheram-Fuller, E. (2011). Social networks and friendships at school: Comparing children with and without Autism. *Journal of Autism and Developmental Disorders, 41*, 533–544.

Kendall, P. C., & Hedtke, K. A. (2006). *Cognitive-behavioral therapy for anxious children: Therapist manual* (3rd ed.). Ardmore, PA: Workbook Publishing.

Koegel, R. L., & Frea, W. D. (1993). Treatment of social behavior in autism through the modification of pivotal social skills. *Journal of Applied Behavior Analysis, 26*, 369–377.

Lang, R., Regester, A., Lauderdale, S., Ashbaugh, K., & Haring, A. (2010). Treatment of anxiety in autism spectrum disorders using cognitive behavior therapy: A systematic review. *Developmental Neurorehabilitation, 13*, 53–63.

Lickel, A., MacLean, W., Blakely-Smith, A., & Hepburn, S. (2012). Assessment of the prerequisite skills for cognitive behavioral therapy in children with and without autism spectrum disorders. *Journal of Autism and Developmental Disorders, 42*, 992–1000.

Lovaas, O. (1987). Behavioral treatment and normal educational and intellectual functioning in young autistic children. *Journal of Consulting and Clinical Psychology, 55*, 3–9.

Lyneham, H. J., Abbott, M. J., Wignall, A., & Rapee, R. M. (2003). *The Cool Kids family program—therapist manual.* Sydney: Macquarie University.

Mancil, G. (2006). Functional communication training: A review of the literature related to children with Autism. *Education and Training in Developmental Disabilities, 41*, 213–224.

McCabe, M. P., McGillivray, J. A., & Newton, D. C. (2006). Effectiveness of treatment programmes for depression among adults with mild/moderate intellectual ability. *Journal of Intellectual Disability Research, 50*, 239–247.

McEachin, J., Smith, T., & Lovaas, O. (1993). Long-term outcome for children with autism who received early intensive behavioral treatment. *American Journal of Mental Retardation, 97*, 359–372.

McGregor, E., & Campbell, E. (2001). The attitudes of teachers in Scotland to the integration of children with autism intro mainstream schools. *Autism, 5*, 189–207.

McNally Keehn, R. H., Lincoln, A., Brown, M., & Chavira, D. (2013). The Coping Cat Program for children with anxiety and autism spectrum disorder: A pilot randomized controlled trial. *Journal of Autism and Developmental Disorders, 43*, 57–67.

Mifsud, C., & Rapee, R. M. (2005). Early intervention for childhood anxiety in a school setting: Outcomes for an economically disadvantaged population. *Journal of the American Academy of Child and Adolescent Psychiatry, 44*, 996–1004.

Muris, P., Steerneman, P., Merckelbach, H., Holdrinet, I., & Meesters, C. (1998). Comorbid anxiety symptoms in children with pervasive developmental disorders. *Journal of Anxiety Disorders, 12*, 387–393.

Oathamshaw, S. C., & Haddock, G. (2006). Do people with intellectual abilities and psychosis have the cognitive skills required to undertake cognitive behavior therapy? *Journal of Applied Research in Intellectual Disabilities, 19*, 35–46.

Padesky, C. A., & Greenberger, D. (1995). *Clinician's guide to mind over mood.* New York, NY: Guilford Press.

Paul, R. (2003). Promoting social communication in high functioning individuals with autistic spectrum disorders. *Child and Adolescent Psychiatric Clinics of North America, 12*, 87–106.

Puleo, C. M., & Kendall, P. C. (2011). Anxiety disorders in typically developing youth: Autism spectrum symptoms as a predictor of cognitive-behavioral treatment. *Journal of Autism and Developmental Disorders, 41*, 275–286.

Rao, P. A., Beidel, D. C., & Murray, M. J. (2008). Social skills interventions for children with Asperger's syndrome or high-functioning autism: A review and recommendations. *Journal of Autism and Developmental Disorders, 38*, 353–361.

Reaven, J. A. (2011). The treatment of anxiety symptoms in youth with high-functioning autism spectrum disorders: Developmental considerations for parents. *Brain Research, 1380*, 255–263.

Reaven, J., Blakeley-Smith, A., Leuthe, E., Moody, E., & Hepburn, S. (2012). Facing your fears in adolescence: Cognitive-behavioral therapy for high-functioning autism spectrum disorders and anxiety. *Autism Research and Treatment, 2012*, 1–13.

Reaven, J. A., Blakeley-Smith, A., Nichols, S., Dasari, M., Flanigan, E., & Hepburn, S. (2009). Cognitive-behavioral group treatment for anxiety symptoms in children with high-functioning autism spectrum disorders: A pilot study. *Focus on Autism and Other Developmental Disabilities, 24*, 27–37.

Reaven, J., Blakeley-Smith, A., Nichols, S., & Hepburn, S. (2011). *Facing your fears: Group therapy for managing anxiety in children with high-functioning autism spectrum disorders.* Baltimore: Paul Brookes Publishing.

Reaven, J., & Hepburn, S. (2003). Cognitive-behavioral treatment of obsessive-compulsive disorder in a child with Asperger syndrome: A case report. *Autism, 7*, 145–164.

Rogers, S. (2000). Interventions that facilitate socialization in children with autism. *Journal of Autism and Developmental Disorders, 30*, 399–409.

Rotheram-Fuller, E., Kasari, C., Chamberlain, B., & Locke, J. (2010). Social involvement of children with autism spectrum disorders in elementary school classrooms. *Journal of Child Psychology and Psychiatry, 51*, 1227–1234.

Rutter, M. (1983). Cognitive deficits in the pathogenesis of autism. *Journal of Child Psychology and Psychiatry, 24*, 513–531.

Shirk, S. R., Kaplinksi, H., & Gudmundsen, G. (2009). School-based cognitive behavioral therapy for adolescent depression: A benchmarking study. *Journal of Emotional and Behavioral Disorders, 17*, 106–117.

Simpson, R. L., de Boer-Ott, S. R., & Smith-Myles, B. (2003). Inclusion of learners with autism spectrum disorders in general education settings. *Topics in Language Disorders, 23*, 116–133.

Smith, T. (2001). Discrete trial training in the treatment of autism. *Focus on Autism and Other Developmental Disabilities, 16*, 86–92.

Sofronoff, K., Attwood, T., & Hinton, S. (2005). A randomised controlled trial of a CBT intervention for anxiety in children with Asperger syndrome. *Journal of Child Psychology and Psychiatry, 46*, 1152–1160.

Storch, E. A., Arnold, E. B., Lewin, A. B., Nadeau, J. M., Jones, A. M., De Nadai, A. S., et al. (2013). The effect of cognitive-behavioral therapy versus treatment as usual for anxiety in children with autism spectrum disorders: A randomized, controlled trial. *Journal of the American Academy of Child and Adolescent Psychiatry, 52*, 132–142.

Sturmey, P. (2005). Against psychotherapy with people who have mental retardation. *Mental Retardation, 43*, 55–57.

Sung, M., Ooi, Y. P., Goh, T. J., Pathy, P., Fung, D. S. S., Ang, R. P., et al. (2011). Effects of cognitive-behavioral therapy on anxiety in children with autism spectrum disorders: A randomized controlled trial. *Child Psychiatry and Human Development, 42*, 634–649.

Sze, K. M., & Wood, J. J. (2007). Cognitive behavioral treatment of comorbid anxiety disorders and social difficulties in children with high-functioning autism: A case report. *Journal of Contemporary Psychotherapy, 37*, 133–143.

Sze, K. M., & Wood, J. J. (2008). Enhancing CBT for the treatment of autism spectrum disorders and concurrent anxiety. *Behavioural and Cognitive Psychotherapy, 36*, 403–409.

Taylor, J., Lindsay, W., & Willner, P. (2008). CBT for people with intellectual disabilities: Emerging evidence, cognitive ability and IQ effects. *Behavioural and Cognitive Psychotherapy, 36*, 723–733.

Vismara, L. A., & Rogers, S. J. (2010). Behavioral treatments in autism spectrum disorder: What do we know? *Annual Review of Clinical Psychology, 6*, 447–468.

Weiss, J. A., & Lunsky, Y. (2010). Group cognitive behaviour therapy for adults with Asperger syndrome and anxiety or mood disorder: A case series. *Clinical Psychology & Psychotherapy, 17*, 438–446.

White, S. W., Albano, A. M., Johnson, C. R., Kasari, C., Ollendick, E., Klin, A., et al. (2010). Development of a cognitive-behavioral intervention program to treat anxiety and social deficits in teens with high-functioning autism. *Clinical Child and Family Psychology Review, 13*, 77–90.

White, S. W., Keonig, K., & Scahill, L. (2007). Social skills development in children with autism spectrum disorders: A review of the intervention research. *Journal of Autism and Developmental Disorders, 37*, 1858–1868.

Wood, J. J., & Drahota, A. (2005). *Behavioral interventions for anxiety in children with autism.* Los Angeles, CA: University of California–Los Angeles.

Wood, J. J., Drahota, A., Sze, K., Har, K., Chiu, A., & Langer, D. A. (2009). Cognitive behavioral therapy for anxiety in children with autism spectrum disorders: a randomized controlled trial. *The Journal of Child Psychology and Psychiatry, 50,* 224–234.

Wood, J. J., & McLeod, B. (2008). *Child anxiety disorders: A family-based treatment manual for practitioners.* New York, NY: Norton.

Yoder, P., & Stone, W. L. (2006). A randomized comparison of the effect of two prelinguistic communication interventions of the acquisition of spoken communication in preschoolers with ASD. *Journal of Speech, Language and Hearing Research, 49,* 698–711.

Chapter 11
Pediatric Elimination Disorders

Camilo Ortiz and Alex Stratis

Pediatric elimination disorders are poorly understood by parents and teachers and often mistreated by medical and mental health professionals. Most children with these problems do not even receive treatment, often suffering for years (Foxman, Valdez & Brook, 1986). Fishman, Rappaport, Schonwald, and Nurko (2003) found that approximately one third of parents mistakenly believed that the cause of their child's encopresis was "emotional" in nature, while other parents believed that attention seeking and laziness were causes. This is unfortunate because the consequences of having enuresis or encopresis can be profound for the child and his family. Psychologists working in schools have a tremendous opportunity to alter these inaccurate and unhelpful beliefs and consequently change the trajectory of the lives of these children.

The dearth of high-quality research in the area of pediatric elimination disorders is also responsible for the lack of knowledge on how to work effectively with these children. One particularly troubling deficit in the literature is that little work has been done to identify treatment modifications for the subtypes of these disorders (Butler, Heron, & The ALSPAC Study Team, 2006). Another somewhat mystifying shortfall in the literature, given that these problems often manifest at school, is that almost no work has been published addressing how educational professionals, including school psychologists, can effectively assess and treat elimination problems. Using a detailed case example, the current chapter aims to provide a clear picture of encopresis and enuresis while focusing on the assessment and treatment of the subtypes of each disorder that would typically be encountered by a psychologist in a school setting. It is important to note that these two disorders share little in terms of presentation, etiology, assessment, and treatment. However, there are some common issues that psychologists may face. When possible, a discussion of these issues for both disorders will be integrated.

C. Ortiz, Ph.D. (✉) • A. Stratis, Psy.D.
Clinical Psychology Program, Long Island University, C.W. Post, Brookville, NY, USA
e-mail: drcamilo.ortiz@gmail.com; strats@umich.edu

© Springer Science+Business Media New York 2015
R. Flanagan et al. (eds.), *Cognitive and Behavioral Interventions in the Schools*, DOI 10.1007/978-1-4939-1972-7_11

Encopresis is defined by the Diagnostic and Statistical Manual of Mental Disorders (5th ed.; DSM–5; American Psychiatric Association, 2013) as the "repeated passage of feces into inappropriate places (e.g., clothing or floor) whether involuntary or intentional" (p. 357)[1]. To meet the DSM-5 criteria, the child must experience at least one event per month, for at least three months (criterion B), and be at least four years old (criterion C). Encopresis affects approximately 1.5–7.5 % of children aged six to 12 (McGrath, Mellon, & Murphy, 2000). It is up to six times as common in boys as it is in girls (Schonwald & Rappaport, 2008; Van der Wal, Benninga, & Hirasing, 2005). Once a practitioner has made a diagnosis, the most important question to be answered is whether the passage of feces (fecal incontinence) is *retentive* or *non-retentive* because the treatment for each subtype is quite different. Retentive encopresis almost always involves constipation and comprises approximately 85 % of cases, while the remaining cases are categorized as nonretentive, which refers to inappropriate soiling without evidence of fecal constipation and retention (McGrath et al., 2000).

Enuresis is somewhat more common, affecting 5–10 % of five-year-olds and decreasing to about 1 % of people over the age of 15. It is defined by the Diagnostic and Statistical Manual of Mental Disorders (5th ed.; DSM–5; American Psychiatric Association, 2013) as the "repeated voiding of urine into bed or clothes, whether involuntary or intentional" (p. 355). To meet the DSM-5 criteria, the voiding must occur at least twice per week, for at least 3 months (criterion B), and the child must be at least 5 years old (criterion C). The DSM-5 (2013) describes three subtypes of enuresis. The most common form is nocturnal enuresis, commonly known as bedwetting, which accounts for approximately 85 % of cases. The remaining 15 % consists of the remaining two subtypes: diurnal enuresis, in which the child voids inappropriately during waking hours, and a combined subtype for children who void during waking hours and during nighttime sleep (5th ed.; DSM–5; American Psychiatric Association, 2013). Recently, research has suggested that nocturnal enuresis can be further divided into monosymptomatic enuresis, which is not associated with any daytime incontinence or urological symptoms, and polysymptomatic (or non-monosymptomatic) enuresis, which *is* associated with bladder dysfunction, such as urgency or toileting frequency (Butler & Holland, 2000; Djurhuus, 1999). Boys have a higher prevalence (between 50–100 % higher) of nocturnal enuresis than girls do (Chiozza et al., 1998; Foxman, Valdez, & Brook, 1986). Diurnal enuresis has a more even prevalence among girls and boys, with some studies finding it to be slightly more common in girls (Lee, Sohn, Lee, Park, & Chung, 2000; Ozden et al., 2007; Serel et al., 1997).

Another important distinction that has treatment implications is whether enuresis and encopresis are considered primary or secondary. Primary enuresis and encopresis, which are more common, refer to cases in which a child has never established a history of urinary or fecal continence (control). Secondary refers to children who

---

[1] No significant changes were made to the elimination disorders from DSM-IV to DSM-5. The disorders were previously classified under *disorders usually first diagnosed in infancy, childhood, or adolescence* in DSM-IV and exist now as an independent classification in DSM-5.

have established and maintained a minimum of six months of continence during the day and night (5th ed.; DSM–5; American Psychiatric Association, 2013). Whether primary or secondary, a psychologist working in a school setting is most likely to encounter cases of diurnal enuresis or the combined type, since both of these subtypes involve daytime accidents. With respect to encopresis, a psychologist working in a school setting is most likely to treat the retentive type because it is much more common in general. As such, the chapter will focus on the assessment, treatment, and other important considerations of these subtypes of each disorder. The information that follows is most relevant for children ages 5–12.

Etiology

A biopsychobehavioral model of retentive encopresis is summarized by Cox and colleagues (2003), who describe the ten steps that typically (although not always) occur in the development of this most common subtype. The first is a preceding event, either physical or psychological, such as a change in diet or an environmental stressor. This contributes to constipation and the formation of hard, impacted stool (2), the passing of which is painful and challenging for the child (3). Subsequently, the child anticipates future attempts will be painful (4) and begins to ignore physiological urges to defecate (5). As such, the child may avoid using the toilet entirely, which results in chronic constipation (6). However, some fecal matter above the developing impaction will move around it and leak out (typically outside of the child's awareness) (7), and parents may respond with an ineffective intervention, such as punishing the child (8). A conflict of parent intervention and child resistance typically occurs, along with continued fecal soiling (9). Ultimately, the child experiences shame, rejection, and confusion and may engage in deception to hide accidents (10). This can occur at home and in the school setting.

School factors can play a role in the etiology and maintenance of retentive encopresis. Some children (and adults for that matter) are anxious about using public toilets. Children may fear being teased at school for defecating, with the sounds and smells that are associated with this necessary activity (Har & Croffie, 2010). Schools can also contribute to the problem by limiting the amount of time children may spend in the bathroom, restricting the activity to certain times of day, and not having doors on bathroom stalls. Specifically, these factors may exacerbate fecal withholding, which may contribute to step 6, chronic constipation.

Significantly less is known about the etiology of diurnal enuresis. According to Fritz et al. (2004), genetics plays a major role. Forty-four percent of children with one enuretic parent developed one of the subtypes of the disorder, whereas 77 % of children with two enuretic parents did. The genetic transmission of enuresis may be mediated by developmental immaturity, including but not limited to lower average height and bone density as well as delayed language and sexual development. In addition, a reduced functional bladder capacity (the volume of urine in the bladder that signals the need to void to the brain) has been found in children with diurnal enuresis. Children suffering from diurnal enuresis are at increased risk of developing several comorbid disorders, including attention deficit hyperactivity disorder (ADHD), depression, and generalized anxiety. While children suffering from diurnal enuresis are more likely to have experienced parental divorce, sexual abuse, and coercive toilet training (Fritz et al., 2004), primary diurnal enuresis is rarely a result of a single environmental factor. However, diurnal enuresis in a previously continent child (secondary enuresis) can be caused by a single environmental stressor (Action, 2004).

In a cruel twist of physiology, 40 % of children who suffer from chronic constipation also have enuresis because the digestive mass in the rectum creates pressure on the bladder, leading to incontinence (Har & Croffie, 2010; Yazbeck, Schick, & O'Regan, 1987). One recent study found that 100 % of children treated for enuresis at a university urology clinic demonstrated rectal distention and 80 % were constipated (Hodges & Anthony, 2012). Amazingly, only 10 % of the parents of these children reported that their child was constipated, suggesting that constipation is often a hidden cause of enuresis.

Assessment

The proper assessment of either elimination disorder is absolutely necessary in order to determine how to proceed with treatment. Skimping on the time and care required for assessment is a surefire way to sabotage one's attempts to help these children. Because constipation is by far the most common mechanism in the development of encopresis, the assessment of encopresis must focus on constipation. Therefore, a physical examination by a physician (preferably including an abdominal x-ray) must be the first step.

A physical exam is also important because there are several rare congenital causes of encopresis. Hirschsprung's disease is the most commonly cited example of an organic cause for encopresis. Children with this disorder are born with a lack of enervation in a section of the colon, hampering peristalsis of fecal material through the large intestine. The treatment of Hirschsprung's disease is surgical, and thus attempting to treat encopresis without first obtaining medical clearance can be premature and ineffective. Other congenital problems, such as structural abnormalities of the lower digestive tract, metabolic conditions, and cystic fibrosis, can lead to encopresis.

If in fact the child is experiencing retentive encopresis, sometimes a parent will already have seen to it that a medical evaluation is completed and will provide the school psychologist with an extensive workup by a pediatric gastroenterologist. However, in most cases, the school psychologist will meet with the parent before a workup by a physician has been completed. It is important to clarify for the parent that the referral to the physician is a consult and that you, as the psychologist, will maintain responsibility for carrying out the treatment. Physicians can be indispensable in the assessment stage of treatment, but they are rarely trained to carry out the intricate functional analysis and behavioral interventions required to maximize the chances of a successful outcome. Primary care physicians in particular do not typically employ behavioral strategies that are important in preventing recurrences of encopresis. Philichi and Yuwono (2010) studied the treatment strategies suggested by pediatric primary care providers and found medications and high-fiber diets to be the most common strategies used. It is not uncommon for a pediatrician to take a history and simply put the child on a course of a laxative, which may not be sufficient to produce long-term relief.

Once congenital causes have been ruled out, a physician will typically disimpact the fecal blockage (described later) and put the child on a course of laxatives. This is a necessary step but treatment will often fail if further steps are not taken. During the time that the child is waiting to see a physician, the psychologist should be conducting his or her own assessment. Proper assessment of elimination disorders should include broadband scales of childhood psychopathology (e.g., Child Behavior Checklist; CBCL, Achenbach & Rescorla, 2001; Behavior Assessment System for Children; BASC-2, Reynolds & Kamphaus, 2006). While the evidence that children with elimination disorders are at increased risk for comorbid psychological disorders is equivocal (e.g. Cox, Morris, Borowitz, & Sutphen, 2002), such scales are nonetheless an important preparation for roadblocks that can occur during treatment.

In addition to broadband measures of psychopathology, more focused measures of encopresis symptoms can be useful. Unfortunately, objective, evidence-based measures of pediatric elimination disorders are virtually nonexistent. One notable exception is the Virginia Encopresis-Constipation Apperception Test (VECAT; Cox et al., 2003). The VECAT consists of several drawings of children, each consisting of two parts. Children (or their parents) are asked to choose the drawing that best represents them. For example, one drawing depicts a child having a painful bowel movement and a child having a bowel movement that is not painful. The scale demonstrates good test-retest reliability and internal consistency. Encopretic children who responded to treatment were found to have significantly improved VECAT scores.

In lieu of objective measures, school psychologists should collect detailed information from parents and teachers about the child's current and past stooling habits (including accidents). The frequency, timing, size, and consistency of bowel movements should be assessed, at least over a two-week period, to get a clear sense of the severity of the problem. Older children can take a more active role during this assessment phase. Christophersen and Friman (2010) suggest that children who are old enough to estimate stool volume be asked to track the number of cups of stool they produce per week. Psychologists should pay particular attention to a history of constipation (to establish a pattern of withholding). Parents often deny constipation, stating that the child has a bowel movement every day. It is important to remember that constipation can still be present, even with daily bowel movements. Passing small, pebble-like stools can indicate incomplete evacuation of the rectum and constipation. On the other hand, passing very large stools can indicate purposeful withholding, as fecal matter will build up in the colon when children withhold (Har & Croffie, 2010). Any straining, bleeding, or pain associated with bowel movements, as well as any avoidance of going to the bathroom, should also be noted (Garman & Ficca, 2012).

Since diet has been implicated in the etiology of encopresis, a detailed dietary history, including an estimate of the number of grams of dietary fiber consumed per day and an estimate of dairy and clear fluid intake, should be taken. Because exercise is related to better digestive motility and in turn softer stools (since stools that move through the large intestine more quickly have less opportunity to lose water), an account of the frequency and intensity of exercise should be recorded. Because some common medications (anticholinergics, antidepressants, antacids, iron) can contribute to constipation, they should be inquired about. Finally, information on toilet training history and on prior intervention attempts (by professionals *or* parents) should be gathered. In particular, information on the child's response to accidents is important, as hiding soiled underwear or other evidence of an accident can suggest a prior history of punishment by adults.

Once a comprehensive assessment has been conducted, the psychologist should speak with school personnel, parents, and the child to ascertain each party's motivation to participate in treatment. Parenting styles and family functioning should be assessed as well, both to understand parents' ability to institute a treatment and to assess for stressors in the child's life that may be contributing to the problem. In particular, signs of anger or blaming the child are in our experience a poor prognostic indicator for treatment. Teachers should be asked about their policies on bathroom breaks and whether they would be willing to adjust those rules.

Much of the above information also applies to enuresis. An assessment of the timing and frequency of accidents is more difficult with an enuretic child because others often do not notice an odor when an accident happens. However, timing and frequency of accidents can be estimated by the wetness of the underwear or by having a child perform a "dry check" at lunch or any other convenient time to see if an accident had occurred prior to that time. The timing of accidents can be an important indicator of treatment success as having accidents later in the day can be the first sign that treatment is working. Professionals, parents, and children alike can become disheartened if the focus is exclusively on the frequency of accidents. As described above, assessing the presence of constipation is also quite important when working with an enuretic child, as recent research suggests that a high percentage of children suffering from enuresis are constipated and that often, parents are completely unaware (Hodges & Anthony, 2012).

Intervention

Encopresis

While several strategies have been employed to treat pediatric encopresis, including cognitive behavioral play therapy (Knell & Moore, 1990), biofeedback (Loening-Baucke, 1995), paradoxical instruction (Bornstein, Sturm, Retzlaff, Kirby, &

Chong, 1981), and punishment (Edelman, 1971), most commonly, the treatment of encopresis involves four steps: education, clearing the colon of obstruction, initiating regular bowel movements, and maintaining regular bowel movements. The research literature on this comprehensive approach is sparse, however, as the vast majority of studies have only examined the components of the four-step method and few randomized controlled trials have been conducted. However, this approach is believed to be the one with the highest likelihood of success (Har & Croffie, 2010; Mikkelsen, 2001). While no studies have examined the effect of child age on treatment success, in our experience, treatment takes longer with older children. The reasons are unclear but one hypothesis is that older children tend to present with more severe symptoms that have been resistant to previous interventions. The families of older children have also had more time to build up resentment and frustration, often making a focus on family dynamics more integral to treatment than is typical with younger children.

Education

The most important goal for school psychologists in the education phase is to get across to all parties involved that the child is *almost never* soiling on purpose. This can require quite a bit of clinical skill, as it is common for parents (and teachers) to be angry and frustrated at the child by the time a psychologist becomes involved. The second goal of the education phase is to explain the functioning of the bowel in normal and encopretic children (see above) and to explain the treatment (e.g., "in order for the colon to heal, we must clean it out so it regains its natural shape and muscle tone. This will allow you to feel when you have to poop"). During the education phase, parents and the child should be praised liberally for addressing the situation proactively as there is little evidence that children "grow out of" this problem (Bernard-Bonnin, Haley, Belanger, & Nadeau, 1993; Staiano, Andreotti, Greco, Basile, & Auricchio, 1994). It is also important to communicate to parents, teachers, and the child that treatment is a difficult and time-intensive proposition. Treatment can fall apart if any of the parties involved does not remain committed for the long term. We have found it useful to actively assess and plan for barriers to treatment success. For example, sometimes an initial improvement can lead to reduced motivation, or logistical barriers such as vacations or visits to a noncustodial parent can halt progress.

Disimpaction

There are a number of commonly used methods of emptying the colon of fecal obstruction. Little research has directly compared the different methods, so a discussion with the family about *their* preferences with respect to the different methods is a sound approach. Parents can choose to (1) administer enemas, which push fluid into the rectum, softening the stool and stretching the rectum walls, creating an overwhelming urge to pass a bowel movement; (2) administer suppositories, which typically work by irritating the bowel, causing it to contract; (3) administer oral laxatives, which generally cause the retention of water in the colon, softening the stool and causing diarrhea; (4) have the child take oral stool softeners, which moisten the stool; and (5) have the child take oral lubricants, which grease the stool, enabling it to move through the colon more easily. All of these methods require over-the-counter medication and can generally taken without a physician's supervision. These options are all safe and each has its own guidelines for administration, which are beyond the scope of this chapter. In general, parents often prefer to attempt a "clean out" over the course of a weekend, when any subsequent diarrhea can be more easily dealt with. This step is important because if the impaction is not fully cleared, the treatment as a whole is unlikely to succeed.

Initiating Regular Bowel Movements

In many cases, as soon as the colon is completely evacuated, the encopresis improves dramatically. However, some children experience a new impaction soon after the colon has been cleaned out. In particular, children who have had constipation for a long time are at greater risk for a reoccurrence. For some children, it takes time (up to a year) for the colon to "heal" and regain muscle tone after it has been stretched out by constipation. The stretching can cause habituation to the feeling of distention (McGrath et al., 2000), which may be why children continue to be at risk for further impacted stools.

There are two components to initiating regular bowel movements. The first is scheduled toilet sits and the second is continued use of laxatives. Children should get in the habit of sitting on the toilet for 5–15 minutes after breakfast and again after dinner. Many families have busy schedules and their children are not in the habit of making time to pass bowel movements. By establishing regular "bathroom times" after meals, we take advantage of the gastrocolic reflex, which are intestinal contractions that occur in response to eating. This explains why some people have bowel movements every morning after breakfast or every evening after dinner. To ensure enough time in the morning to have a bowel movement, the child should be instructed to eat breakfast as close to awakening as possible. Another reason that it is useful to establish regular bathroom times after breakfast and dinner is that some children are unwilling to pass bowel movements at school (just as many adults are unwilling to pass bowel movements at work).

Praises, tangible rewards, and allowing a special toy only while the child is on the toilet are ways to increase compliance. School psychologists can also use imagery techniques to help the child imagine a relaxed and pain-free bowel movement. General stress reduction strategies can also be helpful as there is some evidence that high stress levels contribute to constipation (Philichi, 2008). In conjunction with scheduled bathroom visits, laxatives are administered regularly to produce soft, painless bowel movements. While some parents worry about "addiction" to laxatives, there is no evidence to support this fear (Müller-Lissner, Kamm, Scarpignato, & Wald, 2005).

Maintaining Regular Bowel Movements

The changes required to help prevent a reoccurrence of constipation are perhaps the most difficult to maintain. Fundamental changes to the child's lifestyle are required. These include (1) Consuming more fiber: The American Academy of Pediatrics recommends a daily intake of dietary fiber equivalent to the child's age plus 5 g. Parents can be provided with a handout listing the fiber content of foods. In general, insoluble fiber, such as corn, promotes motility better than does soluble fiber, since it does not dissolve in water. (2) Drinking more water: Significantly increasing fiber consumption without also increasing clear fluid intake can lead to a worsening of constipation. In particular, children should consume water and not clear sugary liquids, such as fruit juice (Kuhl, Felt, & Patton, 2009). Research has demonstrated that if water intake is specifically targeted in a multifaceted intervention, it can be increased significantly for encopretic children (Kuhl et al., 2010). (3) Consuming fewer dairy products: Because dairy products take more time to digest, they can worsen constipation. Constipation may also be caused by intolerance to cow's milk (Iacono et al., 1998). Therefore, children should consume the equivalent of one pint *or less* of milk. Parents and teachers can work together to reduce dairy intake. (4) Doing more exercise, since it promotes intestinal motility (Dobson, 2009). In some ways, these lifestyle changes are easier to implement with younger children, since parents and teachers have more control over what children eat. However, we have found that for these changes to be maintained, a commitment from all family members to change their habits is necessary. It is difficult to convince a child to eat more vegetables if the rest of the family often eats highly processed food.

In addition, school psychologists can suggest to parents that they model sitting on the toilet in a relaxed manner for their children. Parents can also be instructed to purchase a small step stool so that the child can increase leverage to push more effectively during a bowel movement (Schonwald & Sheldon, 2006). The psychologist can also work closely with teachers and the school nurse to establish a toileting schedule and to allow bathroom breaks in a nonjudgmental manner. Parents should be instructed to provide teachers with clean clothing, wet wipes, and plastic bags to store soiled clothing (Garman & Ficca, 2012). Because laxatives are employed after the child is disimpacted, there may still be episodes of fecal incontinence early on. Teachers should be made aware of this and have a plan in place for managing accidents.

The treatment of children with non-retentive encopresis varies considerably from the description above. Because these children are by definition not constipated, disimpaction of the colon is unnecessary. While that modification is clear, little else about the treatment of these children is. Unfortunately, not a single controlled study has been published on the assessment and treatment of these children, and to our knowledge, no manualized treatments exist. In a recently published and quite outstanding book on elimination disorders (Christophersen & Friman, 2010), roughly ten pages are devoted to the description of treatments for retentive encopresis, while only *one paragraph* covers the treatment of non-retentive encopresis.

What is a psychologist working in the schools to do with an encopretic child who gets a clean bill of health from a physician? The consensus among researchers seems to be that the soiling behavior in these cases should be assessed in a similar way to any problem behavior. In other words, while soiling is a particularly unappealing problem behavior, it is in many ways no different than any other inappropriate child behavior. The implication of this approach is that a psychologist should use behavioral assessment skills to develop a careful functional analysis of the behavior. While a description of functional analysis is beyond the scope of this chapter, the psychologist's goal should be to identify the controlling variables of the behavior. If the soiling appears to be positively reinforced (e.g., by adult attention) or negatively reinforced (e.g., by escape from classroom demands), psychologists would seek to modify those operant processes by reducing or eliminating the reinforcers and instead reinforcing incompatible (the absence of accidents) behaviors. If, on the other hand, a functional analysis reveals that the soiling does not principally function to obtain reinforcement and instead is a respondent behavior (e.g., a conditioned response to the presence of a barking dog in the schoolyard), the psychologist might use stimulus control (e.g., removing the dog) or exposure (to the dog) to reduce the behavior. It is important to keep in mind that if the soiling is an operant behavior, it is likely that the child exhibits other problematic behavior (e.g., defiance, tantruming) that serves the same function. School psychologists may want to employ broader behavioral interventions, such as parent management training or school-based behavioral interventions, and not focus simply on the soiling. One last caution is that school psychologists should avoid jumping to conclusions about the meaning of soiling behavior. We have experienced quite a few school personnel proclaiming that soiling is "a sign" of trauma or sexual abuse. Research does not support this claim (Mellon, Whiteside, & Friedrich, 2006). Behavioral assessment works best when clinicians have an open mind about controlling variables and actively look for disconfirming evidence.

A psychologist working with a child with encopresis will want to stay involved even after the child's condition has improved or been cured because the negative consequences of having had accidents at school or at home in the presence of classmates can last far longer than the symptoms of encopresis do. Psychologists will often need to shift gears from solving the elimination problem to preventing and dealing with teasing or ostracizing of the encopretic child.

Enuresis

The evidence-based treatment of enuresis has several distinct steps as well. As with the treatment of encopresis, the first step is education. Education on how common enuresis is and why it happens will often serve to reduce guilt in parents and shame in children. Children can also be taught the difference between the feeling of a full and empty bladder by having them describe the pressure, discomfort, and other sensations they feel in each state. One may be tempted to skip this step with children under 7, assuming that they will not understand the physiology of urination, but even a simple stick drawing showing that the brain and the bladder "talk to each other" and sometimes the bladder fails to communicate to the brain that it is full can bring an enormous sense of relief to a child.

There are two treatment components for diurnal enuresis that are supported by the literature and are often used in combination (Christophersen & Friman, 2010). The first is the urine alarm, which has, by far, the most empirical support, although the vast majority of studies have demonstrated its effectiveness with nocturnal enuresis (e.g., Friman, 2008). Three published studies have found the urine alarm to be effective for diurnal enuresis (Halliday, Meadow, & Berg, 1987; Friman & Vollmer, 1995; Van Laecke et al., 2006). However, only the Halliday study was a group-based experiment. The most common type of urine alarm has a sensor that goes in the underwear and sets off an audible alarm when it comes into contact with liquid. When used at night, the alarm wakes the child so that he or she can use the bathroom. An audible alarm is not desirable for a child with diurnal enuresis, since it would alert others to an accident, so in recent years, a number of vibrating urine alarms have been developed. The exact mechanism of action of the alarm is not fully understood, but the consensus among researchers seems to be that it works to negatively reinforce the behavior of walking to the bathroom because the alert is aversive to the child.

The second treatment component with empirical support is teaching children to perform Kegel exercises, in which the child practices initiating and interrupting the flow of urine (and maintaining the contraction for 5 s). The activity can be made more pleasurable by allowing the child to drink his or her favorite drink in order to produce urine. Having boys aim for a Cheerio in the toilet bowl can also make this activity more enjoyable. The practice is theorized to strengthen the muscles around the pelvic organs. Only one study has examined this treatment component with children suffering with diurnal enuresis. Schneider, King, and Surwit (1994) found that with fewer than two hours of professional intervention time, having children practice Kegel exercises three times per day eliminated daytime wetting in 60 % of the 79 children in the sample. Interestingly, children who had both diurnal and nocturnal enuresis tended to show improvements in both problems.

While pharmacological agents (e.g., DDAVP) are often used in the treatment of nocturnal enuresis, they are not well studied in children with diurnal enuresis and remain controversial due to their side effects and lack of effectiveness when withdrawn.

As with the treatment of encopresis, teachers should be incorporated into the treatment of diurnal enuresis. The main way that teachers can help is by allowing children to use the bathroom as often as needed. Care must be taken that this does not become a distraction. Children can be asked to construct a number of "bathroom passes" that allow them to use the bathroom. The child is instructed to hand a pass to the teacher, without fanfare, so that he can silently be excused to use the bathroom. A small incentive can be provided for unused passes at the end of the day so that children only use them when necessary (Christophersen & Friman, 2010). If parents cannot afford to purchase a vibrating urine underwear alarm or a vibrating wristwatch, the teacher will need to help remind the child to use the bathroom at predetermined times. The school psychologist can work with the teacher or school nurse to gradually extend the intervals between bathroom visits and to praise the child for making it to the next scheduled bathroom break. Intervention components that can be done at home, such as having the child put soiled clothes in the laundry basket (a mildly aversive activity) and overlearning, where the child drinks extra liquid to consolidate treatment gains, can be added to promote generalization.

Case Example

Max was a 7-year-old, second-grade boy when the school nurse referred him to the school psychologist for treatment. An initial description from the nurse revealed that he was having bowel movements in his pull-ups (he had never fully transitioned to underwear) one to two times per week in school. The school nurse also reported that Max was urinating in his pull-ups about twice per week. Max's teacher reported that he was inattentive, impulsive, and occasionally exhibited tantrums in class. Max lived with his parents and an 11-year-old sister who attended the nearby middle school.

The psychologist asked Max's parents to meet with her at school without Max present. Max's parents reported that he had never fully established fecal or urinary continence and that while the fecal incontinence was limited to the daytime, the urinary incontinence happened at night as well. Max's parents were embarrassed and frustrated but believed that he would outgrow these problems. They stated that in frustration, they had begun to use time-outs to try to limit the episodes at home. In addition, they mentioned that Max was being teased in school about these problems and he had started resisting getting on the school bus in the mornings. The psychologist did some psychoeducation during this meeting, explaining to Max's parents that typically developing children with incontinence rarely soil themselves on purpose. Max's parents were asked to cease using pull-ups at night, time-outs at home, and obtain a workup from a nearby pediatric gastroenterologist and a urologist before the following meeting. In addition, a number of assessments were to be completed before the next session, including a Child Behavior Checklist (CBCL), Virginia Encopresis-Constipation Apperception Test (VECAT), and a detailed monitoring of urination and bowel movements. Although they admitted that Max's problems were putting a strain on their relationship, since they argued about how to handle them, Max's parents appeared committed and eager to participate in his treatment and complete these necessary preliminary steps.

Max, his mother, and father all attended the following session, which sought to gather additional information, review assessments, and deliver further psychoeducation about his conditions. While Max fidgeted and moved around the office, his parents reported that the pediatric gastroenterologist and urologist could not find any congenital causes for Max's incontinence. However, Max's parents reported that the gastroenterologist had palpated a sizable mass of solidified fecal matter in Max's rectum. They were confused as to how this could happen, as Max had bowel movements most days. Max became tearful and said that most mornings and evenings, very little stool ended up in the toilet. His parents asked why he hadn't told them, and Max responded that he didn't like talking about it. Results from the CBCL revealed clinically significant scores on the social problems and attention problem syndrome scales and an elevated score for the depressed syndrome scale. Over the course of the week, bowel movements were either absent or very small on most days, and Max had two enuretic episodes during the day and one at night. Max completed the VECAT with the help of his mother, and a score of 24 indicated significant problems with bowel movements.

For the remainder of this session, a psychoeducational approach was taken while continuing to understand Max's perspective. The biopsychobehavioral models of retentive encopresis and enuresis were explained to Max and his parents, using child-friendly illustrations. It was imperative to convey to Max and his parents that his presentation was common. Max appeared to feel liberated, knowing that these were truly accidents, not his fault, and that he wouldn't receive time-outs as a result.

Prior to the next session, his parents were instructed to buy commercially available enemas and administer them for three days in order to fully disimpact fecal matter and proceed with treatment. In addition, they were asked to purchase a vibrating urine alarm for Max to wear during the daytime and nighttime, as well as a wristwatch with a vibrate setting to remind Max to go to the bathroom.

At the next session, Max's parents reported success with using the enema, and they checked on him after each time he sat on the toilet. He returned to having regular bowel movements by the day before this session. Although the frequency of urinary incontinence decreased once the constipation was resolved, he continued to have some episodes during school and on weekends. This session focused on maintaining the progress made toward the treatment of encopresis and implementing strategies to reduce Max's persisting urinary incontinence. A schedule of bathroom visits was created for the home and school, as well as corresponding sticker charts. He was able to place up to six stickers per day on his chart, each as a reward for sitting on the toilet and attempting to void urine and feces. This occurred after breakfast, three times throughout the school day or weekend, after dinner, and at bedtime. After the session, Max decorated the chart and picked out his favorite kind of stickers from the supermarket. After Max had collected 35 stickers (average of five completed bathroom sits per day), he was rewarded with a weekend trip to the local dinosaur museum with his father (no sisters allowed!). In addition, the schedule during school was coordinated with Max's teacher, who agreed to review progress with him discretely at the end of each day. She also agreed to let Max use up to five bathroom passes per day. Max was allowed to use the bathroom in the school nurse's office, which was more private.

Learning how to affix the vibrating urine alarm was challenging, as Max had a difficult time deciding where it would be most comfortable to have it vibrate. However, he ultimately found a nonintrusive position that alerted him well enough, and his parents agreed to help him put it on for the first week before school and place it appropriately at bedtime. For the remainder of the session, an emphasis was placed on a new diet that included significantly more water and fiber, as well as fewer dairy items. This served to limit the possibility of hard and painful stools in the future.

In the following session, Max and his parents reported some success but a number of difficulties. Max had earned a trip to the museum and per his homeroom teacher's report, Max enthusiastically completed his bathroom visits. He had no accidents that involved stool, but did have an incident in which he voided a noticeable amount of urine at school, which resulted in significant embarrassment. This occurred because he found the urine alarm uncomfortable during recess, removed it, and put it in his backpack. Max became excited during recess and forgot to perform one of his scheduled bathroom visits. He also had two bed-wetting incidents (late in his sleep cycle, as evidenced by the wetness of the bed upon waking), but Max was not uncomfortable with the alarm at night so no intervention was necessary. In addition to the accident at school, Max exhibited tantrums during snack after school because his parents told him he could not have cheese, one of his favorite snacks.

At this point, there was considerable rapport built with Max, and the next session was started without his parents. The first intervention was to discuss Max's sadness about his accident during the week. He told the story of what happened and after some empathic listening, the story was used as a rationale for trying to use the urine alarm more effectively and completing his bathroom visits in the future. The enuresis diagram was reviewed with Max, and the goal of strengthening the connection between the brain and bladder was reinforced. Max reported to the therapist that his stools did not hurt at all in the past week and asked to have cheese again. His parents were brought back into the room and the whole family agreed upon a new contingency; if Max wore the urine alarm during the day, regardless of accident occurrence, 1.5 ounces of cheese would be allowed for a snack in the afternoon. Max's parents agreed to follow this plan closely and monitor Max for any hard stools throughout the week.

By the next session, Max's parents were less frustrated and reported decreased tantrums and no accidents at home. They even reported less marital strain and healthier eating themselves. The small amount of cheese each day was working well as a reward for wearing the urine alarm, and his parents reported no hard stools. The daily increase of water and fiber appeared to compensate for the small but rewarding amount of dairy. Max was continuing to use his sticker chart to track bathroom visits and received another trip with dad. However, a small accident occurred at school, and Max voided some urine into his pants before being able to stop from the vibration of the alarm.

At this point in the treatment, all of the contingencies for maintaining regular bowel movements and decreasing urinary incontinence were in place, and the final four sessions focused on how to respond to continued teasing from classmates (although it had decreased). In addition, progress with continence and adherence to the behavioral and diet plan continued to be tracked. Max had no encopretic incidents throughout this time and averaged one small urinary accident per week, usually at school. He improved his ability to use his pelvic floor muscles when the vibration from the urinary alarm began at the onset of wetness. At a six-month follow-up, Max maintained his success with the treatment of encopresis and averaged one enuretic incident per month. Max maintained a clinically significant score on the CBCL attention problem syndrome scale, but his score in the social problem scale was reduced to elevated, and depression was in the normal range. Max's score on the VECAT was consistent with peers who had only minor encopresis problems. He reported less sadness and was working toward having play dates with a number of peers with whom he had grown friendlier. Max's parents even reported planning a sleepover for Max at a friend's house.

Special Topic: Working With Comorbid Problems

While many children with elimination disorders do not exhibit clinically significant comorbid problems (Cox et al., 2002), treating children who do can be particularly challenging. Clinicians often have questions about whether to treat the elimination problem or the comorbid problems first. There is also often confusion about how to handle the barriers to treatment success that these co-occurring problems pose. While research has not conclusively demonstrated whether elimination disorders are a risk factor for the development of comorbid conditions or whether the mechanism is reversed (Shaffer, 1973), it is clear that these problems often occur in tandem. For example, Levine, Mazonson, and Bakow (1980) found that encopretic children who were classified as "uncured" after treatment showed more aggressive behaviors, on average, before treatment than did the group who would go on to experience treatment success. Van Hoecke, De Fruyt, De Clercq, Hoebeke, and Walle (2006) found that enuretic children (with combined nocturnal and diurnal enuresis) were, on average, less conscientious and more neurotic than typically developing children. Significant differences were also observed between the two groups on the Child Behavior Checklist, internalizing and externalizing scales, and on ADHD problems.

Comorbid conditions can seriously interfere with the treatment of elimination disorders. For example, in encopretic children, significant noncompliance can be a barrier to disimpaction and scheduled toilet visits. In a similar way, dysfunctional family dynamics can interfere with treatment. For instance, encopretic children are more likely than typically developing children to come from families with low levels of organization (Cox et al., 2002). Treatment for both encopresis and enuresis requires a compliant child and a consistent, organized approach from parents and teachers.

Attention problems are also fairly common in children with elimination disorders. For example, Mellon et al., (2013) found that children with ADHD were 2.1 times as likely to meet the DSM-IV criteria for enuresis and 1.8 times as likely to meet the criteria for encopresis than were non-ADHD controls. Not only might attention issues contribute to the development of an elimination disorder (Johnston & Wright, 1993), they may also hamper treatment. In our experience, children with attention problems tend to have difficulty experiencing the urge to urinate and defecate. They can even have full accidental bowel movements and not even realize it, even when it is apparent to everyone else in the room! Not only does inattention make treatment more difficult, it can cause adults to lose empathy and suspect that the child is incontinent on purpose, since it doesn't seem possible that he wouldn't notice his accidents. In such situations, it is particularly important to have the child evaluated for possible concurrent treatment for inattention. In addition, the treatment for the elimination disorder itself will often require adjusting. In particular, reminders and cues for using the bathroom must be made even more vivid and clear. For example, as described in the case study above, instead of having the child remember to make a scheduled toilet visit during the day, parents can send their child to school with a wristwatch or a urine alarm that vibrates or beeps at the appropriate time. Teachers can set reminders for themselves to tell the child (subtly of course) that it is time for a scheduled bathroom visit. A brightly colored Post-it (that only the enuretic child knows is a cue for a bathroom break) can be placed in a prominent place in the classroom.

There are no objective data about how best to approach these complicated cases. As a result, psychologists working in schools who are faced with such a client are strongly urged to develop and be guided by a clear case conceptualization (e.g., Murphy & Christner, 2006). Our experience has been that, in general, the elimination disorder should be treated first, because it is often so disruptive to every aspect of family functioning, that its resolution can have positive cascading effects on the child's other problems, the parent-child relationship, academic performance, the child's physical health, and even the marital relationship. However, if one's case conceptualization identifies clear barriers to treatment success (Linehan, 1993), those should be prioritized and resolved before the elimination disorder is addressed. As heart breaking as it may be, some co-occurring situations such as peer ridicule can serve to increase commitment on the part of the child, teacher, and parent to comply with treatment. Of course, for other children, teasing from peers can reduce motivation. A thorough case conceptualization will help the clinician to understand what co-occurring issues are exacerbating the elimination disorder and which ones are unfortunate sequelae of the problem and are likely to improve with its resolution.

In conclusion, the treatment of elimination problems within a school setting remains an uncertain proposition, due in part to the lack of high-quality research in this area. Table 11.1 contains information on the stronger available studies. However, a school psychologist who is armed with the right information and who has a solid foundation in case conceptualization, behavioral assessment, and treatment can save many of these children from the frustration and anguish that result from dealing with an elimination disorder.

Table 11.1 Experimental Research for Assessment and Intervention of Elimination Disorders

Reference	Sample	Measures	Results
Cox, D. J., Ritterband, L. M., Quillian, W., Kovatchev, B., Morris, J., Sutphen, J., & Borowitz, S. (2003). Assessment of behavioral mechanisms maintaining encopresis: Virginia encopresis-constipation apperception test. *Journal of Pediatric Psychology, 28*(6), 375-382	87 encopretic 27 non-encopretic siblings 35 non-encopretic controls	*VECAT*: Virginia Encopresis-Constipation Apperception Test	Encopretic children scored higher on the VECAT, reduction in posttreatment scores
Cox, D. J., Morris, J., Borowitz, S. M., & Sutphen, J. L. (2002). Psychological differences of children with and without chronic encopresis. *Journal of Pediatric Psychology, 27*, 585–591	86 encopretic 62 non-encopretic controls	*CBCL*: Child Behavior Checklist *TRF*: Teacher Rating Form *WRAT*: Wide Range Achievement Test *PH*: Piers-Harris Self-Perception	Increased anxiety, depression, family problems, social problems, disruptive behavior Decreased school performance, attention, and self-esteem
Kuhl, E. S., Felt, B. T., & Patton, S. R. (2009). Brief report: Adherence to fluid recommendations in children receiving treatment for retentive encopresis. *Journal of Pediatric Psychology, 34*, 1165–1169	26 encopretic children	Chart review of mean daily fluid intake during group behavioral treatment	Mean fluid intake increased by 30 %, but only 48 % of children met fluid intake goals
Kuhl, E. S., Hoodin, F., Rice, J., Felt, B. T., Rausch, J. R., & Patton, S. R. (2010). Increasing daily water intake and fluid adherence in children receiving treatment for Retentive Encopresis. *Journal of Pediatric Psychology, 35*(10), 1144–1151	18 encopretic in enhanced intervention (EI) 19 encopretic in standard care (SC)	Comparison of diet diary over the course of 7-week treatment	Mean fluid intake significantly greater in EI, and EI participants 4–6 times more likely to meet fluid intake goals
Johnston, B.D., & Wright, J.A. (1993). Attentional dysfunction in children with Encopresis. *Journal of Developmental and Behavioral Pediatrics*, 14(6), 381–385	167 child clinic patients	*CBCL*: Child Behavior Checklist, hyperactivity scale	Children with encopresis were 10 times more likely to have clinically significant hyperactivity on CBCL
Levine, M. D., Mazonson, P., & Bakow, H. (1980). Behavioral symptom substitution in children cured of encopresis. *American Journal of Diseases of Children*, 134, 663–667	47 previously encopretic children		No symptom substitution was found in a three-year follow-up of treated encopretic children

(continued)

Table 11.1 (continued)

Reference	Sample	Measures	Results
Van Hoecke, E., De Fruyt, F., De Clercq, B., Hoebeke, P., & Walle, J. V. (2006). Internalizing and externalizing problem behavior in children with nocturnal and diurnal enuresis: A five-factor model perspective. *Journal of Pediatric Psychology, 31*(5), 460–468	85 combined-type enuretics 56 nocturnal enuretics 155 healthy controls	*HiPIC*: Hierarchical Personality Inventory for Children *CBCL*: Child Behavior Checklist *DBDRS*: Dutch Disruptive Behavior Disorder Rating Scale	Combined-type children are less conscientious and more neurotic Combined-type children increased internalizing, externalizing, attentional, and hyperactivity difficulties

References

Achenbach, T. M., & Rescorla, L. A. (2001). *Manual for the ASEBA school-age forms and profiles*. Burlington, VT: University of Vermont, Research Center for Children, Youth, and Families.

Action, A. O. (2004). Practice parameters for the assessment and treatment of children and adolescents with enuresis. *Journal of the American Academy of Child and Adolescent Psychiatry, 43*, 1540–1550.

American Psychiatric Association. (2013). *Diagnostic and statistical manual of mental disorders* (5th ed.). http://dx.doi.org/10.1176/appi.books.9780890425596.910646

Bernard-Bonnin, A. C., Haley, N., Belanger, S., & Nadeau, D. (1993). Parental and patient perceptions about encopresis and its treatment. *Journal of Developmental and Behavioral Pediatrics, 14*(6), 397–400.

Bornstein, P. H., Sturm, C. A., Retzlaff, P. D., Kirby, K. L., & Chong, H. (1981). Paradoxical instruction in the treatment of encopresis and chronic constipation: An experimental analysis. *Journal of Behavior Therapy and Experimental Psychiatry, 12*(2), 167–170.

Butler, R. J., & Holland, P. (2000). The three systems: a conceptual way of understanding nocturnal enuresis. *Scandinavian journal of urology and nephrology, 34*(4), 270–277.

Butler, R. J., Heron, J., & The ALSPAC Study Team. (2006). Exploring the differences between mono- and polysymptomatic nocturnal enuresis. *Scandinavian Journal of Urology and Nephrology, 40*, 313–319.

Chiozza, M. L., Bernardinelli, L., Caione, P., Del Gado, R., Ferrara, P., Giorgi, P. L., … & Vertucci, P. (1998). An Italian epidemiological multicentre study of nocturnal enuresis. *British Journal of Urology, 81*(s3), 86-89.

Christophersen, E. R., & Friman, P. C. (2010). *Elimination disorders in children and adolescents (2010)*. Cambridge, MA: Hogrefe.

Cox, D. J., Morris, J., Borowitz, S. M., & Sutphen, J. L. (2002). Psychological differences of children with and without chronic encopresis. *Journal of Pediatric Psychology, 27*, 585–591.

Cox, D. J., Ritterband, L. M., Quillian, W., Kovatchev, B., Morris, J., Sutphen, J., et al. (2003). Assessment of behavioral mechanisms maintaining encopresis: Virginia encopresis-constipation apperception test. *Journal of Pediatric Psychology, 28*(6), 375–382.

Djurhuus, J. C. (1999). Definitions of subtypes of enuresis. *Scandinavian Journal of Urology and Nephrology Supplement, 202*, 5–7.

Dobson, P. (2009). Assessing and treating faecal incontinence in children. *Nursing Standard, 24*, 49–56.

Edelman, R. I. (1971). Operant conditioning treatment of encopresis. *Journal of Behavior Therapy and Experimental Psychiatry, 2*(1), 71–73.

Fishman, L., Rappaport, L., Schonwald, A., & Nurko, S. (2003). Trends in referral to a single encopresis clinic over 20 years. *Pediatrics, 111*(5), e604–e607.

Foxman, B., Valdez, R. B., & Brook, R. H. (1986). Childhood enuresis: prevalence, perceived impact, and prescribed treatments. *Pediatrics, 77*, 482–487.

Friman, P. C. (2008). Evidence-based therapies for enuresis and encopresis. In R. G. Steele, T. D. Elkin, & M. C. Roberts (Eds.), *Handbook of evidence-based therapies for children and adolescents* (pp. 311–333). New York, NY: Springer.

Friman, P. C., & Vollmer, D. (1995). Successful use of the nocturnal urine alarm for diurnal enuresis. *Journal of Applied Behavior Analysis, 28*(1), 89–90.

Fritz, et al., (2004). Practice parameter for the assessment and treatment of children and adolescents with enuresis. *Journal of the American Academy of Child & Adolescent Psychiatry, 43*(12), 1540-1550.

Garman, K., & Ficca, M. (2012). Managing encopresis in the elementary school setting: The school nurse's role. *The Journal of School Nursing, 28*(3), 175–180.

Halliday, S., Meadow, S. R., & Berg, I. (1987). Successful management of daytime enuresis using alarm procedures: A randomly controlled trial. *Archives of Disease in Childhood, 62*(2), 132–137.

Har, A. F., & Croffie, J. M. (2010). Encopresis. *Pediatrics in Review, 31*, 368–374.

Hodges, S. J., & Anthony, E. Y. (2012). Occult megarectum–A commonly unrecognized cause of enuresis. *Urology, 79*(2), 421–424.

Iacono, G., et al. (1998). Intolerance of cow's milk and chronic constipation in children. *New England Journal of Medicine, 339*(16), 1100–1104.

Johnston, B. D., & Wright, J. A. (1993). Attentional dysfunction in children with encopresis. *Journal of Developmental and Behavioral Pediatrics, 14*, 381–385.

Knell, S. M., & Moore, D. J. (1990). Cognitive-behavioral play therapy in the treatment of encopresis. *Journal of Clinical Child Psychology, 19*(1), 55–60.

Kuhl, E. S., Felt, B. T., & Patton, S. R. (2009). Brief report: Adherence to fluid recommendations in children receiving treatment for retentive encopresis. *Journal of Pediatric Psychology, 34*, 1165–1169.

Kuhl, E. S., Hoodin, F., Rice, J., Felt, B. T., Rausch, J. R., & Patton, S. R. (2010). Increasing daily water intake and fluid adherence in children receiving treatment for retentive encopresis. *Journal of Pediatric Psychology, 35*(10), 1144–1151.

Lee, S. D., Sohn, D. W., Lee, J. Z., Park, N. C., & Chung, M. K. (2000). An epidemiological study of enuresis in Korean children. *BJU International, 85*(7), 869–873.

Levine, M. D., Mazonson, P., & Bakow, H. (1980). Behavioral symptom substitution in children cured of encopresis. *American Journal of Diseases of Children, 134*, 663–667.

Linehan, M. (1993). *Cognitive-behavioral treatment of borderline personality disorder*. New York, NY: The Guilford Press.

Loening-Baucke, V. (1995). Biofeedback treatment for chronic constipation and encopresis in childhood: Long-term outcome. *Pediatrics, 96*(1), 105–110.

McGrath, M. L., Mellon, M. W., & Murphy, L. (2000). Empirically supported treatments in pediatric psychology: Constipation and encopresis. *Journal of Pediatric Psychology, 25*(4), 225–254.

Mellon, M. W., Natchev, B. E., Katusic, S. K., Colligan, R. C., Weaver, A. L., Voigt, R. G., et al. (2013). Incidence of enuresis and encopresis among children with Attention Deficit Hyperactivity Disorder in a population-based birth cohort. *Academic Pediatrics, 13*(4), 322–327.

Mellon, M. W., Whiteside, S. P., & Friedrich, W. N. (2006). The relevance of fecal soiling as an indicator of child sexual abuse: A preliminary analysis. *Journal of Developmental and Behavioral Pediatrics, 27*(1), 25–32.

Mikkelsen, E. J. (2001). Enuresis and encopresis: Ten years of progress. *Journal of the American Academy of Child and Adolescent Psychiatry, 40*(10), 1146–1158.

Müller-Lissner, S. A., Kamm, M. A., Scarpignato, C., & Wald, A. (2005). Myths and misconceptions about chronic constipation. *The American Journal of Gastroenterology, 100*(1), 232–242.

Murphy, V. B., & Christner, R. W. (2006). A cognitive-behavioral case conceptualization approach for working with children and adolescents. In R. B. Mennuti, A. Freeman, & R. W. Christner (Eds.), *Cognitive behavioral interventions in educational settings: A handbook for practice.* New York, NY: Routledge.

Ozden, C., Ozdal, O. L., Altinova, S., Oguzulgen, I., Urgancioglu, G., & Memis, A. (2007). Prevalence and associated factors of enuresis in Turkish children. *International Brazilian Journal of Urology, 33*(2), 216–222.

Philichi, L. (2008). When the going gets tough. *Gastroenterology Nursing, 31*, 121–130.

Philichi, L., & Yuwono, M. (2010). Primary Care: Constipation and encopresis treatment strategies and reasons to refer. *Gastroenterology Nursing, 33*(5), 363.

Reynolds, C. R., & Kamphaus, R. W. (2006). *BASC-2: Behavior assessment system for children* (2nd ed.). Upper Saddle River, NJ: Pearson.

Schneider, M. S., King, L. R., & Surwit, R. S. (1994). Kegel exercises and childhood incontinence: A new role for an old treatment. *The Journal of Pediatrics, 124*(1), 91–92.

Schonwald, A. D., & Rappaport, L. A. (2008). Elimination conditions. In M. L. Wolraich, D. D. Drotar, P. H. Dworkin, & E. C. Perrin (Eds.), *Developmental-behavioral pediatrics* (pp. 791–804). Philadelphia, PA: Mosby.

Schonwald, A. D., & Sheldon, G. G. (2006). *The pocket idiot's guide to potty training problems.* Royersford, PA: Alpha.

Serel, T. A., Akhan, G., Koyuncuoglu, H. R., Öztürk, A., Dogruer, K., Ünal, S., et al. (1997). Epidemiology of enuresis in Turkish children. *Scandinavian Journal of Urology and Nephrology, 31*(6), 537–539.

Shaffer, D. (1973). The association between enuresis and emotional disorder: A review of the literature. In I. Kolvin, R. C. McKeith, & S. R. Meadow (Eds.), *Bladder control and enuresis* (pp. 118–136). London: William Heinemann Medical Books.

Staiano, A., Andreotti, M. R., Greco, L., Basile, P., & Auricchio, S. (1994). Long-term follow-up of children with chronic idiopathic constipation. *Digestive Diseases and Sciences, 39*(3), 561–564.

Van der Wal, M. F., Benninga, M. A., & Hirasing, R. A. (2005). The prevalence of encopresis in a multicultural population. *Journal of Pediatric Gastroenterology and Nutrition, 40*(3), 345–348.

Van Hoecke, E., De Fruyt, F., De Clercq, B., Hoebeke, P., & Walle, J. V. (2006). Internalizing and externalizing problem behavior in children with nocturnal and diurnal enuresis: A five-factor model perspective. *Journal of Pediatric Psychology, 31*(5), 460–468.

Van Laecke, E., Wille, S., Vande Walle, J., Raes, A., Renson, C., Peeren, F., et al. (2006). The daytime alarm: A useful device for the treatment of children with daytime incontinence. *The Journal of Urology, 176*(1), 325–327.

Yazbeck, S., Schick, E., & O'Regan, S. (1987). Relevance of constipation to enuresis, urinary tract infection and reflux. A review. *European Urology, 13*(5), 318–321.

Part III
Interventions: The Practitioner's Tool-Kit

Chapter 12
Cognitive Interventions

**Prerna Arora, Patrick Pössel, Allison D. Barnard, Mark Terjesen,
Betty S. Lai, Caroline J. Ehrlich, Kathleen I. Diaz, Rebecca Rialon Berry,
and Anna K. Gogos**

Cognitive Restructuring : As per Beck

Prerna Arora

Cognitive-behavioral interventions are founded on the principle that individuals' thoughts about their experiences and themselves influence their affect and behavior (Beck, 1967). When these thoughts are distorted, they can trigger maladaptive information processing, leading to the development of pathological symptoms.

P. Arora, Ph.D. (✉)
Division of Child and Adolescent Psychiatry, University of Maryland School of Medicine,
Baltimore, MD, USA
e-mail: arorapm@gmail.com

P. Pössel, Dr. rer. soc. (✉) • A.D. Barnard, M.S.
Department of Educational & Counseling Psychology, Counseling, and College
Student Personnel, University of Louisville, Louisville, KY, USA
e-mail: patrick.possel@louisville.edu; Allisondbarnard@gmail.com

M. Terjesen, Ph.D. (✉)
Department of Psychology, St. John's University, Jamaica, NY, USA
e-mail: terjesem@stjohns.edu

B.S. Lai, Ph.D. (✉)
Division of Epidemiology and Biostatistics, School of Public Health, Georgia State
University, P.O. Box 3984, Atlanta, GA 30302-3984, USA
e-mail: bettylai10@yahoo.com; blai@gsu.edu

C.J. Ehrlich, M.S. • K.I. Diaz, B.A. • A.K. Gogos, B.A.
Department of Psychology, University of Miami, Coral Gables, FL, USA
e-mail: caroline.ehrlich@gmail.com; kathleen.diaz18@gmail.com; akgo914@gmail.com

R.R. Berry, Ph.D.
Department of Psychiatry and Behavioral Sciences, Stanford School of Medicine,
Stanford, CA, USA
e-mail: Rrialon@stanford.edu

© Springer Science+Business Media New York 2015
R. Flanagan et al. (eds.), *Cognitive and Behavioral Interventions
in the Schools*, DOI 10.1007/978-1-4939-1972-7_12

The central tenet underlying cognitive-based treatments is that therapeutic change occurs when individuals successfully transform their dysfunctional cognitions and behaviors (Curry & Reinecke, 2003). Cognitive restructuring methods are used to address dysfunctional cognitions, including expectations, beliefs, and self-statements (Beck, Shaw, Rush, & Emery, 1979).

Generally, cognitive restructuring techniques include a variety of procedures intended to modify cognitions and cognitive processes. These techniques are employed with the goal of encouraging the student to: (1) monitor automatic thoughts or cognitions; (2) identify the relationship between thoughts, emotions, and behaviors; (3) evaluate the evidence for and against distorted cognitions; (4) replace maladaptive thinking with more accurate cognitions; and (5) detect and modify those dysfunctional core beliefs tainting the perception of experiences and maintaining pathology (Beck et al., 1979). Following a brief outline of cognitive restructuring techniques (Beck, 1995), the efficacy of cognitive interventions for mental health disorders in children and adolescents is addressed.

Cognitive Restructuring Techniques

Eliciting Automatic Thoughts

An early step in implementing cognitive interventions is identifying thoughts that are often slightly outside of one's consciousness and that occur in certain situations. If the student is challenged by this task, the therapist may assist by directly eliciting the thought, eliciting related imagery, role-playing with the student, or offering possible hypotheses as to the cognition, as appropriate considering the developmental needs of the student. This is either accomplished in session or between sessions, with the student noting their cognitions as they arise or following a pre-allotted period of time (Beck et al., 1979). This activity is conducted with greater ease as the student becomes proficient in detecting such thoughts and understanding situations that may elicit them (Beck, 1995). For example, consider a depressed 14-year-old girl. Her therapist asks, "I noticed your mood changed when we were talking about your math class. What was going through your mind?"

Relationship Between Thoughts and Feelings

Once accurately differentiated, the connection between cognitions and emotions is underscored. This is accomplished by eliciting those cognitions experienced in the context of affective states. The student then realizes that when a situation is interpreted negatively, this will lead to a negative feeling. The degree to which the student believes the thought is also important and can be assessed with a rating scale, further underscoring the connection between emotions and cognitions (Beck, 1995). For example, the therapist asks, "You said that when you think about your math class you have the thought, 'I'm going to fail.' How does having that thought make you feel?…On a scale from 1-10, how sad do you feel?"

Exploring Personal Meaning

In order to discover the student's schema or their established pattern of thinking that shapes their understanding of events, the therapist delves into the automatic thoughts (e.g., "I'm going to fail," in the above example) that are believed to stem from underlying beliefs. The therapist then elicits the personal meaning of the thought from the student. At times, this will result in the disclosure of the student's intermediate beliefs (e.g., assumptions and rules) and core beliefs (Beck, 1995). For instance, in our example, exploring the personal meaning of the automatic thought might lead to disclosure of the beliefs, "I must not disappoint anyone," and, "If I disappoint people, they won't love me."

Exploring Underlying Assumptions

The student and therapist collaborate to explore thinking patterns underlying the student's negative thoughts, behaviors, and emotions across contexts (Beck, 1995). This can also be viewed as a unique set of rules the student applies to himself (e.g., "I should always get the highest grade in the class") that likely result in negative affective states.

Development of Underlying Assumptions

The therapist promotes the exploration of the student's developmental experiences and their contribution to underlying beliefs and assumptions. This is accomplished by examining and reframing the original experiences, which support the current dysfunctional beliefs, unearthing evidence invalidating the assumptions the student currently holds, and identifying core beliefs (Beck, 1995).

Recognizing Cognitive Errors

The therapist helps the student identify cognitive disorders or "thinking traps." Twelve common cognitive errors exist, including catastrophizing, overgeneralizing, and dichotomous thinking, among others (see Beck, 1995, p. 119). The therapist applies interventions to such cognitive distortions with the purpose of modifying dysfunctional thinking, thus improving affective symptoms.

Distancing from Thoughts

The therapist further prepares the student for engaging in cognitive restructuring techniques by underscoring the subjective nature of cognitions. The therapist discourages the student from viewing the cognitions as established fact (Stark, 2008). Various strategies are used to accomplish this, including eliciting feedback that one would give to a best friend were they in the same situation, using of metaphors to assist the student in getting perspective, and conceptualizing the cognition as a subjective and distorted one (Beck, 1995).

Examining Available Evidence

After identifying the automatic thought and underscoring its relationship to the affective symptoms, the therapist and student collaboratively discover evidence from the students' experiences to either support or disconfirm the cognition. The therapist's goal here is to help the student more accurately and objectively assess the situation (Beck, 1995). In our example, the therapist might ask the student, "What is the evidence that you will fail your math class?"

Searching for Alternative Explanations

The therapist uses the knowledge gained from the exploration of evidence for and against the dysfunctional thought to help the student consider more adaptive and accurate alternative explanations (Beck, 1995). This is done by asking such questions as, "What is another way of looking at it?" and "What is the new thought?"

Realistic Consequences of Negative Cognitions

The therapist, in an effort to address cognitive distortions and weaken the strength of negative thoughts, encourages the student to consider the realistic consequences of the cognition if it were true. The therapist may use such inquiries as, "So what if it is true?" and "What is the worst that could happen?" (Beck, 1995).

Testing Beliefs Prospectively

The therapist may use behavioral experiments with the goal of assessing of the accuracy of the student's beliefs (Beck, 1995). Here, the therapist might elicit from the student predictions about the outcome of the experiment, reviewing the accuracy of the outcome after the experiment is over.

Adaptive Functional Value of Beliefs

The therapist encourages the student to assess how useful having the cognition is by considering the advantages and disadvantages of the dysfunctional thought. When the student better appreciates the negative consequences of the belief, the therapist helps in developing more adaptive cognitions (Beck, 1995).

Guided Discovery and Empiricism

The cognitive therapist embraces both guided discovery and empiricism throughout the use of these techniques. The therapist refrains from debating with the student or trying to convince the student to think differently. Rather, the therapist collaboratively guides the student in investigating beliefs, gathering evidence, and testing hypotheses. The student then, more independently, reaches increasingly adaptive conclusions (Beck, 1995).

Practicing Rational Responses

Collaboratively, in an effort to disturb certain patterns of thinking and improve the student's mood, the therapist and student practice more adaptive responses to the student's negative cognitions. This may be done by encouraging the student to talk back to the negative thought (Beck, 1995).

Recording Thoughts

The therapist encourages the student to record thoughts as they occur. With certain students, this can even be accomplished as homework between sessions. To assist with cognitive restructuring, the student monitors the thought, the context in which the thought occurred, the degree to which the thought was believed, the resultant feelings, and the intensity of those feelings. When the student more adeptly modifies thoughts, instruction is given in recording cognitive restructuring attempts and their outcomes (Beck, 1995).

Building a Positive Schema

While removing dysfunctional beliefs, the therapist also helps the student to develop positive, though realistic, beliefs about the self (Beck, 1995). The therapist and student work together to identify positive qualities supporting the student's new beliefs about the self, world, and future.

Empirical Support for Cognitive Interventions

Cognitive restructuring is only one of the many techniques used in CBT. As cognitive restructuring techniques are mostly used alongside other related interventions in the context of CBT treatment, their individual effects are challenging to ascertain. Those studies that have attempted to address the effectiveness of cognitive interventions with children and adolescents are described below.

Kendall and Braswell (1982) evaluated a cognitive-behavioral treatment in which 27 8–12-year-olds were treated for concerns related to impulsivity, hyperactivity, and aggression and were randomly assigned for 12 weeks to one of three conditions. The attention-control condition incorporated psychoeducation and interpersonal contact, while the behavioral condition included modeling and contingency management; the cognitive-behavioral condition included, in addition to the above, a cognitive component, namely, cognitive modeling in problem resolution, as well as problem-solving training. Treatment did not impact parent ratings of behavior; however, both the CBT and behavioral conditions resulted in improvements in teachers' ratings of hyperactivity. The CBT condition had the additional impact of improving teachers' ratings of self-control. CBT and behavioral treatments, further, improved academic achievement, though only CBT resulted in improved self-assessment of self-concept. Results were maintained at ten-week follow-up but were no longer apparent at one-year posttreatment. This study provides some support for the inclusion of cognitive interventions, though the latter is confounded with the inclusion of a problem-solving component.

Jaycox, Reivich, Gillham, and Seligman (1994) assessed the efficacy of a depression prevention treatment with youth aged 10–13 years. The treatment was composed of two components. Based both on Ellis (1962) and Beck's (1967) cognitive models, the cognitive component included the identification of negative attributions regarding problematic events and the evaluation of the accuracy of such beliefs. The second component included the instruction of social problem-solving and coping skills. One hundred and forty-three participants were randomly assigned to either the cognitive, social problem-solving, combined treatment, or control conditions. Results indicated that, when compared with control, all treatment groups were comparably more efficacious at reducing existing depressive symptoms, as well as diminishing externalizing conduct problems. The relative contribution of each component was not studied and, despite data that supported the use of a deconstructed version of the program, follow-up studies of the program continue to combine treatment components (Shirk & Karver, 2006).

In a trial of a group cognitive restructuring depression prevention program, Clarke et al. (2001) randomized at-risk adolescents to either usual care or usual care plus a 15-session cognitive restructuring therapy program. The experimental condition, an abbreviated version of a previously assessed depression prevention program (Clarke, Rodhe, Lewinsohn, Hops, & Seeley, 1999), involved numerous cognitive restructuring techniques, including having the adolescents identify and challenge irrational or unrealistic thoughts. Those in the experimental condition had a significant advantage in terms of being at a reduced risk for developing a depressive disorder up to 15 months following the completion of the prevention trial (Clarke et al., 2001).

Examining only those randomized controlled trials evaluating treatments of depressed youth, in an effort to parse their relative contribution, Weisz, McCarty, and Valeri (2006) compared the mean effect size of treatments that incorporated a cognitive change component to the mean effect size of those treatments that did not (e.g., relaxation training). The mean effect size of both groups, while significantly different from zero, were comparable and did not differ to a significant degree, leading the authors to conclude that treatment for youth depression may not require a focus on cognitive change (Weisz et al., 2006).

McCarty and Weisz (2007) conducted a meta-analysis of nine treatment studies of depressed children and adolescents, including studies with an effect size of 0.50 or greater. Frequently included components of the studies were cognitive behavioral with measurable goals: psychoeducation, self-monitoring, interpersonal skills, cognitive restructuring, problem-solving, and behavioral activation. As these components were combined in those studies examining effective treatments, it remains unclear which particular component directly influences treatment outcome, though the study provided preliminary support for the use of cognitive restructuring in the treatment of childhood and adolescent depression.

Rosenberg, Jankowski, Fortuna, Rosenberg, and Mueser (2011) explored the feasibility and efficacy of a manualized cognitive restructuring intervention for treating PTSD in adolescents. Nine adolescents engaged in 12–16 sessions of a primarily cognitive restructuring intervention; some psychoeducation about PTSD and relaxation training was also incorporated. Following treatment, the adolescents demonstrated statistically significant reductions in both PTSD and depression symptoms, with gains maintained at three-month follow-up. While not examining the role of cognitive restructuring as a stand-alone treatment, this study does provide some evidence for the use of cognitive restructuring as a major aspect of treatment for PTSD in youth (Rosenberg et al., 2011).

As such, in those few studies that have been conducted in which cognitive interventions are examined in isolation, results have been mixed, with cognitive interventions demonstrating a positive association with improved outcome in many, with others indicating no effect. The latter studies conclude that change is attributed to other factors, resulting in some questions about the importance of inclusion of cognitive interventions with child and adolescent populations. Overall, CBT interventions, including those incorporating a cognitive component, have demonstrated significant success in addressing concerns in youth populations (David-Ferdon & Kaslow, 2008; Silverman & Hinshaw, 2008; Silverman, Pina, & Viswesvaran, 2008).

Developmental Considerations

While CBT is widely used with children and adolescents, some uncertainty remains regarding the efficacy and effectiveness of cognitive components with children of a certain developmental level (Spence, 1994). Evidence suggests that, while the level of cognitive development plays a key role in the efficacy of CBT, CBT can be effective with use in younger children if treatment delivery is developmentally appropriate (Grave & Blissett, 2004). Methods of adapting CBT for youth include the use of simpler, less verbally based cognitive restructuring techniques, concrete examples (e.g., visual devices), frequent summaries and reviews, mnemonic aids, metaphors, experiential learning, and frequent practice (Grave & Blissett, 2004; Weersing et al. 2006).

Stress-Inoculation Training (SIT) per Meichenbaum

Patrick Pössel Allison D. Barnard

Description of the Stress-Inoculation Training (SIT)

Meichenbaum's (1975) Stress-Inoculation Training (SIT) is a cognitive intervention for overcoming anger, anxiety, pain, and stress. The general treatment goals of SIT are to increase a student's skills that help him/her to cope with stressful situations by allowing for a normalization of emotional and psychological adaptation and to increase his/her self-confidence to master stressful situations. SIT provides the therapist with a set of principles and clinical procedures and includes three flexible interlocking phases: the conceptual-educational phase, the skills acquisition and consolidation, and rehearsal phase, and the application phase (Meichenbaum, 2008).

Theoretical Underpinnings of SIT

SIT is based on two perspectives of stress, transactional and strengths-based. The transactional approach maintains that the best way to cope with some stressors is to change the stress-generating situation. For example, if a specific classroom situation creates the stress for a student, the best way to reduce the stress may be to work collaboratively with a teacher to change the situation. Cohen, Mannarino, and Deblinger (2006) used this approach to treat sexually abused children by working with the nonoffending parents.

"Inoculation" as the core idea of SIT is rooted in the strengths-based approach. In other words, the theoretical consideration underlying SIT is that the exposure to mildly stressful situations can make the student stronger. Teaching the student how to use coping skills in mildly stressful situations increases the coping skills used in more severe stressful situations. Further, by gradual exposure and rehearsal in imagination and real life, the self-confidence to master stressful situations is bolstered. A more detailed description of the theoretical underpinnings of SIT can be found in Meichenbaum (2007).

Mechanics of SIT

Meichenbaum recognized that only some stressful situations can be changed or avoided. Further, some of the remaining stressors cannot be mastered with active problem-solving strategies. Thus, the coping skills trained in SIT, and therefore, the length of SIT, vary widely. Meichenbaum (2008) includes versions that range from 20 min (preparation of patients for surgery) to 40 sessions (patients with chronic medical and psychiatric conditions), but in most cases SIT includes 8–15 sessions plus booster sessions. The length of SIT in empirical studies with students ranges from 8 to 15 to sessions and a duration of 20–60 min per session (Table 12.1).

Table 12.1 List of empirical studies applying SIT to students in schools

Authors	Sample	Measures	SIT conditions	Outcomes
Hains (1992)	6 males, 15–17 years old, 5 European A, 1 Asian A	STAI; STAXI; CSEI; RADS; APES	15 individual sessions (40 min), multiple baseline design	Pre-post-intervention: 5 of 6 youths showed decrease in anxiety Pre-3-month follow-up: lower levels of anxiety scores for 3 youths
Hains and Ellmann (1994)	21 youths (16 girls, 5 boys), 9th–12th grades, 19 European A, 1 Hispanic, 1 Asian A	STAI; STAXI; RADS; APES; health problems; school absences; GPA	13 group and individual sessions (50 min)	Pre-post-intervention: high emotional arousal youths decrease in trait and state anxiety and depression SIT vs. control: lower trait anxiety in high emotional arousal youths in SIT at post-intervention
Hains and Szyjakowski (1990)	21 males, 16–17 years old, 20 European A, 1 African A	STAI; Anger Inventory; CSEI; BDI	Each phase began with a 60-min group session followed by two individual sessions (30–40 min)	Pre-post-intervention and pre-10-week follow-up: decrease in trait anxiety and anger and increase in self-esteem SIT vs. control: lower anxiety and anger and higher self-esteem in SIT at post-intervention

(continued)

Table 12.1 (continued)

Authors	Sample	Measures	SIT conditions	Outcomes
Kiselica, Baker, Thomas, and Reedy (1994)	48 European A (26 male, 22 female), 9th grade students	STAI Trait Anxiety Scale; Symptoms of Stress Inventory; GPA	SIT + assertiveness training, 8 sessions (60 min)	Pre-post-intervention: decrease in anxiety and stress in SIT SIT vs. control: lower anxiety and stress in SIT at post-intervention and 4-week follow-up
Walker and Clement (1992)	6 1st/2nd grade boys, diagnosed with ADHD, 5 African A, 1 Hispanic	Behavioral observations; Pupil Evaluation Inventory	8–10 sessions (20 min), half individually and half in group, multiple baseline design	Pre-post-intervention: effect size collapsing observations and peer evaluation = 1.07
Wolmer, Hamiel, and Laor (2011)	1,488 Israeli students, 4th–5th grades, exposed to continuous rocket attacks	UCLA-PTSD Reaction Index; Stress/Mood Scale	14 sessions (45 min), delivered by teachers regulation	Pre-post-intervention: decrease in PTSD symptoms and stress/mood in SIT among intervention group SIT vs. control: less PTSD symptoms and stress mood in SIT at post-intervention

Note. APES = Adolescent Perceived Events Scale; BDI = Beck Depression Inventory; CSEI = Coopersmith Self-Esteem Inventory; RADS = Reynolds Adolescent Depression Scale; STAI = State-Trait Anxiety Inventory; STAXI = State-Trait Anger Expression Inventory

As mentioned above, SIT consists of the flexible interlocking conceptual-educational phase, skills acquisition and consolidation, and rehearsal phase, and application phase (Meichenbaum, 2008). The conceptual-educational phase includes multiple steps and purposes. The aims of this phase include (a) to disaggregate global stressors and to describe the stressful situation in behaviorally relevant and specific terms, (b) to identify the determinants of the problem or stressors, (c) to motivate the student to observe himself/herself to identify his/her stress responses and to learn the associations between his/her own cognitions, emotions, behaviors, and responses from others, and (d) to identify which difficulties are related to deficits in coping skills versus performance failures. The main purpose of this phase is to collect the necessary information about the stressful situation and the student's coping skills and to cognitively prepare the student for the therapeutic work to come. To reach these aims, the therapist uses different strategies including interviews with the student and relevant others (e.g., caregivers, teachers), student's imaginative reconstruction of a typical stressful situation, and psychological and behavioral assessments.

In the skills acquisition and consolidation, and rehearsal phase, the therapist tailors the SIT by considering what coping strategies the student already uses, how they can be used in the problematic stressful situations, and what prevents them so far from being used. Further, during this phase emotion-focused (including acceptance skills, cognitive reframing, perspective taking) and problem-focused coping skills (including assertiveness training, problem-solving, social support) are trained and rehearsed using imaginative and behavioral exercises. Finally, generalization procedures are developed and possible barriers of using the trained coping skills are anticipated and addressed.

In the application phase, the student is encouraged to apply the trained coping skills to gradually more demanding stressful situations. Another important element of the application phase is to bolster the student's self-efficacy. Ideally, the student uses self-attributions for improvements and she/he coaches someone with a similar stressful situation. This also helps the student to generalize the learned strategies to other stressful situations in their life. Finally, relevant others (e.g., caregivers, teachers) are involved in the treatment to allow for a restructuring of environmental stressors. Please see Meichenbaum (2007) for a detailed description of the mechanics of SIT and some examples with adult clients. At this point, we are not aware of published example cases in students.

In schools, SIT was implemented in group and individual settings (Table 12.1) and seems appropriate for Tier II (targeted) or Tier III (intensive) interventions (Ysseldyke et al., 2006). Tier II interventions address "specific academic or social-emotional skill or performance deficits" in students that do not benefit from programs offered to all students in a school (Ysseldyke et al., 2006, p. 13). Thus, SIT may be offered to students that academically struggle in group sessions. As Tier III interventions target individual students, SIT may be administered by a school psychologist to a specific student in one-to-one sessions. As with any intervention, school psychologists are obligated to consider if SIT is the most appropriate approach to help students to be successful in the general education program and to use data-based problem-solving processes to plan the implementation of SIT, monitor its effects, and modify SIT if necessary (Jacob, Decker, & Hartshorne, 2011).

Research Support

Meichenbaum (1993) identified approximately 200 published empirical studies using SIT with populations as different as psychiatric patients (e.g., addiction, anger-control problems in students and adults, PTSD), medical patients (e.g., cancer, childhood asthma, hypertension), individuals having a stressful occupation (e.g., nurses, soldiers, teachers), parents of children with cancer, and many more. However, studies in the school setting are much less common. Our own search revealed only six published studies with SIT in schools. Besides the limited number of studies, further limiting is that only three of the six (Hains & Ellmann, 1994; Hains & Szyjakowski, 1990; Wolmer et al., 2011) include a control group, only three studies provided follow-up data (Hains, 1992; Hains & Szyjakowski, 1990; Kiselica et al., 1994), and the small sample size in five of the six studies. Thus, while it seems clear that SIT is effective in children and adolescents outside the school setting (Maag & Kotlash, 1994) and it is likely that SIT is similarly effective in schools, the lack of empirical findings of SIT within schools is unsatisfactory, and no final conclusions about the effects of SIT implemented in schools can currently be drawn.

Changing Unhealthy Patterns of Thinking—An REBT Approach

Mark Terjesen

Conceptual Model of Rational Emotive Behavior Therapy

Rational Emotive Behavior Therapy (REBT), like other cognitive-behavioral approaches (CBT), is based on the notion that unhealthy affect and behavior are influenced by an individual's cognitive processing and that a modification of maladaptive cognitive processes can promote healthier emotional and behavioral responses (David & Szentagotai, 2006). While the different CBT approaches are in conceptual agreement about the role of cognitive variables in the development of cognitive, emotional, and behavioral problems (Hyland & Boduszek, 2012), there are variations in the intervention approaches of each model.

The REBT approach is based on Ellis (1962) ABC model: individuals experience undesirable activating events (A), and they have beliefs/cognitions (B) about these events that may be irrational/dysfunctional or rational/functional. The model proposes that these beliefs in turn lead to either dysfunctional or functional behavioral or emotional consequences (C). For example, a child receives a poor grade on a school assignment (A) and thinks, "My teacher thinks I am stupid" (B), which, in turn, may leave the child feeling sad and/or lead to negative behaviors in the classroom (C) (these are examples of dysfunctional emotional and behavioral consequences, respectively).

Rational beliefs are healthy, pragmatic, flexible, logical, and empirically consistent with reality. Irrational beliefs are rigid and absolutist, dysfunctional/non-pragmatic, and, in general, not consistent with reality (Hyland & Boduszek, 2012; Szentagotai & Freeman, 2007). The REBT model proposes that if a child holds healthy, logical, rational beliefs about a negative activating event they experience, this increases the likelihood that they will experience "healthy" negative emotions (e.g., concern, frustration, sadness) and will engage in adaptive behaviors in response to stressors (Hyland & Boduszek, 2012). Alternatively, if a person holds irrational beliefs about the negative activating event, they are likely to experience unhealthy negative emotions (e.g., anxiety, anger, depression) and to engage in maladaptive behavioral responses (Hyland & Boduszek, 2012). Core to the treatment model is the identification and replacement of these unhealthy, maladaptive thoughts to reduce emotional difficulties experienced and the problematic behavior of children and adolescents (David, Szentagotai, Eva, & Macavei, 2005).

Cognitive Restructuring in REBT

Ellis identified 11 types of irrational beliefs that he proposed were endorsed by clients (Ellis, 1962). Subsequently, the model has been refined, and these beliefs were then organized into four primary belief categories: (1) demandingness of self or others (demands) (e.g., "I *have* to succeed"; "She *must* treat me with respect"), (2) frustration intolerance (e.g., "I *can't stand* homework"), (3) awfulizing or catastrophizing (e.g., "It would be *horrible* if I made a mistake"), and (4) global evaluations of human worth of self or others (ratings of worth) (e.g., "If I fail the test, I am a loser/failure") (DiGiuseppe, Doyle, Dryden, & Backx, 2013; Ellis & Blau, 1998).

A key component of the REBT model is helping the student to identify and challenge these irrational beliefs and assist children in adopting a new set of beliefs that are functional, rational, and logical (Sava, Maricutoiu, Rusu, Macsinga, & Virga, 2011). There are a number of strategies used to facilitate this change to reduce both the influence of their irrational beliefs and the emotional and behavioral problems experienced (Hyland & Boduszek, 2012). The replacement of these maladaptive thoughts has been proven effective in reducing emotional disturbance and problem behavior in children and adolescents (David et al., 2005; Esposito, 2009; Gonzalez et al., 2004).

Challenging these irrational beliefs is at the core of the cognitive restructuring component of REBT; this process is called "disputation." Disputation debates or challenges the irrational beliefs that a student is holding to allow for the newer, healthier belief system to have an opportunity to develop. These disputation strategies can be cognitive, imaginal, and/or behavioral in nature (DiGiuseppe et al., 2013) and are described below as they relate to specific beliefs that students may endorse.

A necessary prerequisite to disputing is to make sure that the student understands the connection between their irrational beliefs and the consequences (emotional, behavioral, or cognitive) that they experience (DiGiuseppe et al., 2013). This is referred to as the B-C connection. There are a number of ways that this connection can be made with children and adolescents, such as the use of analogies, or social/situational examples. Demonstrating the REBT model by focusing on someone other than the student can be particularly helpful, as the student can remain more detached from the situation and the accompanying affective state. An additional strategy to promote the B-C connection is to have the student keep a thought log where they track what happened (the "A"), what emotion they felt at that moment ("the C"), what they did at that moment ("the behavioral C"), and what they were thinking ("the B"). With younger students this visual model may help reinforce the connection. Finally, role-plays in session may be done to further support understanding of the model.

Disputation Types

What follows is an overview of the core cognitive disputation techniques and behavioral approaches used to challenge the evaluative irrational beliefs in the REBT framework.

Empirical disputation involves working with the student to evaluate the reality of their inferences and evaluations: "Where is the evidence to support your idea that the teacher does not like you?" or "Where is the proof that you are a complete failure because you did not make the team?" DiGiuseppe and Bernard (2006) provide the rationale for this approach when working with youth when one considers that "children between the approximate ages of 7 and 11 structure their world in an empirical and inductive manner" (p. 87). Given this, we will then work with children on developing healthier beliefs by intensive analyses of the situation that they are getting themselves upset about. Part of this approach that may in fact be more "user-friendly" in working with children would be to have them engage in some actual data collection to test the accuracy of their conclusions. The clinician could work with the student and design an experiment where they test their beliefs. If a student believes that "no one in my class likes me," you could go through the class list and seek specific examples as to how each and every other student has demonstrated that they do not like him/her. It is more likely than not that the student overgeneralized to all students not liking him from perhaps a few students. The student can then work on generating a new rational self-statement such as: "Even though some people don't like me, I still have friends." At the same time it is important to consider the developmental level of the student and use language in your work that is consistent with their level of understanding. Children are likely to use and express their ideas in a manner that is related to the REBT model but not exactly consistent with the REBT jargon. The consideration of their level of understanding and language used is also important when the clinician presents challenges to their unhealthy beliefs. That is, the term "evidence" may not exactly be in the child's vocabulary, and we may want to use a word or phrase that is something they can relate to. Asking the child to work with you to help see if that idea is true or not and where the proof for it is may be helpful.

Bernard, Ellis, and Terjesen (2006) offer another approach to empirical disputation in having students provide examples of behaviors that others might engage in that either support or "debunk" the belief "no one likes me." For example, the student could list behaviors indicative that someone is liked (e.g., people say hello, sit with you at lunch, play with you at recess). Then over the course of the next week, they would record each time that they notice a classmate engaging in these behaviors. This provides more objective data as to the number of positive peer behaviors and may provide the evidence to challenge the thinking that "no one likes me."

The REBT practitioner does not just concern themselves with the challenging of the inferences but will also target deeper irrational evaluations that may accompany these beliefs. Potential irrational evaluations that may accompany the thought of "no one likes me" would be that "it is awful that no one likes me. I can't stand it. I am a loser." Practitioners would work on empirically challenging these deeper evaluations by helping the client develop healthier thoughts such as: "while unlikely, it would be disappointing if no one liked me, but may not be truly awful," or, "even if no one likes me, I am made up of more positive than negative traits, and, most importantly, this one area (not being liked) does not define who I am."

Logical disputation involves working with the student to examine whether the conclusions that they have drawn sensibly and logically follow from the facts. Examples of logical disputes would be: "Just because you want to succeed at sports, does it follow logically that it *must* happen?" "Does it make sense to conclude you are never going to be able to pass the test?" "You have many good traits, does it follow that when you do not succeed in a desired area that you are a complete and total failure?"

Semantic disputation involves working with the student at coming up with an objective definition (i.e., operationalized in behavioral terms) of the emotionally charged words and phrases that they use. For example, examining when a person defines something as "awful" or someone (perhaps themselves) as a complete loser or an idiot. By working with the student to define awful as "one of the absolute very worst things that could happen to them," this may provide the student with a reference point for their view of a specific event (e.g., failing a test) as being awful. The event is reframed as negative or undesirable but not as meeting the true definition "awful." The use of an emotional thermometer (DiGiuseppe & Bernard, 2006) is often implemented to assist students in developing a better understanding of the emotion that they experience and see the varying levels of affect and accompanying outcomes of their emotions. Clinicians may want to consider adding a cognitive component to this thermometer to better represent the relationships between affect, beliefs, and behavior. Clinicians can help students construct an "awfulness scale" from 1 to 100, whereby 100 is the worst possible scenario (i.e., "death of a loved one"). This scale can help students gain perspective, that perhaps the things or people that they thought were truly awful are most accurately placed at a lower number. Similarly, the following is an example of using a semantic dispute to counter a student's belief that they are a "total loser":

> The word 'loser' means that you have and always will lose in everything you do. You have not succeeded and never will. From what I know of you, you have had some successes and some failures. Given this definition, is your labeling yourself a loser consistent with this meaning?

Pragmatic disputing involves educating the student about how their beliefs are not helping them function effectively and are in fact stopping them from working toward their goals. If a student is experiencing anxiety about a test because they are thinking: "If I fail the test, this would be awful" or "If I fail the test I am an idiot," these types of beliefs would serve to contribute to the anxiety the student is experiencing. The practitioner would work with the student to challenge these ideas by asking: "Where will it get me if they keep thinking that if they did not pass the test it would be awful? How does it help me to succeed on the test by thinking I will be an idiot if I fail this test?" The answers to these questions most likely would be that it does not help but actually make things worse for the student. This then provides an opportunity for the clinician to reinforce the idea that unhealthy ways of thinking lead to maladaptive/unhealthy behaviors and that individuals then would benefit from working on developing a new, healthy, rational alternative.

Behavioral Approaches to Cognitive Restructuring

The abovementioned approaches to cognitive restructuring were primarily cognitive in nature because via verbal exchanges and some exercises in data collection, specific cognitions were directly targeted for change. The clinician then works with the child to develop healthy alternative beliefs. Behavioral activities are also common within the REBT approach to reinforce the newly developed adaptive ways of thinking and/or to indirectly challenge the unhealthy irrational beliefs. Harrington (2011) describes a number of behavioral activities that could be used as part of the REBT approach. These involve: (a) "risk-taking activities" that encourage a student to challenge themselves to do something they normally would avoid (e.g., speak in front of the whole class), (b) "staying in there" or remaining in a situation until the emotional arousal subsides, (c) "shame attacks," which involve students concerned with others thinking poorly are encouraged to act in an embarrassing way and tolerate the discomfort, and (d) "behavioral and imagery methods" (Harrington, 2011, p. 14).

Developmental Considerations

The use of cognitive restructuring with youth, much like the overall model of REBT, considers the child's age, developmental level, and intelligence (Bernard, 1990). Because REBT was developed initially for adults, it would be a mistake to assume it is applicable to youth without considering their developmental level. Developmental milestones are relevant to the child's presenting problem as well as which approaches for cognitive restructuring are the most developmentally appropriate.

The practice of REBT with children may involve the use of visual aids or mnemonic devices than one might see in practice with adults. Further, to help engage the child or adolescent and build on their understanding of concepts, the cognitive restructuring approach may be seen to be more hands-on (Bernard & Pires, 2006a; Ellis & Bernard, 2006). Depending upon the linguistic level and cognitive maturity of the child, the types of cognitive techniques used (e.g., rational self-statements, disputing of irrational beliefs) may vary (Bernard et al., 2006). With younger students, practitioners may focus on building their emotional vocabulary to increase the range of emotional responses and helping them distinguish emotions and understand their differences. The linguistic groundwork for eventual cognitive disputation is laid by helping them differentiate thoughts and feelings and become aware of the connection between thoughts and feelings. Regarding cognitive restructuring, the rehearsal of more adaptive ways of thinking rather than directly challenging and disputing dysfunctional thoughts is recommended for younger students. Adolescents, in contrast, are often at the formal operational stage and are able to grasp abstract, big picture attempts at cognitive restructuring ("why must you be liked by all"); with younger students it is better to focus on more concrete examples ("why must you be liked by her").

Summary and Conclusions

REBT is a cognitive-behavioral approach that may be presented to youth to assist with managing disruptive behavioral and emotional patterns. By fostering their understanding of the relationship of thinking with emotion and behaviors, students will learn to accept emotional responsibility for their own emotions and behaviors. The specific interventions employed in this model include a variety of cognitive, emotional, and behavioral strategies (e.g., empirical, logical, semantic, and pragmatic disputation strategies and other emotive-evocative and active behavioral approaches). The goal of these interventions is to guide students in changing their unrealistic, irrational, and dysfunctional beliefs into healthy alternatives that will reduce their unhealthy feelings and behaviors. Through the application of the interventions presented, students will be better prepared to manage adversity and increase their potential for academic, social, and personal success.

Covert Conditioning

Betty S. Lai Caroline J. Ehrlich Kathleen I. Diaz

Covert conditioning refers to a set of therapy procedures developed in the 1970s by Joseph Cautela (Kazdin, 1977). Based on the principles of operant conditioning, covert conditioning techniques involve imagining responses and their consequences (Cautela & Baron, 1977). Covert conditioning aims to change overt (i.e., public) behavior, covert psychological behavior (e.g., private behaviors such as thoughts and feelings), and physiological behavior (Cautela & Kearney, 1990).

Covert conditioning is based upon three basic assumptions (Cautela & Baron, 1977; Cautela & Kearney, 1990): (1) *homogeneity* between overt and covert behaviors, (2) *interaction* between overt and covert events, and (3) the idea that *learning* principles are similar for overt and covert events. Elaborating further, the *homogeneity* assumption implies that there is no difference between overt or covert behaviors. Under the *interaction* assumption, covert behaviors may influence overt behaviors and vice versa. For example, if an adolescent imagines smoking a cigarette and vomiting as a result (covert behavior), this imagined behavior may change their actual smoking patterns (overt behavior). Similarly, when a child stops seeing a neighborhood dog (overt behavior), his or her feelings about dogs may change (covert behavior). The *learning* assumption implies that overt and covert behaviors are learned in the same way. Thus, although behavior principles were derived from observing overt behavior, those principles apply directly to covert behaviors.

Specific procedures used in covert conditioning are ostensibly direct applications of operant learning principles (Cautela, 1973; Cautela, Flannery, & Hanley, 1974; Kazdin, 1977). When using covert conditioning with children, clinicians should conduct an assessment of a child's ability to manipulate imagery. Specifically, clinicians should consider a child's ability to carry out verbal instructions, learn by observing a live model, and a child's ability to accurately describe past and future experiences (Cautela, 1982). Also integral to covert conditioning is a behavioral analysis that identifies the antecedents and consequences of the student's target behavior. For example, if a 12-year-old girl presents with test anxiety, her treatment plan should include information about what she worries will happen if she performs poorly on a test, whether there are certain subjects that elicit more test anxiety than others, and if exam test formats are equally anxiety provoking.

Covert processes differ depending on whether the desired effect is to change target behaviors so that they increase (e.g., covert reinforcement, negative reinforcement, and modeling) or decrease (e.g., covert sensitization, extinction, and response cost); thus, these are versatile because they can be used to increase positive behaviors and decrease negative behaviors. Details on these strategies are provided below, but in general, each process advances along the same set of steps, outlined in Table 12.2. Clinicians should provide psychoeducation and a rationale for utilizing covert conditioning techniques with children. As opposed to the detailed description for adults, clinicians working with youth can present covert conditioning as a game that will help them get over their fears or help them make new friends (Cautela, 1982; Cautela & Bennett, 2001). Also important early on, clinicians should explain that tape-recording each covert conditioning trial permits practicing the described scenes at home, which may be especially important for youth.

These steps may also be used with other types of covert conditioning. For example, in covert sensitization, the clinician would provide rationale. Then, the clinician would

Table 12.2 Covert conditioning techniques

	Technique	Sample script for covert positive reinforcement
Step 1	Introduce covert conditioning and provide rationale	*Today, we are going to play a pretend game that will help you overcome your fear of writing on the chalkboard*
Step 2	Describe scene in as much detail, using as many sensory modalities as possible. Record covert conditioning trial for child to listen to at home	*When you are ready, imagine yourself standing at the chalkboard. You can smell the chalk and feel the dry powder on your hands. You hear your teacher ask you to write your name on the board. You pick up the chalk and slowly write each letter*

(continued)

Table 12.2 (continued)

	Technique	Sample script for covert positive reinforcement
Step 3	Once the child has obtained clear imagery of the scene described, discuss something reinforcing or transition into playtime	*Now imagine all of your friends clapping and cheering. They are hugging you and congratulating you. Your teacher awards you with a star and a good grade. You show this grade to your parents, when you get home, and they take you out for your favorite dinner*
Step 4	Instruct child to listen to covert conditioning trial for 15–20 min per day at home	*You've done a great job today, and you worked hard to imagine that scene. Now, I want you to listen to the recording of that scene every night before you go to bed. Don't forget to work hard to imagine every detail with all of your senses*

describe a scene in which the student is engaging in the target behavior, followed by an aversive consequence. Finally, the clinician would instruct the student to listen to the trial at home. This technique, while applicable to adolescent smoking behaviors mentioned above, is generally not utilized with youth populations or in school settings.

Similarly, in covert extinction, the clinician would provide rationale. Then, the clinician would guide the student toward imagining himself or herself engaging in the target behavior. However, instead of an aversive consequence, the student would imagine that positive reinforcements for that behavior, or the maintaining factors, are removed. The clinician would then instruct the student to listen to the trial at home. The ethical concerns, which apply to both covert extinction and sensitization and are addressed below, impede the use of these techniques in younger populations.

During covert conditioning trials, students may experience anxious symptoms. Clinicians can rely on basic relaxation techniques before beginning a covert conditioning trial; in fact, children taught relaxation techniques in the context of covert conditioning sessions have been shown to be more cooperative in the process overall (Cautela, 1982).

Empirical support for utilizing covert conditioning with young populations comes mainly from Krop, Calhoon, and Verrier's (1971) study. Krop and colleagues studied 36 children ($M = 10.5$ years old) with various behavior problems. The experiment used covert and overt reinforcement to modify children's self-concept. Subjects were randomly assigned to one of three groups: (1) covert reinforcement group, (2) overt reinforcement group, and (3) control group. The covert reinforcement group was rewarded with a pleasant scene after giving a response indicating positive self-concept. The overt conditioning group was rewarded with gum and a token when they indicated positive self-concept. Lastly, those in the control group were provided with no reinforcement. Only the covert reinforcement group reported significantly increased positive self-concept. These differences were maintained at two-week follow-up. Of note, applications of covert conditioning have also been conducted with adult populations (Kazdin, 1973, 1975, 1980; Manno & Marston, 1972; Marshall, Boutilier, & Minnes, 1974).

Ethical questions can arise around the use of covert conditioning, especially in light of the sensitization techniques that mimic aversive conditioning. Although there is support for using aversive stimuli and similar techniques in the treatment of adult substance use, ethical guidelines of non-maleficence render the use of such strategies in youth populations questionable. Working with children requires adherence to stricter guidelines. Specifically, while fulfilling the ethical obligation to select effective behavioral change procedures, school psychologists are faced with several options. First-line treatments include positive behavioral interventions like differential reinforcement, followed secondly by strategies relying on extinction. The removal of desirable stimuli ranks third, while the presentation of aversive stimuli is considered the least acceptable (Jacob et al., 2011). However, to remain within their fields' ethical guidelines, clinicians are urged to use discretion when considering covert sensitization with young clients, because covert sensitization is not a component of probably efficacious treatments for child depression (Kaslow & Thompson, 1998), phobias, or anxiety (Ollendick & King, 1998).

Reframing

Betty S. Lai, Rebecca Rialon Berry, Anna K. Gogos

Reframing is a therapeutic technique that shifts the frame of reference for a problem behavior from a negative perspective to a more neutral or positive interpretation (Kass & Fish, 1991). The goal of reframing includes changing how a client interprets the meaning of a situation or behavior by offering another view or "frame" for the situation (Eckstein, 1997), typically one that is less troublesome for the client. Once the meaning attributed to a situation or behavior changes, the person's response to it is also likely to change (Cormier, Nurius, & Osborne, 2012).

Reframing is a cornerstone technique for family therapy (e.g., systemic family therapy, structural family therapy) and cognitive-behavioral therapies (Cohen & Mannarino, 2000; Eckstein, 1997; Reynaert & Janne, 2011). In the context of family therapy, reframing techniques are sometimes termed "rewording," "relabeling," or "redefining the problem" (Reynaert & Janne, 2011). The goal of reframing in family therapy is to help families move toward a new way of viewing its interactions. For example, if a child's maladaptive behavior requires such constant care and parental attention that it becomes difficult for the parent to be employed, the child is likely to become the "identified patient" (i.e., viewed as the "problem" in the family). Reframing the concern or problem in terms of what actions need to take place in order for the parent to return to work may be a more productive course of action. In the context of cognitive-behavioral therapy, reframing techniques are sometimes termed "cognitive restructuring" techniques (Eckstein, 1997). The goal of reframing in cognitive-behavioral therapy is to "rewrite" automatic, self-defeating thoughts (Beck, 1993; Eckstein, 1997).

Reframing can yield substantial benefits for students, teachers, parents, and other school personnel, particularly when addressing problematic child behavior. Many children may exhibit disruptive classroom behaviors (Cholewa, Smith-Adcock, & Amatea, 2010), and these children are more likely to be considered troublemakers in school. However, acting out behaviors may, in fact, reflect underlying learning challenges or nonacademic-related conflicts and problems (e.g., exposure to community violence, poor sleep, poor nutrition). In considering alternative explanations for a child's disruptive classroom behavior, educational staff members often become amenable to problem-solving and are more likely to generate effective behavior modification solutions. Increasing the overall use of positive behavioral descriptions (e.g., labeling the child's behavior as the "positive opposite," for example, praising and labeling times when a child sits in their seat versus calling attention to when the child is out of their seat) can help foster improved parent-child and parent-teacher interactions (Brinkmeyer & Eyberg, 2003; McIntosh, Rizza, & Bliss, 2000).

According to Seaward (2006), the steps for reframing involve: (1) identifying internal thoughts and beliefs in a situation or about a specific behavior, (2) evaluating the content of these thoughts and perceptions, and (3) questioning the validity of negative perceptions (Hughes, Gourley, Madson, & Le Blanc, 2011). The following model explains how reframing can be implemented as a coping technique to reduce client stress (Table 12.3).

For many individuals, developing alternative thoughts and behaviors does not come easily; clients often assume that there are risks involved in changing habitual

Table 12.3 Reframing as coping technique to reduce client stress

Steps	Rationale and examples
Identification of client internal thoughts and beliefs about a situation (increasing awareness).	The first step in the reframing process involves identifying and acknowledging the client's stressors (e.g., *giving a presentation in class*). This includes having the client write down all thoughts, frustrations, and worries about the particular event (e.g., *"The speech is too long and the topic is hard. I will say something wrong and mess up during the presentation. The teacher will give me a bad grade"*)
Evaluate the content of the thoughts and perceptions.	Clients are often unaware of what features or details they turn their attention to in a situation and what information about the situation they encode (Cormier et al., 2012). Therefore, the second part of reframing is to identify what the client automatically attends to in the problem situation and what emotional attitudes are associated with each (e.g., *"I might get called on first because I sit in the front row…my heart will race, I will speak too quickly and no one will understand me…everyone will be staring at me and think I am an idiot if I mess up. The teacher will be disappointed; he will think I didn't practice and give me a bad grade. I will feel sad"*)
Question the validity of negative perceptions (reappraisal of the situation).	Next, clients are guided toward challenging erroneous beliefs or negative thoughts, and clients are asked to examine the issue from multiple perspectives. The former method involves helping clients identify "thinking mistakes" (irrational patterns of thinking) that are occurring for them in each stressful situation, such as <u>catastrophizing</u> (predicting the future negatively without considering other, more likely outcomes) or <u>mind reading</u> (predicting what others are thinking). Clients are also taught to determine the advantages and disadvantages of maintaining the negative perception (e.g., by asking, "Is this thought/worry helping me achieve my goal or feel better?") and to consider alternative explanations and outcomes (e.g., "What are other, more likely outcomes of the situation?"). In doing so, clients learn to "reappraise" the situation by choosing a neutral, or preferable (positive), stance to interpret or deal with the issues at hand. For example, an individual giving a presentation in class might think, *"I do not know what order the teacher will call students, but if I did have to present first, I can handle it; I practiced this three times and have given a lot speeches before and did fine. If I mess up, I will pause, take a deep breath, and keep trying… Instead of negatively evaluating me, my classmates and teacher might be impressed by my topic and oratory skills"*

(yet often pessimistic and troublesome) thought patterns and behaviors. To help sustain motivation, therapists provide education about what clients can expect during and after the reframing process (i.e., that substituting a positive attitude for a negative perception may make the client feel uncomfortable or vulnerable at first, but like other skills that improve with practice, a new comfort will emerge) (Seaward, 2006). With cognitive reframing the new approaches to information processing must be repeatedly substituted when stress is encountered and practiced again and again to demonstrate their effectiveness. Research supports the use of reframing among families (Bugental & Schwartz, 2009) and students (Hughes et al., 2011) in improving mood and relationships. Research supports the use of reframing among families and students in improving mood and relationships (See Table 12.4).

Table 12.4 Research support for reframing among families and students

Researchers	Sample	Measures (assessment and/or outcome)	Treatment conditions	Follow-up data
Bugental and Schwartz (2009)	102 families with infants identified as being born at medical risk (*M* age of infants at intake = 9.37 weeks).	Parents were assessed using the following measures: Conflict Tactics Scale, Framingham Safety Survey, Child Injury Survey, and Perceived Power.	Parents were randomly assigned to receive either the enhanced home visitation program, which included the cognitive reframing intervention, or an unenhanced home visitation program.	Families assigned the home visitation program had fewer incidences of corporal punishment, fewer reported child injuries, and greater safety maintained at home. There was a lower prevalence of harsh tactics to discipline the child in the group assigned the cognitive reframing-enhanced home visitation program.
Hastings, Allen, McDermott, and Still (2002)	41 mothers of children with intellectual disabilities (*M* age = 41.40 years old).	Mothers completed a self-report questionnaire that measured demographic factors, child demographics (i.e., caregiving demand), social support, coping strategies, and dimensions of positive perceptions.	No treatment conditions.	Mothers' positive perceptions were related to coping strategies, in particular reframing coping strategies. Mothers who viewed their child in a positive light were better able to cope.

(continued)

Table 12.4 (continued)

Researchers	Sample	Measures (assessment and/ or outcome)	Treatment conditions	Follow-up data
Hughes et al. (2011)	143 students from a midsize southwestern university (79 female, 61 male, 3 unidentified; *M* age = 19 years).	Students were given a number of stressful scenarios and were given the opportunity to respond on paper to the situation as well as provide advice for a fellow peer.	Participants attended either a lecture about reframing or a reframing activity which included responding to scenarios on their own, pairing with another student to practice challenging negative thoughts, and merging with another pair to discuss the activity.	Participants in the reframing activity condition were more likely to suggest that the other person actively challenges their beliefs and thoughts and to examine a given stressor from multiple perspectives in order to reframe a negative thought. They were more likely to encourage active coping techniques, responded more positively, and learned more than students who received the lecture.
Kass and Fish (1991)	60 students in the third grade and fourth grade (30 high test anxious and 30 low test anxious; 34 girls, 26 boys; *M* age for girls = 9.53 years, *M* age for boys = 9.46 years). 30 students with the highest levels of test anxiety and 30 students with the lowest levels of test anxiety were included in this study, out of an original pool of 127 children.	Students were given an arithmetic word problem test immediately followed by a state anxiety measure. Measures included the Test Anxiety Scale for Children, the Lie Scale for Children, the Arithmetic Word Problem Test, and the State Anxiety Scale for Children.	Children received one of three forms of instruction before the exam: neutral, reassuring, or positive reframing.	The form of instruction assigned to the child had no effect on test performance. Contrary to hypotheses, all children who received positive reframing instructions before the exam scored noticeably higher on the state anxiety measure. Positive reframing appears to have an emotional impact but was ineffective in aiding arithmetic test performance for high test anxiety students.

(continued)

Table 12.4 (continued)

Researchers	Sample	Measures (assessment and/ or outcome)	Treatment conditions	Follow-up data
Morris et al. (2011)	153 children from preschool through second grade (67 girls, 86 boys; *M* age = 6 years, 2 months).	Data were collected during 1.5–2-h home visits. Mothers were asked to complete questionnaires about their child and home environment. The mother and child worked together to complete a series of tasks, and the parent-child relationship was assessed. In an emotion-inducing task, anger and sadness intensity were measured via the expression of the child, followed by the mother's attempts to aid the child regulating emotions.	No treatment conditions.	Mothers using attention refocusing and mother-child use of cognitive reframing were associated with lower intensity of expressed anger and sadness. Younger children expressed higher intensity of sadness than older children, and mothers' use of attention refocusing was less helpful among older children than it was among younger ones.
Pottie and Ingram (2008)	93 parents of children with autism spectrum disorders. 69 of these families were represented by one parent (60 mothers and 33 fathers); 24 of the families were represented by both parents.	Use of a repeated daily measure was employed in this study. Twice weekly over a period of 12 weeks, parents reported their daily stress, coping responses (i.e., seeking support, positive reframing), and end-of-day mood.	No treatment conditions.	Five coping responses, including positive reframing and seeking support, were associated with a positive mood at the end of the day. Gender did not appear to be a moderating factor in the daily coping and mood relationship. The child's symptoms and time since the diagnosis was made did not predict the daily mood of the parent.

(continued)

Table 12.4 (continued)

Researchers	Sample	Measures (assessment and/or outcome)	Treatment conditions	Follow-up data
Stoeber and Janssen (2011)	149 students (33 male, 116 female; *M* age = 20.8 years).	Students completed daily reports for 3 to 14 days. Each day they reported the most bothersome failure they had, what coping strategies they employed, and how satisfied they felt at the day's end.	No treatment conditions.	Positive reframing acceptance and humor predicted higher satisfaction for all students. For students high in perfectionistic concerns, positive reframing was reported to be particularly helpful.

References

Beck, A. T. (1967). *Depression: Clinical, experimental, and theoretical aspects*. New York: Hoeber.

Beck, A. T. (1993). The past and future of cognitive therapy. *The Journal of Psychotherapy Practice and Research, 6*, 276–284.

Beck, J. S. (1995). *Cognitive therapy: Basics and beyond*. New York: Guilford Press.

Beck, A. T., Shaw, B. F., Rush, A. J., & Emery, G. (1979). *Cognitive therapy of depression*. New York: Guilford Press.

Bernard, M. E. (1990). Rational-emotive therapy with children and adolescents: Treatment strategies. *School Psychology Review, 19*, 294–303.

Bernard, M. E., Ellis, A., & Terjesen, M. D. (2006). Rational emotive behavior approaches to childhood disorders: History, theory, practice and research. In A. Ellis & M. E. Bernard (Eds.), *Rational emotive behavior approaches to childhood disorders*. New York, NY: Springer.

Bernard, M. E., & Pires, D. (2006a). Emotional resilience in children and adolescence: Implications for rational-emotive behavior therapy. In A. Ellis & M. E. Bernard (Eds.), *Rational emotive behavioral approaches to childhood disorders: Theory, practice and research* (pp. 156–174). New York, NY: Springer Science and Business Media.

Brinkmeyer, M., & Eyberg, S. M. (2003). Parent-child interaction therapy for oppositional children. In A. E. Kazdin & J. R. Weisz (Eds.), *Evidence-based psychotherapies for children and adolescents* (pp. 204–223). New York: Guilford.

Bugental, D. B., & Schwartz, A. (2009). A cognitive approach to child mistreatment prevention among medically at-risk infants. *Developmental Psychology, 45*, 284–288.

Cautela, J. R. (1973). Covert processes and behavior modification. *Journal of Nervous and Mental Disease, 157*(1), 27–36.

Cautela, J. R. (1982). Covert conditioning with children. *Journal of Behavior Therapy and Experimental Psychiatry, 13*(3), 209–214.

Cautela, J. R., & Baron, M. G. (1977). Covert conditioning: A theoretical analysis. *Behavior Modification, 1*(3), 351–368.

Cautela, J. R., & Bennett, A. K. (2001). Covert conditioning. In R. J. Corsini (Ed.), *Handbook of innovative therapy* (2nd ed., pp. 125–136). New York, NY: Wiley.

Cautela, J. R., Flannery, R. B., & Hanley, S. (1974). Covert modeling: An experimental test. *Behavior Therapy, 5*, 494–502.

Cautela, J. R., & Kearney, A. J. (1990). Behavior analysis, cognitive therapy, and covert conditioning. *Journal of Behavior Therapy and Experimental Psychiatry, 21*(2), 83–90.

Cholewa, B., Smith-Adcock, S., & Amatea, E. (2010). Decreasing elementary school children's disruptive behavior: A review of four evidenced-based programs for school counselors. *Journal of School Counseling, 8*, 1–35.

Clarke, G. N., Hornbrook, M., Lynch, F., Polen, M., Gale, J., Beardslee, W., et al. (2001). A randomized trial of a group cognitive intervention for preventing depression in adolescent offspring of depressed parents. *Archives of General Psychiatry, 58*, 1127–1134.

Clarke, G. N., Rodhe, P., Lewinsohn, P. M., Hops, H., & Seeley, J. R. (1999). Cognitive-behavioral treatment of adolescent depression: Efficacy of acute group treatment and booster sessions. *Journal of American Academy of Child and Adolescent Psychiatry, 38*, 272–279.

Cohen, J. A., & Mannarino, A. P. (2000). Predictors of treatment outcome in sexually abused children. *Child Abuse & Neglect, 24*, 983–994.

Cohen, J. A., Mannarino, A. P., & Deblinger, E. (2006). *Treating trauma and traumatic grief in children and adolescents*. New York: Guilford.

Cormier, S., Nurius, P., & Osborne, C. J. (2012). *Interviewing and change strategies for helpers: Fundamental skills and cognitive behavioral interventions* (7th ed.). Belmont, CA: Brooks/ Cole.

Curry, J. F., & Reinecke, M. A. (2003). Modular cognitive behavior therapy for adolescents with major depression. In M. Reinecke, F. Durrilio, & A. Freeman (Eds.), *Cognitive therapy with children and adolescents* (2nd ed., pp. 95–127). New York: Guilford Press.

David, D., & Szentagotai, A. (2006). Cognition in cognitive-behavioral psychotherapies: Toward an integrative model. *Clinical Psychology Review, 26*(3), 284–298.

David, D., Szentagotai, A., Eva, K., & Macavei, B. (2005). A synopsis of rational-emotive behavior therapy (REBT): Fundamental and applied research. *Journal of Rational-Emotive & Cognitive-Behavioral Therapy, 23*(3), 175–221.

David-Ferdon, C., & Kaslow, N. J. (2008). Evidence-based psychosocial treatments for child and adolescent depression. *Journal of Clinical Child & Adolescent Psychology, 37*(1), 62–104.

DiGiuseppe, R., & Bernard, M. E. (2006). REBT assessment and treatment with children. In A. Ellis & M. E. Bernard (Eds.), *Rational emotive behavioral approaches to childhood disorders: Theory, practice and research* (pp. 85–114). New York, NY: Springer Science and Business Media.

DiGiuseppe, R., Doyle, K., Dryden, W., & Backx, W. (2013). *A practitioner's guide to rational-emotive behavior therapy*. Oxford: Oxford University Press.

Eckstein, D. (1997). Reframing as a specific interpretive counseling technique. *Individual Psychology, 53*, 418–428.

Ellis, A. (1962). *Reason and emotion in psychotherapy*. Secaucus, NJ: Citadel.

Ellis, A., & Bernard, M. E. (Eds.). (2006). *Rational emotive behavior approaches to childhood disorders*. New York: Springer.

Ellis, A., & Blau, S. (1998). Rational emotive behavior therapy. *Directions in Clinical and Counseling Psychology, 8*, 41–56.

Esposito, M. A. (2009). REBT with children and adolescents: A meta-analytic review of efficacy studies. *Dissertation Abstracts International: Section B. The Sciences and Engineering, 70*(5-B), 138.

Gonzalez, J. E., Nelson, J. R., Gutkin, T. B., Saunders, A., Galloway, A., & Shwery, C. S. (2004). Rational emotive therapy with children and adolescents: A meta-analysis. *Journal of Emotional and Behavioral Disorders, 12*(4), 222–235.

Grave, J., & Blissett, J. (2004). Is cognitive behavior therapy developmentally appropriate for young children? A critical review of the evidence. *Clinical Psychology Review, 24*(4), 399–420.

Hains, A. A. (1992). A stress inoculation training program for adolescents in a high school setting: A multiple baseline approach. *Journal of Adolescence, 15*, 163–175.

Hains, A. A., & Ellmann, S. W. (1994). Stress inoculation training as a preventative intervention for high school youths. *Journal of Cognitive Psychotherapy, 8*, 219–232.

Hains, A. A., & Szyjakowski, M. (1990). A cognitive stress-reduction intervention program for adolescents. *Journal of Counseling Psychology, 37*, 79–84.

Harrington, N. (2011). Frustration intolerance: Therapy issues and strategies. *Journal of Rational-Emotive & Cognitive-Behavioral Therapy, 29*, 4–16.

Hastings, R. P., Allen, R., McDermott, K., & Still, D. (2002). Factors related to positive perceptions in mothers of children with intellectual disabilities. *Journal of Applied Research in Intellectual Disabilities, 15*, 269–275.

Hughes, J. S., Gourley, M. K., Madson, L., & Le Blanc, K. (2011). Stress and coping activity, reframing negative thoughts. *Teaching of Psychology, 38*, 36–39.

Hyland, P., & Boduszek, D. (2012). Resolving a difference between cognitive therapy and rational emotive behavior therapy: Towards the development of an integrated CBT model of psychopathology. *Mental Health Review Journal, 17*(2), 104–116.

Jacob, S., Decker, D. M., & Hartshorne, T. S. (2011). *Ethics and law for school psychologists* (6th ed.). New York, NY: Wiley.

Jaycox, L., Reivich, K., Gillham, J., & Seligman, M. (1994). Prevention of depressive symptoms in school children. *Behaviour Research and Therapy, 32*(8), 801–816.

Kaslow, N., & Thompson, M. (1998). Applying the criteria for empirically supported treatments to studies of psychosocial interventions for child and adolescent depression. *Journal of Clinical Child Psychology, 27*(2), 146–155.

Kass, R. G., & Fish, J. M. (1991). Positive reframing and the test performance of test anxious children. *Psychology in the Schools, 28*, 43–52.

Kazdin, A. E. (1973). Covert modeling and the reduction of avoidance behavior. *Journal of Abnormal Psychology, 81*(1), 87–95.

Kazdin, A. E. (1975). Covert modeling, imagery assessment, and assertive behavior. *Journal of Consulting and Clinical Psychology, 43*(5), 716–724.

Kazdin, A. E. (1977). Research issues in covert conditioning. *Cognitive Therapy and Research, 1*(1), 45–58.

Kazdin, A. E. (1980). Covert and overt rehearsal and elaboration during treatment in the development of assertive behavior. *Behavior Research and Therapy, 18*, 191–201.

Kendall, P. C., & Braswell, L. (1982). Cognitive-behavioral self-control therapy for children: A components analysis. *Journal of Consulting and Clinical Psychology, 50*(5), 672–689.

Kiselica, M. S., Baker, S. B., Thomas, R. N., & Reedy, S. (1994). Effects of stress inoculation training on anxiety, stress, and academic performance among adolescents. *Journal of Counseling Psychology, 41*, 335–342.

Krop, H., Calhoon, B., & Verrier, R. (1971). Modification of the "self-concept" of emotionally disturbed children by covert reinforcement. *Behavior Therapy, 2*, 201–204.

Maag, J. W., & Kotlash, J. (1994). Review of stress inoculation training in children and adolescents. Issues and recommendations. *Behavior Modification, 18*, 443–469.

Manno, B., & Marston, A. R. (1972). Weight reduction as a function of negative covert reinforcement (sensitization) versus positive covert reinforcement. *Behavior Research and Therapy, 10*, 201–207.

Marshall, W. L., Boutilier, J., & Minnes, P. (1974). The modification of phobic behavior by covert reinforcement. *Behavior Therapy, 5*, 469–480.

McCarty, C. A., & Weisz, J. R. (2007). Effects of psychotherapy for depression in children and adolescents: What we can (and can't) learn from meta-analysis and component profiling. *American Academy of Child and Adolescent Psychiatry, 46*(7), 879–886.

McIntosh, D. E., Rizza, M. G., & Bliss, L. (2000). Implementing empirically supported interventions: Teacher-child interaction therapy. *Psychology in the Schools, 37*, 453–462.

Meichenbaum, D. W. (1975). Self-instructional approach to stress management. A proposal for stress inoculation training. In C. D. Spielberger & I. G. Sarason (Eds.), *Stress and anxiety* (Vol. 1). New York, NY: Wiley.

Meichenbaum, D. W. (1993). Stress inoculation training: A 20-year update. In P. M. Lehrer & R. L. Woolfolk (Eds.), *Principles and practice of stress management*. New York: Guilford Press.

Meichenbaum, D. W. (2007). Stress inoculation training: A preventive and treatment approach. In P. M. Lehrer, R. L. Woolfolk, & W. S. Sime (Eds.), *Principles and practice of stress management* (3rd ed.). New York: Guilford Press.

Meichenbaum, D. W. (2008). Stress inoculation training. In W. O'Donohue & J. E. Fisher (Eds.), *Cognitive behavior therapy: Applying empirically supported techniques in your practice* (2nd ed.). New York: Wiley.

Morris, A. S., Silk, J. S., Morris, M. D. S., Steinberg, L., Aucoin, K. J., & Keyes, A. W. (2011). The influence of mother-child emotion regulation strategies on children's expression of anger and sadness. *Developmental Psychology, 47*, 213–225.

Ollendick, T., & King, N. (1998). Empirically supported treatments for children with phobic and anxiety disorders: Current status. *Journal of Clinical Child Psychology, 27*(2), 156–167.

Pottie, C. G., & Ingram, K. M. (2008). Daily stress, coping, and well-being in parents of children with autism: A multilevel modeling approach. *Journal of Family Psychology, 22*, 855–864.

Reynaert, C., & Janne, P. (2011). Reframing "reframing": Another look at "reframing" inspired by a sonnet by Charles Baudelaire. *The American Journal of Family Therapy, 39*, 419–436.

Rosenberg, H. J., Jankowski, M. K., Fortuna, L. R., Rosenberg, S. D., & Mueser, K. T. (2011). A pilot study of a cognitive restructuring program for treating posttraumatic disorders in adolescents. *Psychological Trauma: Theory, Research, Practice, and Policy, 3*(1), 94–99.

Sava, F. A., Maricutoiu, L. P., Rusu, S., Macsinga, I., & Virga, D. (2011). Implicit and explicit self-esteem and irrational beliefs. *Journal of Cognitive and Behavioral Psychotherapies, 11*(1), 97–111.

Seaward, B. L. (2006). *Stress management: Principles and strategies for health and well-being* (5th ed.). Boston, MA: Jones & Bartlett.

Shirk, S., & Karver, M. S. (2006). Process issues in cognitive-behavioral therapy for youth. In P. Kendall (Ed.), *Child & adolescent therapy* (3rd ed.). New York, NY: Guilford Press.

Silverman, W. K., & Hinshaw, S. P. (2008). The second special issue on evidence-based psychosocial treatments for children and adolescents: A ten-year update. *Journal of Clinical Child and Adolescent Psychology, 37*(1), 1–7.

Silverman, W. K., Pina, A. A., & Viswesvaran, C. (2008). Evidence-based psychosocial treatments for phobic and anxiety disorders in children and adolescents: A review and meta-analysis. *Journal of Clinical Child and Adolescent Psychology, 37*, 105–130.

Spence, S. H. (1994). Practitioner review: Cognitive therapy with children and adolescents: From theory to practice. *Journal of Child Psychology and Psychiatry, 35*, 1191–1228.

Stark, K. (2008). Experiences implementing the ACTION treatment program: Implications for preventive interventions. *Clinical Psychology: Science and Practice, 15*(4), 342–345.

Stoeber, J., & Janssen, D. P. (2011). Perfectionism and coping with daily failures: Positive reframing helps achieve satisfaction at the end of the day. *Anxiety, Stress, and Coping, 24*, 477–497.

Szentagotai, A., & Freeman, A. (2007). An analysis of the relationship between irrational beliefs and automatic thoughts in predicting distress. *Journal of Cognitive and Behavioral Psychotherapies, 7*, 1–11.

Walker, C. J., & Clement, P. W. (1992). Treating inattentive, impulsive, hyperactive children with self-modeling and stress inoculation training. *Child and Family Behavior Therapy, 14*, 75–85.

Weersing, V. R., Iyengar, S., Birmaher, B., Kolko, D. J., & Brent, D. A. (2006). Effectiveness of cognitive-behavioral therapy for adolescent depression: A benchmarking investigation. *Behavior Therapy, 37*, 36–48.

Weisz, J. R., McCarty, C. A., & Valeri, S. M. (2006). Effects of psychotherapy for depression in children and adolescents: A meta-analysis. *Psychological Bulletin, 132*(1), 132–149.

Wolmer, L., Hamiel, D., & Laor, N. (2011). Preventing children's posttraumatic stress after disaster with teacher-based intervention: A controlled study. *Journal of the American Academy of Child and Adolescent Psychiatry, 50*, 340–348.

Ysseldyke, J. E., Burns, M. K., Dawson, M., Kelly, B., Morrison, D., Ortiz, S., et al. (2006). *School psychology: A blueprint for the future of training and practice III*. Bethesda, MD: National Association of School Psychologists.

Chapter 13
Cognitive and Behavioral Interventions

Mitchell L. Schare, Kristin P. Wyatt, Rebecca B. Skolnick, Mark Terjesen, Jill Haak Bohnenkamp, Betty S. Lai, Rebecca Rialon Berry, and Caroline J. Ehrlich

Developing an Anxiety Hierarchy

Mitchell L. Schare; Rebecca B. Skolnick; Kristin P. Wyatt

M.L. Schare, Ph.D., A.B.P.P. (✉) • K.P. Wyatt, M.A. • R.B. Skolnick, Ph.D.
Department of Psychology, Hofstra University, Hempstead, NY, USA
e-mail: mitchell.l.schare@hofstra.edu; kp.wyatt@gmail.com; rebeccabskolnick@gmail.com

M. Terjesen, Ph.D.
Department of Psychology, St. John's University, Jamaica, NY, USA
e-mail: terjesem@stjohns.edu

J.H. Bohnenkamp, Ph.D.
Center for School Mental Health, University of Maryland School of Medicine,
Baltimore, MD, USA
e-mail: jbohnenk@psych.umaryland.edu

B.S. Lai, Ph.D.
Division of Epidemiology and Biostatistics, School of Public Health, Georgia State
University, P.O. Box 3984, Atlanta, GA 30302-3984, USA
e-mail: blai@gsu.edu

R.R. Berry, Ph.D.
Department of Psychiatry and Behavioral Sciences, Stanford School of Medicine,
Stanford, CA, USA
e-mail: Rrialon@stanford.edu

C.J. Ehrlich, M.S.
Department of Psychology, University of Miami, Coral Gables, FL, USA
e-mail: caroline.ehrlich@gmail.com

© Springer Science+Business Media New York 2015
R. Flanagan et al. (eds.), *Cognitive and Behavioral Interventions in the Schools*, DOI 10.1007/978-1-4939-1972-7_13

Description

Hierarchy development is an integral component of graded exposure therapy for anxiety disorders. A hierarchy, often referred to as a "fear ladder" (e.g., Kendall & Hedtke, 2006), is a list of anxiety-provoking situations, or stimuli that a child avoids, organized in order of increasing difficulty. Hierarchies can take numerous forms, such as a written list, drawing of a ladder (e.g., Kendall & Hedtke, 2006), picture of a pyramid, or a map of different sized "islands" based on the level of anxiety provoked by each situation (e.g., March & Mulle, 1998). The hierarchy is developed in the beginning sessions of therapy and is used as an assessment tool to aid in case conceptualization and treatment planning. Hierarchies are also guides for determining graduated exposure or desensitization exercises to conduct in therapy.

Theoretical and Research Underpinnings

The concept of a fear hierarchy can be found in literature as early as the famous Little Albert study, (Watson & Raynor, 1920) during which a child conditioned to a white rat also demonstrated various levels of conditioned anxiety to other animals and objects that shared characteristics of the rat. This led to the conceptualization of the anxiety hierarchy as a key component of Wolpe (1958) model of systematic desensitization, one of the first comprehensive scientifically derived, evidence-based models of behavior therapy. In the initiation of systematic desensitization, Wolpe (1990) advocated that hierarchy construction and relaxation training occur at the beginning of therapy. He then had patients relax and imagine increasingly anxiety-provoking situations from the hierarchy (in a step-wise fashion) until the stimuli became associated with a relaxed state and no longer evoked substantial anxiety. Regardless of what CBT protocols are used, a hierarchy-based exposure is often part of the procedure for the treatment of childhood anxiety (see Table 13.3).

Hierarchy development functions to combat anxiety from the start, as discussing anxiety-provoking situations (i.e., conditioned stimuli) can be a form of informal exposure in itself if the child becomes anxious in session. Creating a hierarchy may also begin to provide distance between the child and his/her anxiety, which will facilitate the ability to externalize the disorder during treatment (March & Mulle, 1998). Hierarchy construction can also be used to build rapport (e.g., by making it game-like) so that the child stays in treatment. Once the hierarchy is developed, the therapist is encouraged to work collaboratively with the child to negotiate and plan the order, sequence, and difficulty level of exposure exercises, thus increasing self-efficacy (Kendall et al., 2005).

Table 13.1 Steps for developing a hierarchy

Step	Brief description
1. Interview child	Explore presenting problem, related issues, hypothesized issues, parent(s) may be included dependent upon age/maturity
2. Select and administer appropriate assessment instruments to child and parent	Utilize general and specific self-report and observational measures of fears/anxiety
3. Provide rationale for hierarchy	Psychoeducation about anxiety/avoidance, discuss how hierarchy will be used to guide exposures or "therapy experiments"
4. Explain SUDs rating procedure	Can take many forms, such as fear ladder, and may range from 0 to 8, 0 to 10, or 0 to 100
5. Offer stimuli and obtain SUDs ratings	Present in random order; anchor high and low points near beginning of process; assess presented items and hypothesized cues. Can use post-it or index card methods.
6. Obtain parent ratings and elicit other potential stimuli	Depending on developmental level, parent(s) may be involved in hierarchy construction
7. Check parent contribution with child	If additional information is received from parent, obtain SUDs ratings from child
8. Organize list from highest to lowest intensity	Collaboratively select items to go on hierarchy, and write it out for child. This may take different forms, such as fear ladder, island drawings, or a pyramid. If there are multiple themes, may create more than one hierarchy.
9. Reassess hierarchy throughout treatment	This may be done weekly, bi-weekly, at therapist's discretion

Mechanics

Hierarchy construction involves a number of steps to ensure accurate assessment of the child's fears in order to develop a thorough treatment plan (see Table 13.1). Depending on the child's developmental level, caretakers can be an important source of information as well. Table 13.2 provides an example of a hierarchy for a child with school refusal behavior.

Hierarchy development begins with an interview exploring the nature of the presenting problem, issues related to the problem, hypothesized cues, and other concerns stated by the child. It is important to ascertain what the child thinks will happen when faced with the feared situation. Depending upon the child's developmental level, parent(s) may be involved in this stage. Standardized self-report and behavioral assessment instruments can aid in determining potential stimuli for the hierarchy. The therapist must select anxiety assessment measures that are relevant to the presenting problem. Instruments can include general anxiety measures,

Table 13.2 Example of school refusal hierarchy

Situations or places that scare me	SUDs rating (0–10)
Taking math test (hardest class) where I don't understand material because I missed so much school and other kids are laughing at me	10
Taking math test where I don't understand material but no one notices	9
Peer girls asking why I missed so much school	9
Peer boys asking why I missed so much school	8
Taking social studies test	7
Attending full day of school without tests	6
Attending school basketball game as spectator	5
Walking into school during the day alone	4
Walking into school during the day with therapist	3
Walking into school at night with parent (no one else is around)	2

such as the Fear Survey Schedule for Children-II (FSSC-II; Gullone & King, 1992), and specific measures, such as the Spider Phobia Questionnaire for Children (SPQ-C; Kindt, Brosschot, & Muris, 1996) or the children's Yale-Brown Obsessive-Compulsive Scale (CY-BOCS; Scahill et al., 1997). Behavioral avoidance tests can also be used to assess anxiety symptoms and determine stimuli for the hierarchy.

Following assessment, the rationale for hierarchy development should be provided. This includes psychoeducation about anxiety and avoidance and a discussion of how the hierarchy will be used to guide exposures or "therapy experiments." Specifically, examples of the thoughts, feelings, and behaviors associated with anxiety can be elicited. This may involve drawings of the child's body, circling areas of the body where the child feels anxiety, and/or completing drawings of people with thought bubbles (e.g., Kendall & Hedtke, 2006; Chorpita, 2007). Anxiety can be explained as an alarm (Chorpita, 2007) that is tested by putting oneself in the avoided situation and seeing if the "fear comes true." Metaphors can also be used to enhance the child's comprehension of anxiety and avoidance. For example, an analogy of developing a hierarchy to climbing a ladder or mountain can be used to clarify the process (e.g., Kendall & Hedtke, 2006). Further, hierarchy development can be explained as a tool to help the therapist get to know the child better and aid the child in understanding his/her anxiety so that it can be conquered, thus building rapport. Parents, teachers, etc. need to be aware of this process as well.

Once the rationale is understood, a subjective units of distress (SUDs; Wolpe, 1969) rating procedure for anxiety-provoking situations is introduced. This involves a Likert-type scale ranging from 0 to 100 (0 = *no distress* and 100 = *highest level of distress*), 0 to 10 (e.g., Wolpe, 1990), or 0 to 8 (e.g., Kendall & Hedtke, 2006; Kearny & Albano, 2007). For younger children, a visual analogue scale, such as coloring in a picture of a fear ladder, may be more useful.

The rating procedure is then applied to a range of potential feared stimuli offered by the therapist. Present the stimuli in random order (not as they might fall on the hierarchy) and anchor high and low points at the beginning of the process. Different hierarchies can be created for distinct "themes" or fears, and it is recommended to work on one at a time. Stimuli can be situations, cues, sensations, obsessions, or thoughts. The therapist should try to obtain specific items at different levels and elaborate on stimuli using descriptors or adjectives (e.g., tiny vs. big spider). The stimuli offered should be based both on what the child states and on hypothesized cues (i.e., related stimuli or thoughts not explicitly stated).

A number of researchers suggest that stimuli can be written on index cards or Post-its (Chorpita, 2007; Kearney & Albano, 2007; Kendall & Hedtke, 2006) to make an interactive, game-like task. Once there are at least ten items, record SUDs rating for each stimulus and make sure that almost every level of anxiety is represented. These will be ordered later with the child. The goal is to have a range of items with different intensity levels. Praise the child for hard work and doing well on an important task. For older children, the therapist may just solicit the items, obtain ratings, and organize them on a piece of paper.

Depending on the child's developmental level, it is often useful to meet with the parent(s) alone to obtain information about the child's feared stimuli (Chorpita, 2007; Kearney & Albano, 2007). During this meeting, ensure that the parents understand the SUDs rating procedure, and get their ratings of the stimuli offered by the child (without telling them the child's ratings). Then ask if there are any other feared stimuli that have been omitted, and obtain ratings for these as well. If the parent(s) has provided additional information, meet with the child and parent(s) together, and obtain the child's SUDs ratings for the new items.

Using all of the information obtained, collaboratively select the hierarchy items that will be used to guide subsequent exposure exercises. The items should then be organized from highest to lowest intensity. Chorpita (2007) suggests making a copy of the hierarchy for both the child and the parent(s). At the end of the session, praise the child again and thank the parents. If time permits, end the session on a positive note, such as a game.

As treatment progresses, the ratings of items on the hierarchy will diminish; thus it is important for the therapist to keep checking in with the child and parent(s) regarding ratings for items. This can be done by distributing an unrated copy of the hierarchy to the parent(s) and child as frequently as the therapist deems appropriate and asking for current SUDs. This way, the hierarchy can also be used to assess treatment progress.

Research Support

Hierarchies are key components in many controlled studies of successful anxiety treatment for children (see Table 13.3). For example, hierarchies have been used as part of individual cognitive-behavioral therapy (CBT), group CBT, family CBT, multiple session treatments, and one-session treatments for children with a range of specific phobias, obsessive compulsive disorder, separation anxiety disorder, and/or generalized anxiety disorder. These treatments have demonstrated significantly greater improvements in anxiety disorder symptoms when compared to control groups.

Table 13.3 Examples of controlled research studies that used a hierarchy as part of successful anxiety treatment for children

Researchers	Sample	Primary outcome measures	Treatment conditions	Results	Follow-up data
Barrett (1998)	60 children (ages 7–14) with separation anxiety, overanxious disorder, or social phobia	1. ADIS-C and ADIS-P (Silverman and Nells, 1988) 2. Diagnostic interview 3. Fear Survey Schedule for Children-Revised (FSSC-R; Ollendick, 1983); 4. Child Behavior Checklist (CBCL; Achenbach and Edelbrock, 1991)	1. Group cognitive-behavioral therapy (CBT) 2. Group CBT with family management 3. Waitlist	64.8 % of children no longer met diagnostic criteria for an anxiety disorder (compared to 25.2 % on waitlist)	At 12-month follow-up, 64.5 % in Group-CBT and 84.8 % in Group CBT with family management did not meet diagnostic criteria for an anxiety disorder
The Pediatric OCD Treatment Study Team (POTS; 2004)	112 patients (ages 7–17) with primary OCD diagnoses	1. CY-BOCS (Scahill et al., 1997)	1. CBT alone 2. Sertraline alone 3. CBT and sertraline 4. Pill placebo	Remission rates of 53.6 % for combined treatment, 39.3 % for CBT alone, 21.4 % for sertraline alone, and 3.6 % of placebo. Remission rate for combined treatment was not significantly different from that of CBT alone, but was significantly greater than sertraline alone and placebo.	

Study	Sample	Measures	Conditions	Results	Follow-up
Walkup et al. (2008)	488 children (ages 7–17) with primary diagnoses of separation anxiety disorder, generalized anxiety disorder (GAD), or social phobia	1. Clinician Global Impression-Improvement Scale (National Institute of Mental Health, 1970) 2. Pediatric Anxiety Rating Scale (Research Unit on Pediatric Psychopharmacology Anxiety Study Group, 2002)	1. CBT alone 2. Sertraline alone 3. CBT and sertraline 4. Pill placebo	At 12 weeks, 80.7 % in the combination group, 59.7 % in the CBT group, 54.9 % in the sertraline group, and 23.7 % in placebo group were rated as much or very much improved. Results on the Pediatric Anxiety Rating Scale yielded similar outcomes.	
Kendall, Hudson, Gosch, Flannery-Schroeder, & Suveg (2008)	161 children (ages 7–14) with primary diagnoses of separation anxiety disorder, social phobia, or GAD	1. ADIS-C/P (Silverman and Albano, 1996)	1. Individual CBT 2. Family CBT 3. Family-based control group	Diagnoses were no longer present for 57 % of those in individual CBT, 55 % in family CBT, and 37 % in control group	At 1-year follow-up, 61 %, 58 %, and 44 % of principal diagnoses for individual CBT, family CBT, and control group, respectively, continued to be absent, with no significant differences across conditions
Hudson et al. (2009)	112 children (ages 7–16) with principal anxiety disorder	1. ADIS-IV-C/P 2. Structured interviews	1. Group CBT 2. Group control	At post-treatment, a significantly higher proportion of those in CBT group compared to the control group no longer met anxiety disorder diagnostic criteria	At 6-month follow-up, 68.6 % in CBT and 45.5 % in control group no longer met diagnostic criteria for their principal anxiety disorder

(continued)

Table 13.3 (continued)

Researchers	Sample	Primary outcome measures	Treatment conditions	Results	Follow-up data
Ollendick et al. (2009)	196 children (ages 7–16) with various specific phobias	1. ADIS-C/P including clinician severity rating (CSR) 2. Behavioral Approach Tests (BATs) 3. Treatment satisfaction survey	1. One-session exposure treatment (OST) 2. Education support treatment (EST) 3. Waitlist control (WLC)	At post-treatment, those in OST and EST had significantly lower CSRs and percentages of phobic-free participants than did those in WLC. The OST was superior to EST on CSR, percentage of phobic-free participants, child ratings of anxiety before BAT, and treatment satisfaction.	At 6-month follow-up, OST continued to demonstrate better CSRs and percentage of phobic-free participants than did the EST condition. However, there were no significant differences on other variables.
Kerns, Read, Klugman, & Kendall (2013)	91 children (ages 8–14) with primary diagnoses of social phobia, GAD, or separation anxiety disorder (SAD)	1. ADIS-C/P (Silverman and Albano, 1996) including CSR	1. CBT (Coping Cat; Kendall and Hedtke, 2006) 2. Waitlist control	Those in CBT condition demonstrated significant improvement in anxiety symptoms from pretreatment to post-treatment. Those with social anxiety had significantly higher anxiety levels at pretreatment and post-treatment.	At 1-year follow-up, those in CBT condition continued to improve. At 7.4-year follow-up, those with social anxiety symptoms were significantly less improved than were others.

Exposure Therapy: Application to Childhood Anxiety

Mitchell L. Schare, Kristin P. Wyatt, Rebecca B. Skolnick

Description

Exposure therapy is a most efficacious procedure to treat anxiety disorders in children ranging from specific phobias to complex issues involving school refusal, obsessive compulsive disorder, and posttraumatic stress reactions. It entails systematic exposure to a feared stimulus or a representation of that stimulus, repeatedly over a prolonged time period to elicit anxiety, with the ultimate goal of decreasing the anxiety and related avoidance behaviors. Stimuli may be presented in a graduated or non-graduated manner (e.g., flooding), using imagery or in vivo experiences to facilitate exposure to the stimulus without allowing avoidance or escape behaviors (i.e., response prevention) which maintain problematic behavior.

Exposure therapy for children and adolescents is described as the key element of cognitive-behavioral treatment (CBT) for childhood anxiety (Foa, Chrestman, & Gilboa-Schechtman, 2008; Kazdin & Weisz, 1998) yet is often applied in the context of a multicomponent CBT package, such as the widely utilized Coping Cat (Kendall, 2000). Components may include awareness of physiological signs of anxiety, cognitive restructuring, and relaxation (Chorpita, 1998; Kendall et al., 2005; Kingery et al., 2006). Exposure is also used with mindfulness-based approaches for teens and children (Greco & Hayes, 2008), including dialectical behavior therapy (Miller, Rathus, & Linehan, 2007; Perepletchikova et al., 2011).

Theoretical and Research Underpinnings

The earliest uses of exposure-like procedures with children are initially found in the pioneering work of Mary Cover Jones (1924). Animal models of anxiety induction (Estes & Skinner, 1941) and subsequent extinction (Page & Hall, 1953; Solomon, Kamin, & Wynne, 1953) demonstrated procedures which were later applied to humans experiencing serious phobias (e.g., Malleson, 1959). Mowrer (1947, 1960) contributed a two-factor theoretical model explaining the acquisition (fear is established via classical conditioning) and maintenance of anxiety (instrumentally through negative reinforcement of escape and avoidance responses), which was subsequently extrapolated into procedures for its treatment. Modern exposure therapy grew out of implosive therapy (Stampfl, 1961), flooding (Rachman, 1966), and response prevention (Baum, 1970).

Mechanics

Effective implementation of exposure involves several phases: assessment, preparation for exposure, exposure, and postexposure processing. Each phase may require tailoring to a child's individual developmental level, and a greater emphasis should be placed on making sessions appealing or fun (while not avoiding) to enhance treatment engagement for younger children (Bouchard, Mendlowitz, Coles, & Franklin, 2004).

Assessment

Thorough conceptualization of childhood anxiety consists of a functional assessment of the anxious behaviors, which may be conducted through clinical interviews of the child and parent, in a structured or unstructured format. The use of additional assessment tools such as multi-rater rating scales (e.g., Multidimensional Anxiety Scale for Children; March, Parker, Sullivan, Stallings, & Conners, 1997) and diagnosis-specific inventories (e.g., Social Phobia and Anxiety Inventory for Children; Beidel, Turner, & Morris, 1995; Revised Children's Manifest Anxiety Scale, 2nd ed; Reynolds & Richmond, 2008) is encouraged.

Brief problem history as well as a thorough functional analysis of the anxiety and associated avoidance and/or escape behaviors needs to occur. Identification of the initial triggering events for the fear (e.g., for dog phobia: child chased by German Shepherd) is helpful but not imperative. A detailed evaluation of fear-inducing stimuli (and variations) is particularly helpful for exposure. Introduction of subjective ratings of distress (SUDs; Wolpe, 1969) during assessment is beneficial for case conceptualization and use during exposure, although a visual or truncated scale, such as 8- or 10-point scale is suggested. The same scale may be used as a treatment process measure, which will be discussed later. An anxiety hierarchy may be constructed to guide exposures but is not necessary.

The pattern of overt escape and avoidance behaviors warrants particular focus as these behaviors will be targeted during exposure. When parents' or other significant persons' (e.g., teacher, peer) behavior inadvertently maintains anxiety, training is required to inhibit presentation of escape and avoidance opportunities to the child.

Preparing for Exposure

Preparation for exposure includes psychoeducation, rationale for exposure, and motivational components. Explanations of anxiety, avoidance, and exposure will vary based on the child's cognitive (reasoning skills) and emotional development (e.g., emotion understanding, regulation). Younger children will benefit from the use of simpler phrasing (e.g., "Not facing things which scare us makes them seem even worse. We have to face the things that scare us"). Adolescents may feel more respected with more complex explanations using scientific terminology (e.g., extinction, habituation), which may help foster rapport and treatment compliance (Kendall et al., 2005). Comparing exposure to other experiences that are initially scary, difficult or improve with practice and time is often helpful as well (e.g., watching a scary scene in a movie; getting into a cold swimming pool). Younger children may benefit from identifying imaginary characters or superheroes to help them cope with the anxiety during an exposure (Bouchard et al., 2004).

Motivation is important to elicit from children to help them tolerate exposures. A good starting point is, "What is your anxiety keeping you from doing that you want to do?" For example, if a child is afraid to get on an airplane but it is stopping them from going to Disney World, the ultimate goal of getting to Disney is worth enduring flight exposures. Tangible motivation through positive reinforcement for engaging in exposures (i.e., rewards for effort) both in and out of session is encouraged by some protocols (Bouchard et al., 2004; Chorpita, 1998; Kendall, 2000) and may be especially helpful when working with younger children. Rewards should be meaningful and presented immediately after the exposure. Lastly, exposure tasks work best when they are collaboratively chosen and planned (Bouchard et al., 2004), using stimuli that evoke an optimal level of anxiety. For cases in which imaginal exposure is utilized, assessment of imagery skills and subsequent imagery training may be conducted as needed.

Exposure

Based on the nature of the stimulus (e.g., accessibility, practicality) and patient factors (e.g., ability to immersively imagine, willingness to confront fear in vivo), a modality of exposure must be chosen to represent the targeted feared stimuli. Ultimately, all forms of exposure immerse the client in the feared situation using multiple sensations, real or generated environmental contexts, and assess for anxiety (SUDs), feelings, thoughts, and physiological responses throughout.

In virtual reality and in vivo environments, the presentation of the stimulus in context requires little effort from the therapist. In these exposures, the therapist must guide the child's attention, using verbal cues, to relevant aspects of the environment (e.g., "look at the yellow flowers and listen to the buzzing sounds of the bee"). During imaginal exposure, the therapist is completely responsible for generating relevant cues through words and thus must present a cohesive scene that incorporates the feared cues in a way that is relatable to the child or adolescent. As such, the therapist must build all sensory aspects of the scene to make it feel real (i.e., simulate in vivo) by drawing the child's attention beyond visual cues to include auditory, olfactory, tactile and even gustatory cues to aid immersion. It is important that verbal construction of imagery is paced slowly to allow the patient to process the information. Younger children may have more difficulty with imaginal exposure (Davis, Whiting, & May, 2012); thus tangible elements may be helpful, such as using props to act out aspects of the fear (Kendall et al., 2005) or writing a story of the feared event with the child. Kendall (2000) suggests that imaginal exposure may be utilized to prepare for subsequent in vivo exposures.

Table 13.4 Steps for conducting exposure

Step	Brief description
Assessment	– Interview the child and parent(s) – Administer structured assessment tools – Conduct thorough functional assessment of anxiety and related behaviors for hierarchical conceptualization and, if desired, hierarchy construction
Prepare for exposure	– Psychoeducation – Exposure rationale – Motivation: discuss reasons to conquer fear, possible behavior plan
Exposure	– Choose modality (e.g., imaginal or in vivo) – Add elements to personalize scene/environment – Assess for and reflect feelings, physiological response, thoughts, and SUDs back to the patient
Postexposure processing	– Summarize experience and emphasize changes in anxiety and fulfillment of feared consequences – Normalize possible memory recall and sensitization – Homework exercises

Once in contact with the stimulus in vivo, in imagery or in virtual reality, the therapist's role is to continue the client's engagement with the scene and to personalize it with aspects of their patient's experience. As such, level of anxiety (using SUDs), thoughts, feelings, bodily responses, and behaviors should be intermittently assessed and reflected to the child (e.g., "That's right. Your heart is beating very quickly, and you're afraid the spider will bite you."). Check-in questions should be paced at a frequency at which they do not detract from immersion and should be phrased in a developmentally appropriate manner. For example, an adolescent may be able to answer questions about physiological signs of anxiety and consequential thinking, while a young child may require questioning about how parts of his or her body feels and what kind of worry thoughts he or she is having. During exposure, it is crucial that escape (i.e., safety) behaviors be attended to through response prevention. A child in vivo is not allowed to look away or turn from feared stimuli. Likewise during imaginal exposure, opening one's eyes is a typical way to avoid concentrating on fearful imagery and is therefore not allowed.

While the length of exposure sessions varies, longer sessions allow for greater in-session habituation and are preferred (Bouchard et al., 2004), with some treatment manuals claiming a 50 % decrease in SUDs reports (Davis, Ollendick, & Öst, 2009; Kendall, 2000). In a single-session protocol, Davis et al. (2009) recommend a 3-h massed session. On the other end of the spectrum, some multiple-session exposure protocols recommend a maximum of 30 min (Chorpita, 1998) or as few as 10 min or less procedures (Hedtke, Kendall, & Tiwari, 2009; Tiwari, Kendall, Hoff, Harrison, & Fizur, 2013) (Table 13.4).

Postexposure Processing

Following exposure, the child should receive verbal praise from the therapist and a reinforcer if a behavior plan is in place. The child's attention is directed to relevant aspects of the experience regarding their emotional reactions. It may be helpful to visually display within and across-session changes in SUDs on a graph to increase progress tangibility and be reinforcing to both child and parents. In addition, it is important to revisit what the child thought would happen and if it did or did not occur.

It is important to discuss and normalize what may happen between sessions. They may find themselves thinking about their fear more or remembering related past experiences. In exposure therapy, this is reframed as a continuation of the work from the session which should be attended to in addition to any other exposure exercises agreed upon. Over the course of treatment, the last three steps, preexposure preparation, exposure, and postexposure, are repeated until sufficient extinction in the anxiety response has occurred (e.g., as indicated by SUDs ratings or approach behaviors) (Table 13.4).

Research Support

Numerous studies show support for exposure-based treatments with children (cf. Davis, May & Whiting, 2011; Reynolds, Wilson, Austin, & Hooper, 2012 for reviews), though few studies examine exposure therapy alone (e.g., Bolton & Perrin, 2008; Sreenivasan, Manocha, & Jain 1979).

Recent exposure-related research includes dismantling studies of multicomponent treatments. Kendall's Coping Cat protocol (2000) serves as the gold standard for the treatment of children's anxiety disorders. In this 16–20 session protocol, exposure is introduced around session 7. Research finds that when exposure is introduced earlier, shorter treatment length and greater effect size are found compared to the Coping Cat model (Gryczkowski et al., 2013; Vande Voort, Svecova, Brown Jacobsen, & Whiteside, 2010). Others, using a modular therapeutic approach, which allowed exposure to be introduced earlier, also found efficacy for doing so (Chorpita, 1998; Chorpita, Taylor, Francis, Moffitt, & Austin, 2004).

Davis, Whiting, and May (2012) suggest that in vivo may be better than imaginal exposure for children, because of developmental maturity. Alternatively, virtual reality exposure shows promise for treatment of childhood phobias (Bouchard, 2011; St-Jacques, Bouchard, & Bélanger, 2010). Tiwari et al. (2013) examined the impact of preexposure preparation and postexposure tasks on treatment response, as both are advocated for, but without empirical basis. Postexposure processing, rewards, and homework assignment were associated with improved outcomes while preparation for exposure was not.

Assertion Training for Youth

Mark Terjesen

Childhood and adolescence involves a complex interplay between the development of social relationships, the pressure toward conformity (Coleman, 1980), and the achievement of one's unique social identity (Wise, Bundy, Bundy, & Wise, 1991). Children are constantly faced with challenging interpersonal situations such as refusing the requests of others, giving and receiving compliments, making friends, coping with criticism, and managing stress. Children who are socially skilled in solving these problems are likely to be "well adjusted in many areas of their life, particularly at school" (Rotheram-Borus, 1988, p. 83). Conversely, children who have interpersonal difficulties or exhibit few assertive behaviors are more likely to be bullied, develop aggressive tendencies, and demonstrate lower academic achievement (Malecki & Elliott, 2002; Sarkova et al., 2013). This chapter will review the definition of assertiveness, describe pre-intervention considerations and social skills assessments, and suggest programs that can be carried out with treatment integrity in the school setting.

Conceptual Model of Assertiveness Skill Development

Assertive behavior is the appropriate, respectful expression of feelings (Alberti & Emmons, 1995; Masters & Rimm, 1987). Assertive behavior typically involves making requests of others as well as refusing requests that are deemed unreasonable (Duckworth, 2009). Assertive behavior allows for the expression of strong feelings and opinions, and it can be further conceptualized as a "middle ground" between passivity and aggression, emphasizing self-expression in socially acceptable ways.

Within a cognitive-behavioral framework, passivity and aggression can be described behaviorally as "learned behaviors" subject to reinforcement principles and result from specific cognitive evaluations. Similarly, assertive behaviors are often maintained by reinforcers, are subject to the motivational and affective states of the student, and may develop as a result from these cognitive-evaluative factors. Both nonassertive and assertive behaviors are learned through rewards or punishment, and how the students think about these behaviors influences their motivation to engage in them.

Consideration of history may be important as behaviors that have been regularly reinforced from an early age may be more resistant to change. Moreover, these behaviors are most likely also maintained in the child's current setting. It is beneficial for the clinician to identify reinforcers for nonassertive behaviors prior to implementing an assertion skills training program and be aware that these reinforcers may be covert or overt. As many events occur within a social setting, discerning through observation which ones may be reinforcing the behavior may be challenged. Consultation with parents and teachers may help to reduce the influence of the reinforcers that maintain undesirable behaviors.

A lack of assertive behavior has been linked to the motivational and affective states of the student (Alberti & Emmons, 1995; Duckworth, 2009). The motivational state of the student that may lead him/her to engage in passive or aggressive behaviors (and not assertive behaviors) may be driven by reinforcement expectancies, which can in turn interfere with the student's motivation to learn these new assertive behaviors. For some children, a successful outcome following assertive behavior is likely a receipt of the preferred outcome, with the child getting what he or she wants. To promote the development of assertive behavior, it may be important for the clinician to reframe success to reflect the notion that assertive behavior reflects more personal control and respect (Duckworth, 2009). Schab (2009) refers to this as the "Golden Rule" in that we seek to educate students that they should treat others like they want to be treated themselves. Appropriately asserting oneself is both respect for the individual they are communicating with as well as respect for themselves for demonstrating control in their interaction and not behaving passively or aggressively. In contrast, students may have the false belief that after the training, the act of engaging in the appropriate assertive behavior will consistently lead to the desired outcome. For example, if a child is upset because they are not asked to participate in a game, we may work with them on a good example of something assertive that they may say (e.g., "I do not like when you don't ask me to play with you. I feel unhappy when this happens. I would like to play with you.") but also would want to work with the student on understanding that because they make the request it does not mean that they will get the desired outcome (i.e., getting asked to play with them). Promoting persistence in assertion is a way to increase the likelihood of the receipt of their desired goal can be explained to students through the use of both personal examples and anecdotes. A clinician may point out that the first time the student tried to do a specific mathematical multiplication computation, it may not have been met with success. The only way the student eventually acquired the ability to do multiplication was through practice and persistence. The same would hold true for assertive behavior.

The affective states influencing assertive behaviors involve emotional and physiological experiences that the student may have in relation to the idea of behaving in an assertive manner. If these experiences are heightened, there may be negative impact on behavior, making them less likely to interact assertively with others, because the decrease in unpleasant emotions following non-assertion is reinforcing.

Pre-Intervention Considerations

Assertiveness training has garnered some empirical support in working with anxious/avoidant youth and for delinquency and disruptive behaviors (American Academy of Pediatrics, 2014). However, in reviewing the research, assertiveness training is very often a part of a multicomponent intervention, such as social skills training. Yet, the skills developed during assertiveness training assume the existence of adequate social skills (Duckworth, 2009). Gresham and Elliott (1990) define social skills as "socially acceptable learned behaviors that enable a person to interact effectively with others and to avoid socially unacceptable responses" (p. 1). Malecki and Elliot (2002) highlight that assertion is one of these key skills. Effective assertive behaviors involve nonverbal and verbal components. Among the nonverbal behaviors the clinician may wish to consider are eye contact, posture, facial expressions, and body movements (Rotheram-Borus, 1988). Poor and inconsistent eye contact and a more rigid posture might convey disinterest or anxiety. Facial expressions may also convey a message that is not consistent with the desired assertive behavior. Affective displays may reflect anxiety or anger. Some body movements may be interpreted as tentativeness in making the assertive request. Last, inappropriate regard or awareness of other's "personal space" may also impact how the assertive behavior is received (Duckworth, 2009). Therefore, clinicians may wish to give feedback about the child's nonverbal behavior and use of personal space and to build these skills via practice.

The assertiveness research on youth is limited when considering the extent to which assertiveness training leads to behavioral change in the absence of other social skills targeted for change. Early research (Huey & Rank, 1984; Pentz, 1980; Rotheram & Armstrong, 1980) reported an increase in assertion among aggressive and nonassertive youth when those behaviors were the primary target for intervention. Generalizability is limited because assertive behavior was evaluated using self and other report, role plays, and experimentally manipulated interactions.

The results of two studies that specifically targeted assertiveness warrant some consideration by clinicians. Wise, Bundy, Bundy, and Wise (1991) demonstrated that increased *knowledge* as to assertiveness does not translate to increased effectiveness. Later studies (Thompson, Bundy, & Broncheau, 1995; Thompson, Bundy, & Wolfe, 1996) expanded this 6-week program to 12 weeks and also reported an increase in knowledge, but there was not an accompanying change in assertive behaviors. Yet social skills programs that incorporate assertion training have impressive results. For example, Jones, Brown, and Aber (2011) reported improvement in behavior, affective states, social skills, and children's math and reading achievement in a longitudinal study of the 4Rs Program, "Reading, Writing, Respect, and Resolution," which included assertion training . This research may support the notion that it may not be sufficient to just teach the skill of assertiveness in isolation but to integrate behavioral practice and other social skills as part of the intervention.

Prior to implementing an intervention, the individual's skill should be assessed followed by the development of specific objectives and expected competencies for the student during the training. It is important to assess carefully so as to determine whether the lack of assertive behavior is a skill deficit or a performance deficit (Dow, 1994). Skill deficits are characterized by the lack of the verbal and nonverbal skills needed to behave assertively; moreover, the child may be unable to tell the clinician what would be a good assertive response for a given situation. In contrast, performance deficits are characterized by knowing the appropriate assertive behavior, but the student has difficulty demonstrating it. This may be due to a number of cognitive and evaluative variables that are negatively impacting the students' ability to transfer knowledge to behavior, such as limited self-efficacy (e.g., "I will not be able to do this well."), dysfunctional cognitions (e.g., "If I say this, she may get upset at me."), or negative evaluations (e.g., "If I don't get what I want by assertively requesting this, it would be terrible."). Treatment may benefit from assessing the cognitions related to the lack of assertive behavior and target them for intervention as indicated. These variables may lead to subsequent negative emotions, with consequent anxiety and depression further impacting upon performance of assertive behavior.

Assessment to Guide Intervention

Assessment of social skills via self-report and other informant questionnaires helps identify who would most benefit from assertiveness training. Specific behaviors and their context may be best gathered via observations. School settings offer ideal opportunities to observe assertive social behaviors. Clinicians may also want students to keep a log of situations when the opportunity to demonstrate the assertive behaviors existed and what the students actually did in that situation. Clinicians might use the happening, thinking, feeling, and behaving (HTFB) framework (Ellis & Bernard, 2006) to categorize the data because the student uses this self-monitoring approach to note the specific situation (happening), their thoughts (thinking), the affective state(s) experienced at that moment (feeling), and the behavioral response(s) performed. Listing outcomes permits the student to consider whether the request was effective. This provides the clinician with "data" to guide the intervention and offers an opportunity for the student to consider information and patterns in his/her behaviors that increase (or decrease) the likelihood of a successful outcome. Although developed to assist in data collection and treatment planning within the CBT/REBT framework, this model may also be useful within a problem-solving therapy (PST; Nezu, Nezu, & McMurran, 2009) framework. Defining the problem, looking at the data collected, and generating alternative solutions (i.e., different ways of thinking, feeling, and behaving) may let the student decide which solution gives them the best chance for success. This provides them with an opportunity to be building a skill that is similar in nature to the problem.

Implementing an Assertive Intervention

Assertiveness training programs almost universally follow a hierarchical, systematic skill-training approach. Typically, the first step in assertion training provides education about what is considered an assertive response and its likely consequences. This may involve discussion about assertiveness, passivity, and aggression and correcting inaccurate or distorted beliefs about these behavior categories. It may be helpful for the clinician to offer a rationale as to why engaging in assertive behavior is important and to define "success" in assertiveness. It is important to reinforce that success is not contingent on a tangible outcome (e.g., by having one's request fulfilled) but rather in demonstrating personal control and respect during the assertive exchange.

Next, most programs will define typical types of assertive behaviors, among which is the ability to express one's opinion. Yet, it is important to clarify that the expression of one's opinion is not the same as a statement of fact and that an assertive expression of opinion allows others in the social exchange to express their own point of view comfortably. For example, "The Yankees are the best team ever. No one comes close" is expressing this as a statement of fact rather than an opinion, and it may discourage others from participating in the exchange.

Clinicians may discuss how the assertive behavior can be influenced by the social context and situation (Duckworth, 2009); there are times when subtle assertive behaviors are required and times when firm responses are indicated. For example, the first time a classmate takes something from a student's desk without asking, an assertive communication that brings the attention to the matter may be sufficient. However, after the third occasion of the classmate engaging in this behavior, a more firm assertive response may be called for which may indicate the intent to bring this to the attention of the teacher.

Next, assertiveness interventions often focus on making requests and address the content clarity, the reasonableness of the request, and the degree of the specificity of the request, its importance and its tone. Duckworth (2009) describes a "sandwiching" of an assertive request in between two impact statements. As an example, the student would make a statement that reflects the negative impact of peers' behavior ("when you take things of mine without asking it makes me think you do not respect me") then suggests a reasonable and specific alternative behavior ("I would like you to ask before taking anything of mine") and concludes stating the potential positive impact of the behavioral suggestion for both of them ("I would feel like you respected me and when possible, I would be open to sharing these things with you").

Additional content addressed depends upon the specific areas of deficit or concern for the individual. These skills may involve education and practice in effective nonverbal communication, practicing the ability to make and refuse requests and giving and receiving compliments and/or criticisms. Each session may begin with an introduction of the skill set that will be presented, demonstration/modeling of the behaviors that are linked to that skill set, and practice of those behaviors during the session. Feedback and discussion of the performance of those behaviors should be promoted and reinforced. Progression to role plays of more student-specific contexts should be incorporated upon successful performance of the behavior. When competency in assertion is demonstrated through general situation assertiveness role plays, the practice of these behaviors then should follow in role play situations similar to the situation that the student finds difficult, such as where they typically behave passively or aggressively. This allows the clinician to see what maintains the maladaptive responses and provides an opportunity to give direct feedback about the behaviors and to reinforce appropriate assertive behaviors.

Homework assignments should be collaboratively developed with the student to give them opportunities to achieve skilled performance through practice and to provide experiences designed to develop self-efficacy and the performance of assertive behavior in specific situations; this will also promote generalization. It is important for clinicians to communicate that the performance of even effective assertive behaviors may be influenced by the situational context and individuals involved. Further, discussion of realistic performance expectations and strategies for reinforcement for appropriate behavior by the child, parent, or teacher may be helpful to promote maintenance of the application of these new behaviors. When assertive behavior is impacted upon by unhealthy affective states (typically a performance deficit rather than a skill deficit), clinicians might introduce cognitive restructuring (see Arora, Possel & Barnard..., Terjesen, Chapter 12, this volume) and relaxation training (see Haak, Chapter 13, this volume) where appropriate.

Summary and Conclusions

Assertion is the appropriate expression of feelings. For some, this is a challenging task. The performance of assertive behaviors among youth is influenced by reinforcement history, factors maintaining nonassertive behaviors, the expectations of students, and the outcome(s) following the assertive request. Clarification as to the benefit of engaging in assertive behavior and the impact that it may have on social relationships is important. Intervention sessions should be designed to build on specific skills related to the child's assertiveness deficits and should provide opportunities to practice these skills within their social context. Children have to deal with many social challenges and interpersonal situations. The development of assertive behavior may help students increase their confidence, improve their social skills, and contribute to their social and emotional development and overall welfare.

Progressive Muscle Relaxation

Jill Haak Bohnenkamp

Introduction

Progressive muscle relaxation (PMR) is a widely used behavioral intervention procedure indicated for numerous mental health disorders and symptomatology in children including anxiety, aggression, depression, sleep problems, and chronic pain (Kendall, 2006; Lopata, 2003; Morgenthaler et al., 2006; Palermo et al., 2010; Reynolds & Coats, 1986). PMR aims to reduce physiological symptoms of stress, tension, and arousal through a guided procedure focused on systematically tensing and relaxing muscle groups. PMR teaches awareness of and control over physiological and muscular reactions to distress such as anxiety, anger, or pain (Kendall,

2006). The background and theoretical bases for PMR as well as research support for PMR for different mental health disorders and symptomatology will be reviewed, focusing on school-aged individuals. An overview of how to conduct PMR with students in the school setting will be provided.

Background

Early research on PMR was conducted by Edmund Jacobson and focused on addressing the "nervous element that appears in a large variety of diseases," in addition to addressing anxiety as a psychological construct (Jacobson, 1929). Jacobson found that tension was related to a shortening of muscle fibers and that this tension typically appeared when a person reported the experience of anxiety (1929). Jacobson's research investigated neuromuscular tension and relaxation, and he argued that "to be excited and to be fully relaxed are physiological opposites"; thus progressive relaxation has the potential to address many disorders in which physiological tension impacts functioning. By systematically tensing and releasing muscle groups and attending to the physiological sensations of tension versus relaxation, a person can decrease muscle contractions and resulting tension (Jacobson, 1929).

Joseph Wolpe (1958) adapted Jacobson's progressive relaxation procedure to a shorter, more efficient relaxation program that could be used in conjunction with his systematic desensitization procedure. Weisman, Ollendick, and Horne (1978) studied the use of PMR in children and found that PMR procedures of both Ollendick and Cerny (1981) and Koeppen (1974) resulted in significantly reduced muscle tension as measured by electromyographic (EMG) recordings (see Kendall & Suveg, 2006, for a discussion).

Support from the Literature

PMR has been integrated into a number of cognitive-behavioral interventions for a range of mental health disorders. Few research studies have investigated the effects of PMR in isolation; however, there are numerous studies supporting the effectiveness of cognitive-behavioral therapies that include PMR as a clinical component to treat diverse mental health disorders. Chorpita and Daleiden (2009) reviewed 322 randomized clinical trials for child mental health treatments and found that the practice element of relaxation was present in 42 % of all protocols for the treatment of anxiety, 42 % for the treatment of depressed mood, 13 % for the treatment of oppositional/aggressive behavior, 15 % for the treatment of delinquency, 23 % for the treatment of ADHD, and 17 % for the treatment of truancy/school refusal. This study focused on relaxation generally, as opposed to PMR, but highlights the frequency of and support for the use of relaxation in a number of child mental health treatments.

Anxiety

The initial research (Jacobson, 1929; Wolpe, 1958) on PMR focused on anxiety reduction, and thus from the onset, PMR has been identified as an important thera- peutic technique for the treatment of anxiety disorders. Many cognitive-behavioral interventions for anxiety in children include PMR as a standard component (Barrett, Dadds & Rapee, 1991; Kendall, 2006). In the Chorpita and Daleidan (2007) review, the clinical technique of relaxation (but not PMR specifically) was categorized as having "good support" for the treatment of anxiety as it was more effective in reduc- ing anxiety symptoms than an alternative treatment in one comparison, and no- treatment control conditions in two comparisons. A number of additional studies of individual and group cognitive-behavioral interventions for anxiety conducted in the school setting include PMR as a treatment component. These studies have found significant decreases in anxiety for children of diverse demographic characteristics (Barrett & Turner, 2001; Dadds, Spence, Holland, Barrett, & Laurens, 1997; Jaycox, Kataoka, Stein, Langley, & Wong, 2012; Mifsud & Rapee, 2005). Stallard et al. (2005) evaluated a school-based group cognitive-behavioral universal preventive intervention that included PMR and found significantly reduced symptoms of anxiety and improved self-esteem.

Anger and Aggression

There is strong theoretical support for PMR in the treatment of anger and aggression as physiological reactions, such as skin conductance, have been found to be linked to arousal and aggressive behavior (Hubbard et al., 2002). One of the few studies investigating PMR in isolation found that this discrete clinical technique reduced aggression in elementary school students with emotional and behavioral disorders (Lopata, 2003). Moreover, several research studies investigating school-based group cognitive-behavioral interventions for anger and aggression, which include some variation of PMR as a treatment component, resulted in significantly reduced symp- toms of anger and aggression (Deffenbacher, Lynch, Oetting, & Kemper, 1996; Feindler & Engel, 2011; Sukhodolsky, Solomon, & Perrine, 2000).

Depression

A school-based study of a group intervention for adolescent depression found that training in PMR alone produced comparable effects to a 5-week cognitive-behavioral intervention (Reynolds and Coats, 1986). In the Chorpita and Daleidan (2007) review, the clinical technique of relaxation (but not PMR specifically) was catego- rized as having "good support" for the treatment of depression as it was more effec- tive in decreasing depressive symptoms than no-treatment control conditions in two separate trials. There is also research supporting the effectiveness of school-based cognitive-behavioral interventions, which include PMR as a treatment component, for middle and high school students with and without other comorbid disorders and across diverse demographic samples (Kahn, Kehle, Jenson, & Clark, 1990; Shirk, Kaplinski, & Gudmundsen, 2009; Stark, Reynolds, & Kaslow, 1987).

Sleep Problems and Pain

Research also supports the effectiveness of PMR for the treatment of sleep problems and chronic pain. The American Academy of Sleep Medicine Practice Parameters identified PMR as an effective treatment for insomnia in adults and children (Morgenthaler et al., 2006). A meta-analytic review of randomized controlled trials of psychological therapies for chronic pain included nine relaxation-based therapies; results yielded positive effects for clinically significant pain reduction with an odds ratio of 9.93 (Palermo et al. 2010).

Basic How-To Guide for Using PMR in School Settings

The goal of PMR is to help the student(s) identify and decrease tension in the body and reduce somatic symptoms of distress. The following description provides an overview of the PMR procedure with student(s) in the school setting. Adaptations to this general script should be used based on the developmental level of the student. This relaxation procedure can be used as an individual intervention or adapted for a group or classroom intervention:

1. Clinician preparation: Plan in advance for the PMR session and brainstorm ways to make the therapy or classroom setting more comfortable. This may include bringing in a small lamp to be able to turn off bright overhead lights or a comfortable cushion or yoga mat to lie on. For a classroom exercise, the clinician could encourage students to put their heads down on their desk or find a comfortable position in their chair. The clinician should also try to limit external distractions and consider placing a Do Not Disturb sign on the classroom/office door.
2. Begin the session by introducing the notion that we have different feelings in our bodies when we are upset (sad, anger, anxious, depressed). Ask the student to identify how her/his body feels when upset (e.g., hot, sweaty, tense, shaky).
3. Discuss with the student the difference between how her/his body feels when it is tense and when it is relaxed. Have the student practice the difference between feeling tense and relaxed by squeezing her/his hand tightly to make a fist and holding for 5 s and then noticing the difference when she/he releases his/her fist.
4. Describe that she/he will be learning how to notice some of those feelings in her/his body and how to help herself/himself feel calm and relaxed.
5. Encourage the student to find a comfortable position. Ask the child if she/he prefers the lights dimmed or would like to lie on the floor. (For a group procedure, plan in advance where students will be allowed to sit/find a comfortable

Table 13.5 PMR imagery

Breathing	Smell the roses (breathe in); blow out the birthday candles (breathe out)
	Pretend like you are filling a balloon with air
Feet	Point your toes like a ballerina
	Pretend your feet are squishing in the sand/mud
Legs	Keep your legs straight like a robot
Arms	Make a muscle
Hands	Squeeze lemons/ball/clay/play-dough
	Make a fist
Stomach	Pretend like someone is standing on your stomach
Shoulders/arms	Stretch like a lazy cat
	Squinch your shoulders up to your ears
Neck	Pretend like you are a turtle and pull your head into it's shell
Face	Squinch like you smell something bad
	Squinch like you taste something sour
	Pretend that you have a large jawbreaker in your mouth, bite down hard
	Pretend that there is a fly on your face, squinch your nose to try to make it fly away

Imagery from Koeppen, 1974; Ollendick & Cernry, 1981

    position. Answer all student questions in advance, reminding students that they must be quiet once the procedure has begun.)

6. Next the student will identify and think about a relaxing place. Help the student brainstorm what the place looks like, how it smells, the sounds that she/he hears, and how it feels. (For group sessions, each student can imagine her/his own relaxing place, or the clinician can choose a relaxing place to describe, e.g., the beach, a rainforest.)

7. Encourage the student to close her/his eyes and imagine the relaxing place using the descriptions that the student provides.

8. Tell the student to start by taking a slow deep breath and try to make her/his stomach expand and then slowly let the breath out. Repeat this procedure for three to five deep breaths.

9. Remind the student to continue imagining being in her/his relaxing place and repeat the details of the relaxing place.

10. Tell the student that she/he will start by tensing and relaxing her/his feet. (Descriptions for this can include pointing toes like a ballerina and squishing toes in the sand/mud. See Table 13.5 for additional imagery.) Tell the student to tense her/his feet and hold the tension for 3–5 s and then to release and let her/his feet completely relax. Encourage the student to notice the difference between when her/his feet are tense and when they are relaxed. Have the student repeat tensing and relaxing her/his feet.

11. Remind the student continue her/his deep, slow breathing, breathing in, pause, and breathing out, and enjoy being in her/his relaxing place.

12. Next move on to the next muscle group and have the student practice tensing and relaxing that muscle as described above. It is recommended to begin with three to five muscle groups (e.g., feet, legs, arms, hands, face) and additional muscle groups can be added in future sessions.
13. Continue to remind the student to continue her/his deep, slow breathing, breathing in, pause, and breathing out, and enjoy being in her/his relaxing place. Also, encourage the student to notice the difference in her/his body overall as she/he relaxes additional muscle groups.
14. After progressing through the muscle groups, encourage the student to enjoy the relaxed and calm feeling, and remind the student that she/he can use this strategy to relax any time she/he is feeling upset. Encourage the student to slowly start to bring her/his attention back into the room and open her/his eyes when she/he is ready.
15. After completing the PMR exercise, ask the student to describe her/his experience of PMR, parts that she/he liked and did not like, and how she/he currently feels.
16. Encourage the student to practice the PMR exercise daily and brainstorm when would be a good time to practice (e.g., before going to sleep at night). Give the student an audio recording of the exercise or a script that a parent/guardian can read.
17. Encourage the student to think about when PMR strategies (but potentially not the whole exercise) might be useful in school, such as taking several deep breaths and tensing and relaxing areas of the body that normally become tense when she/he is upset.

Conclusion

PMR is indicated as an effective behavioral therapeutic technique for a number of mental health disorders with the most support for its use in the treatment of anxiety, aggression, and depression (Kendall, 2006; Lopata, 2003; Reynolds & Coats, 1986). There are many variations of the PMR script with the key feature being the systematic tensing and relaxing of muscle groups. PMR for use with children is frequently adapted to include imagery that helps children to better understand the concept of tensing and relaxing muscle groups. PMR's flexibility makes it ideal for the school setting as the procedure length can be adapted to accommodate scheduling needs, and it can be used to address somatic symptoms for a number of mental health problems. PMR is an effective technique for use in school settings and is indicated for individual and group intervention, in addition to universal preventive intervention. PMR can be used on its own as a way to decrease physiological stress, tension, and arousal but is frequently used and recommended as one behavioral technique to help address somatic symptoms in the context of additional cognitive-behavioral strategies.

Systematic Desensitization

Betty S. Lai, Rebecca Rialon Berry, Caroline J. Ehrlich

Systematic desensitization is an exposure-based technique (Saigh, Yule, & Inamdar, 1996) developed by Joseph Wolpe to alter conditioned anxiety responses (Zettle, 2003).

The basic mechanism underlying systematic desensitization is the principle of *reciprocal inhibition* (Goldfried, 1971). This principle asserts that a feared stimulus has been paired with anxiety. When a client learns to utilize incompatible responses (i.e., relaxation techniques) in the presence of a feared stimulus, these incompatible responses suppress or replace anxiety responses through a process *called counter-conditioning* (Ollendick & King, 1998). Over time, this weakens the relationship between a feared stimulus and anxiety.

The essential component to systematic desensitization is repeated exposure to anxiety-evoking situations without the client experiencing any negative consequences (see Schare, Wyatt, & Skolnick, this volume; Bandura, 1969). In its most basic form, systematic desensitization consists of three parts (see Table 13.6; Ollendick & King, 1998): (1) the clinician trains the client to develop *incompatible responses* (i.e., relaxation techniques) to fear or anxiety. Incompatible responses could include meditation or deep breathing. Responses are termed "incompatible" because Wolpe noted that is it not possible to feel both anxious and relaxed at the same time (King, Muris, & Ollendick, 2005). (2) The clinician develops a fear hierarchy with the client (see Schare, Skolnick, & Wyatt, this volume). In this hierarchy, fear-producing stimuli are ranked from least to highest anxiety evoking or fear inducing. (3) Finally, the clinician helps the client systematically move through their fear hierarchy, pairing each feared stimuli with an incompatible response. Thus, in this approach, the client gradually (systematically) becomes less sensitive (desensitized) to the feared situations. Each of these components, as adapted from Spiegler & Guervemont (2003), is described in more detail in the following sections:

1. *Introduce incompatible responses to anxiety.* Relaxation exercises, such as deep breathing and progressive muscle relaxation (see Haak, this volume), are common coping strategies used in systematic desensitization. The latter method involves tensing and then releasing (relaxing) various skeletal muscle groups, arms, face, neck, shoulders, chest, abdomen, and legs, until a calm physical state is achieved. While the client is sitting or reclining comfortably, the therapist guides the client through the relaxation process. *Developing fear hierarchy.* The client is then asked to identify the objects (e.g., dogs) and/or situations (e.g., taking a math test or presenting a speech in class) that are causing anxiety. These items are rank ordered from least to most anxiety producing using the subjective units of distress scales (SUDS). The SUDS allows the client to self-assess and measure subjective levels of discomfort or disturbance (anxiety) experienced in specific situations. Typical SUDS involve anxiety ratings ranging from 0 (completely relaxed or *no anxiety*) to 100 (the worst anxiety imagined). As the word

Table 13.6 Sample systemic desensitization procedure

	Technique	Sample script
Step 1	Introduce incompatible responses to anxiety.	...I want you to practice tensing and releasing the muscles in your face... then focus on tensing and relaxing the muscles in your arms...
Step 2	Developing a fear hierarchy.	What are the pieces of taking a test that are most anxiety provoking for you...Now let's place these stimuli in order.
Step 3	Systematically expose client to items on their fear hierarchy while the client is engaged in incompatible behavior. (In the first session, this will be the first item in the hierarchy. In all other sessions, this will be the last item from the previous session.)	I want you to imagine that you are seated in your 4th period math class on December 15, the day of the algebra exam...
3a	Ask the client to imagine themselves in the anxiety-producing situation for about 15 s. Slowly increase the amount of time the client is asked to imagine the situation on subsequent presentations until he or she can tolerate at least 30 s of exposure.	You are positioned in the second row of the classroom, and can see the teacher's desk and the chalkboard in front of you, and hear your classmates retrieve their pencils from their bags... (pause for about 15 s).
3b	Tell the client to stop imagining the situation and utilize relaxation techniques. Assess SUDS. Re-establish state of relaxation again and instruct the client to relax for about 30 s.	Now, stop imagining that scene and give all of your attention to relaxing. If the scene you imagined disturbed you even in the slightest degree, raise your right index finger. Stop imagining the scene and just think of your muscles. Let go, and enjoy your state of calm.
3c	Re-read the description of the situation. Ask the client to imagine him or herself in the scene for approximately 15 s.	Imagine the same scene again—the day of your algebra test...
3d	Stop, and again determine the patient's level of anxiety. If he or she is experiencing any anxiety, return to Step 3b. If he or she reports no anxiety, go on to next step.	Stop the scene, and now think of nothing but your own body. If you felt any disturbance in the last scene, raise your right index finger... Just keep relaxing.
3e	Move on to the next item of the fear hierarchy. Repeat the above procedure for this next item, beginning with Step 3a.	Imagine that your teacher has placed the exam on your desk and you open the booklet to the first math problem...

subjective implies, SUDS are specific to each individual, and therefore, each client should be encouraged to determine his or her own anchors (numeric or word labels that represent different levels of anxiety) on the scale.

2. *Systematically expose client to items on their fear hierarchy (in order of least to most fear inducing) while the client is engaged in an incompatible behavior (e.g., progressive muscle relaxation)*. In this step, the therapist instructs the client, who is seated or reclining comfortably, to relax all of his or her muscles. The therapist then describes scenes from the anxiety hierarchy for the client to imagine, starting with the lowest item on the hierarchy; scenes are described in vivid detail and are specific to the client. The client imagines each scene for about 15 s at a time. Whenever the client experiences anxiety or discomfort, the client signals the therapist, usually by raising an index finger. When this occurs, the therapist instructs the client to stop visualizing the scene and to continue relaxing. The result is that over time, the relaxation replaces the tension previously associated with the scene. Each scene in the hierarchy is presented repeatedly until the client reports little or no discomfort. Then, the next highest scene in the hierarchy is visualized.

Systematic desensitization is not applicable to all clients, as young children often experience difficulty carrying out the procedures (Silverman & Rabian, 1994). Techniques more suitable for children may include in vivo exposure, flooding, and modeling therapy. In vivo exposure therapy represents a variant of systematic desensitization and involves exposing the client to the actual feared event (in vivo). The exposure is brief and graduated, and clients are encouraged to stay in the feared situation long enough to learn that the bad things they fear will not happen. If the client pulls out of the exercise before the belief is disconfirmed, the anxiety will not reduce and may even increase. Unlike systematic desensitization, complete deep muscle relaxation is not possible during in vivo exposure because the client is using a variety of muscles during the exposure task (McCarthy & Craig, 1995). Furthermore, clients are taught to use relaxation techniques and to challenge worried thoughts and negative thinking patterns via cognitive restructuring (i.e., identifying and replacing automatic irrational thoughts) prior to engaging in the in vivo exposures (Kendall, 1994).

There are a few ethical concerns surrounding the use of systematic desensitization in young populations. Consistent with the American Psychological Association code of ethics as well as the Individuals with Disabilities Education Act (IDEA) and other federal statutes, school psychologists have an obligation to give preference to evidence-based interventions that are appropriate and found to be efficacious (Jacob & Hartshorne, 1994). According to reviews by both Ollendick and King (1998) and Weisz and Jensen (2001), research supports the probable efficacy of systematic desensitization procedures in the treatment of childhood phobias, but systematic desensitization procedures have not been found to be efficacious for the treatment of childhood anxiety disorders (Ollendick & King, 1998; Weisz & Jensen, 2001) (Table 13.7).

Table 13.7 Research support for systematic desensitization (SD)

Researchers	Sample	Measures (assessment and/or outcome)	Treatment conditions	Follow up data
Coldwell, Wilhelm, Milgrom, Prall, Getz, Spadafora, Chiu, Lroux, & Ramsay, 2007	153 youth with specific phobia of dental injections.	Mini-Structured Clinical Interview for DSM Disorders—for specific phobia; the Needle Survey; Dental Anxiety Scale; Heart rate.	Placebo + SD v. 0.5 mg alprazolam + SD v. 0.75 mg alprazolam + SD; H0: alprazolam + SD will not alter effectiveness or time required for therapy.	No difference between placebo and alprazolam during in vivo therapy on self-reported anxiety. Groups did no differ significantly on any measures.
Koegel, Openden, & Koegel, 2004	3 (2 males) with autism.	Number of hierarchical steps completed with anxiety level rated as comfortable (interval recording system with comfortable, mild anxiety, high anxiety and intolerable categories).	SD effects on auditory hypersensitivity using three different stimuli respective to each subject (vacuum, blender, and hand-mixer).	All three subjects rated as comfortable with stimuli at follow-up proves at least 2 weeks after completion of intervention.
Kondas, 1967	23 youth with stage fright.	Fear Survey Schedule (FSS); palmar perspiration ratings.	Relaxation training v. imaginal SD v. presentation of hierarchy items without relaxation training v. no-treatment control.	SD found to be superior to relaxation training, presentation of hierarchy items without relaxation training and no-treatment control.
Luscre & Center, 1996	3 males with autism and marked fear of dental exams.	Reliability observers trained to an 80 % criterion.	All three subjects exposed to SD with guided mastery, video peer modeling and reinforcement.	Treatment in analog setting generalized to in vivo setting. More steps of the dental exam were completed in vivo following analog treatment, as compared to in vivo baseline.
Mann & Rosenthal, 1969	50 youth with high test anxiety.	Test Anxiety Scale; Gates-McGinnitie Reading Test.	Individual desensitization v. vicarious individual SD v. group SD v. vicarious group SD (observing group tx) v. vicarious group SD (observing individual tx) v. no-treatment control.	All five treatment conditions proved superior to no-treatment condition, but no significant differences were found among treatment groups.

Study	Sample	Measures	Design	Results
Miller, Barrett, Hampe, & Noble, 1972	67 phobic youth.	Louisville Behavior Checklist-parent report; Louisville Fear Survey for Children-parent report; Severity scores as rated by parent and evaluator.	SD v. individualized psychotherapy v. wait-list control.	No differences were found between active treatment groups. Researchers theorize parent training was a confounding variable.
Obler & Terwilliger, 1970	30 neurologically impaired youth with phobia of public bus use or dogs, randomly assigned to treatment or control groups.	Wechsler Intelligence Scale for Children (a cutoff Full Scale IQ score of 75). Treatment effectiveness was measured using a parent-rated questionnaire with 10 items regarding the child's functioning in society, one of which was specific to the phobia.	Treatment: $n=15$ received modified Wolpe SD method. Control: $n=15$ matched to subjects in treatment group on age, sex, IQ and phobia diagnosis.	All 15 subjects in the treatment condition were rated as able to ride a bus or touch a dog either alone or with the help of another person, demonstrating that desensitization was significantly superior to no treatment in reducing phobic disturbances. There was no effect for treatment awareness, indicating that both high- and low-IQ subjects responded equally well to treatment.
Ultee, Griffioen, & Schellekens, 1982	24 youth aged 5–10 with specific phobia of water.	Behavioral observation to evaluate water avoidance; Teacher report on swimming behaviors.	In vitro SD treatment group v. in vivo SD treatment group v. control group.	In vivo SD group showed greater gains than in vitro SD and control groups after four sessions. No relative improvement was shown between the control and in vitro groups.
Zettle, 1993	24 college students with math anxiety.	Mathematics Anxiety Rating Scale; Test Anxiety Inventory; Trait Anxiety Inventory; Wide Range Achievement Test.	Acceptance and Commitment Therapy v. SD.	Participants in the SD group saw significant decrease in trait anxiety across treatment. Overall, both groups resulted in clinically significant reductions in math anxiety, and no significant difference emerged at 2-month follow ups.

References

Achenbach, T. M., & Edelbrock, C. S. (1991). *Manual for the child behavior checklist and profile*. Burlington: University of Vermont.

Alberti, R. E., & Emmons, M. L. (1995). *Your perfect right: A guide to assertive living*. Atascadero, CA: Impact Publishers Inc.

American Academy of Pediatrics. (2014). *Evidence based child and adolescent psychosocial interventions*. Retrieved from http://www.aap.org/en-us/advocacy-and-policy/aap-health-initiatives/ Mental-Health/Documents/CRPsychosocialInterventions.pdf.

Bandura, A. (1969). *Principles of behavior modification*. New York, NY: Holt, Rinehart and Winston.

Barrett, P. M. (1998). Evaluation of cognitive-behavioral group treatments for childhood anxiety disorders. *Journal of Clinical Child Psychology, 27*, 459–468.

Barrett, P., Dadds, M., & Rapee, R. (1991). *Coping Koala workbook*. Nathah, Australia: School of Applied Psychology, Griffith University. Unpublished manuscript.

Barrett, P. M., & Turner, C. M. (2001). Prevention of anxiety symptoms in primary school children: Preliminary results from a universal school-based trial. *British Journal of Clinical Psychology, 40*, 399–410.

Baum, M. (1970). Extinction of avoidance responding through response prevention (flooding). *Psychological Bulletin, 74*, 276–284.

Beidel, D. C., Turner, S. M., & Morris, T. L. (1995). A new inventory to assess childhood social anxiety and phobia: The social phobia and anxiety inventory for children. *Psychological Assessment, 7*, 73–79.

Bolton, D., & Perrin, S. (2008). Evaluation of exposure with response-prevention for obsessive compulsive disorder in childhood and adolescence. *Journal of Behavior Therapy and Experimental Psychiatry, 39*, 11–22.

Bouchard, S. (2011). Could virtual reality be effective in treating children with phobias? *Expert Review of Neurotherapeutics, 11*, 207–213.

Bouchard, S., Mendlowitz, S. L., Coles, M. E., & Franklin, M. (2004). Considerations in the use of exposure with children. *Cognitive and Behavioral Practice, 11*, 56–65.

Chorpita B. F. (1998). *Modular cognitive behavior therapy for child and adolescent anxiety disorders: Therapist manual*. Unpublished manuscript.

Chorpita, B. F. (2007). *Modular cognitive-behavioral therapy for childhood anxiety disorders*. Canada: The Guilford Press.

Chorpita, B. F., & Daleiden, E. L. (2007). *2007 biennial report: Effective psychosocialinterventions for youth with behavioral and emotional needs*. Retrieved from Hawaii Department of Health, Child and Adolescent Mental Health Division. http://hawaii.gov/health/mental-health/ camhd/library/pdf/ebs/ebs012.pdf.

Chorpita, B. F., & Daleiden, E. L. (2009). Mapping evidence-based treatments for children and adolescents: Application of the distillation and matching model to 615 treatments from 322 randomized trials. *Journal of Consulting and Clinical Psychology, 77*, 566–579.

Chorpita, B. F., Taylor, A. A., Francis, S. E., Moffitt, C., & Austin, A. A. (2004). Efficacy of modular cognitive behavior therapy for childhood anxiety disorders. *Behavior Therapy, 35*, 263–287.

Coldwell, S. E., Wilhelm, F. H., Milgrom, P., Prall, C. W., Getz, T., Spadafora, A., et al. (2007). Combining alprazolam with systematic desensitization therapy for dental injection phobia. *Journal of Anxiety Disorders, 21*, 871–887.

Coleman, J. C. (1980). Friendship and the peer group in adolescence. In J. Adelson (Ed.), *Handbook of adolescent psychology* (pp. 408–431). New York, NY: John Wiley.

Dadds, M. R., Spence, S., Holland, D. E., Barrett, P. M., & Laurens, K. R. (1997). Prevention and early intervention for anxiety disorders: A controlled trial. *Journal of Consulting and Clinical Psychology, 65*, 627–635.

Davis, T., May, A., & Whiting, S. E. (2011). Evidence-based treatment of anxiety and phobia in children and adolescents: Current status and effects on the emotional response. *Clinical Psychology Review, 31,* 592–602.

Davis, T., Ollendick, T. H., & Öst, L. (2009). Intensive treatment of specific phobias in children and adolescents. *Cognitive and Behavioral Practice, 16,* 294–303.

Davis, T., Whiting, S. E., & May, A. C. (2012). Exposure therapy for anxiety disorders in children. In P. Neudeck & H. Wittchen (Eds.), *Exposure therapy: Rethinking the model—refining the method* (pp. 111–125). New York, NY: Springer.

Deffenbacher, J. L., Lynch, R. S., Oetting, E. R., & Kemper, C. (1996). Anger reduction in early adolescents. *Journal of Counseling Psychology, 43*(2), 149–157.

Dow, M. G. (1994). Social inadequacy and social skill. In L. K. Craighead, W. E. Craighead, A. E. Kazdin, & M. J. Mahoney (Eds.), *Cognitive and behavioral interventions: An empirical approach to mental health problems* (pp. 123–140). Boston, MA: Allyn and Bacon.

Duckworth, M. P. (2009). Assertiveness skills and the management of related factors. In W. T. O'Donohue & J. E. Fisher (Eds.), *General principles and empirically supported techniques of cognitive behavior therapy* (pp. 124–132). New York: John Wiley & Sons.

Ellis, A., & Bernard, M. E. (Eds.). (2006). *Rational emotive behavior approaches to childhood disorders.* New York, NY: Springer.

Estes, W. K., & Skinner, B. F. (1941). Some quantitative properties of anxiety. *Journal of Experimental Psychology, 29,* 390–400.

Feindler, E. L., & Engel, E. C. (2011). Assessment and intervention for adolescents with anger and aggression difficulties in school settings. *Psychology in the Schools, 48*(3), 243–253.

Foa, E. B., Chrestman, K. R., & Gilboa-Schechtman, E. (2008). *Prolonged exposure therapy for adolescents with PTSD: Emotional processing of traumatic experiences. Therapist guide.* New York, NY: Oxford University Press.

Goldfriend, M. (1971). Systematic desensitization as training in self-control. *Journal of Consulting and Clinical Psychology, 37*(2), 228–234.

Greco, L. A., & Hayes, S. C. (2008). *Acceptance and mindfulness treatments for children and adolescents: A practitioner's guide.* Oakland, CA US: New Harbinger Publications.

Gresham, F. M., & Elliott, S. N. (1990). *Social skills rating system.* Pines, MN: American Guidance Service.

Gryczkowski, M. R., Tiede, M. S., Dammann, J. E., Jacobsen, A., Hale, L. R., & Whiteside, S. H. (2013). The timing of exposure in clinic-based treatment for childhood anxiety disorders. *Behavior Modification, 37,* 113–127.

Gullone, E., & King, N. J. (1992). Psychometric evaluation of a revised fear survey schedule for children and adolescents. *Journal of Child Psychology and Psychiatry, 33,* 987–998.

Hedtke, K. A., Kendall, P. C., & Tiwari, S. (2009). Safety-seeking and coping behavior during exposure tasks with anxious youth. *Journal of Clinical Child and Adolescent Psychology, 38,* 1–15.

Hubbard, J. A., Smithmyer, C. M., Ramsden, S. R., Parker, E. H., Flanagan, K. D., Dearing, K. F., et al. (2002). Observational, physiological, and self-report measures of children's anger: Relations to reactive versus proactive aggression. *Child Development, 73,* 1101–1118.

Hudson, J. L., Rapee, R. M., Deveney, C., Schniering, C. A., Lyneham, H. J., & Bovopoulos, N. (2009). Cognitive-behavioral treatment versus an active control for children and adolescents with anxiety disorders: A randomized trial. *Journal of the American Academy of Child and Adolescent Psychiatry, 48,* 533–544.

Huey, W. C., & Rank, R. C. (1984). Effects of counselor and peer-led group assertive training on Black adolescent aggression. *Journal of Counseling Psychology, 31,* 95–98.

Jacob, S., & Hartshorne, T. S. (1994). *Ethics and law for school psychologists* (2nd ed.). Brandon, VT: Clinical Psychology Publishing.

Jacobson, E. (1929). *Progressive relaxation.* Chicago, IL: University of Chicago Press.

Jaycox, L. H., Kataoka, S. H., Stein, B. D., Langley, A. K., & Wong, M. (2012). Cognitive behavioral intervention for trauma in schools. *Journal of Applied School Psychology, 28*(3), 239–255.

Jones, M. C. (1924). The elimination of children's fears. *Journal of Experimental Psychology, 7*, 382–390.

Jones, S. M., Brown, J. L., & Aber, J. L. (2011). Two-year impacts of a universal school-based social-emotional and literacy intervention: An experiment in translational developmental research. *Child Development, 82*(2), 533–554.

Kahn, J. S., Kehle, T. J., Jenson, W. R., & Clark, E. (1990). Comparison of cognitive behavioral, relaxation, and self-modeling interventions for depression among middle-school students. *School Psychology Review, 19*(2), 196–211.

Kazdin, A. E., & Weisz, J. R. (1998). Identifying and developing empirically supported child and adolescent treatments. *Journal of Consulting and Clinical Psychology, 66*, 19–36. doi:10.1037/0022-006X.66.1.19.

Kearney, C. A., & Albano, A. M. (2007). *When children refuse school. A cognitive-behavioral therapy approach* (2nd ed.). Oxford, NY: Oxford University Press.

Kendall, P. C. (1994). Treating anxiety disorders in children: results of a randomized clinical trial. *Journal of Consulting and Clinical Psychology, 62*(1), 100–110.

Kendall, P. C. (2000). *Cognitive-behavioral therapy for anxious children: Therapist manual* (2nd ed.). Ardmore, PA: Workbook Publishing.

Kendall, P. C. (Ed.). (2006). *Child and adolescent therapy: Cognitive-behavioral procedures* (3rd ed.). New York, NY: Guilford Press.

Kendall, P. C., & Hedtke, K. A. (2006). *Coping cat workbook* (2nd ed.). Ardmore, PA: Workbook Publishing.

Kendall, P. C., Hudson, J. L., Gosch, E., Flannery-Schroeder, E., & Suveg, C. (2008). Cognitive-behavioral therapy for anxiety disordered youth: A randomized clinical trial evaluating child and family modalities. *Journal of Consulting and Clinical Psychology, 76*, 282–297.

Kendall, P. C., Robin, J. A., Hedtke, K. A., Suveg, C., Flannery-Schroeder, E., & Gosch, E. (2005). Considering CBT with anxious youth? Think exposures. *Cognitive and Behavioral Practice, 12*, 136–150.

Kendall, P. C., & Suveg, C. (2006). Treating anxiety disorders in youth. In P. C. Kendall (Ed.), *Child and adolescent therapy: Cognitive-behavioral procedures* (3rd ed.). New York, NY: Guilford Press.

Kerns, C. M., Read, K. L., Klugman, J., & Kendall, P. C. (2013). Cognitive behavioral therapy for youth with social anxiety: Differential short and long-term treatment outcomes. *Journal of Anxiety Disorders, 7*, 210–215.

Kindt, M., Brosschot, J. F., & Muris, P. (1996). Spider phobia questionnaire for children (SPQC): A psychometric study and normative data. *Behaviour Research and Therapy, 34*, 277–282.

King, N., Muris, P., & Ollendick, T. (2005). Childhood fears and phobias: Assessment and treatment. *Child and Adolescent Mental Health, 10*(2), 50–56.

Kingery, J., Roblek, T. L., Suveg, C., Grover, R. L., Sherrill, J. T., & Bergman, R. (2006). They're not just "little adults": Developmental considerations for implementing cognitive-behavioral therapy with anxious youth. *Journal of Cognitive Psychotherapy, 20*, 263–273.

Koegel, R. L., Openden, D., & Koegel, L. K. (2004). A systematic desensitization paradigm to treat hypersensitivity to auditory stimuli in children with autism in family contexts. *Research and Practice for Persons with Severe Disabilities, 29*(2), 122–134.

Koeppen, A. S. (1974). Relaxation training for children. *Elementary School Guidance and Counseling, 9*, 14–21.

Kondas, O. (1967). Reduction of examination anxiety and 'stage-fright' by group desensitization and relaxation. *Behavioral Research and Therapy, 5*, 275–281.

Lopata, C. (2003). Progressive muscle relaxation and aggression among elementary students classified as emotionally disturbed. *Behavioral Disorders, 28*(2), 162–172.

Luscre, D. M., & Center, D. B. (1996). Procedures for reducing dental fear in children with autism. *Journal of Autism and Developmental Disorders, 26*(5), 547–556.

Malecki, C. K., & Elliott, S. N. (2002). Children's social behaviors as predictors of academic achievement: A longitudinal analysis. *School Psychology Quarterly, 17*(1), 1–23.

Malleson, N. (1959). Panic and phobia: A possible method of treatment. *Lancet, 1*, 225–227.

Mann, J., & Rosenthal, T. L. (1969). Vicarious and direct counterconditioning of test anxiety through individual and group desensitization. *Behavioral Research and Therapy, 7*, 359–367.

March, J. S., & Mulle, K. (1998). *OCD in children and adolescents: A cognitive-behavioral treatment manual*. New York, NY: The Guilford Press.

March, J. S., Parker, J. A., Sullivan, K., Stallings, P., & Conners, C. (1997). The Multidimensional Anxiety Scale for Children (MASC): Factor structure, reliability, and validity. *Journal of the American Academy of Child and Adolescent Psychiatry, 36*, 554–565.

Masters, J. C., & Rimm, D. C. (1987). *Behavior therapy: techniques and empirical findings*. San Diego, CA: Harcourt Brace Jovanovich.

McCarthy, G. W., & Craig, K. D. (1995). Flying therapy for flying phobia. *Aviation, Space, and Environmental Medicine, 66*(12), 1179–1184.

Mifsud, C., & Rapee, R. M. (2005). Early intervention for childhood anxiety in a school setting: Outcomes for an economically disadvantaged population. *Journal of the American Academy of Child and Adolescent Psychiatry, 44*(10), 996–1004.

Miller, L. C., Barrett, C. L., Hampe, E., & Noble, H. (1972). Comparison of reciprocal inhibition, psychotherapy, and waiting list control for phobic children. *Journal of Abnormal Psychology, 79*(3), 269–279.

Miller, A. L., Rathus, J. H., & Linehan, M. M. (2007). *Dialectical behavior therapy with suicidal adolescents*. New York, NY: Guilford Press.

Morgenthaler, T., Kramer, M., Alessi, C., et al. (2006). Practice parameters for the psychological and behavioral treatment of insomnia: An update. *Sleep, 29*, 1415–1419.

Mowrer, O. (1947). On the dual nature of learning—a re-interpretation of 'conditioning' and 'problem-solving'. *Harvard Educational Review, 17*, 102–148.

Mowrer, O. (1960). Two-factor learning theory: Versions one and two. In *Learning theory and behavior* (pp. 63–91). Hoboken, NJ: John Wiley & Sons Inc.

National Institute of Mental Health. (1970). CGI: clinical global impressions. In W. Guy & R. R. Bonato (Eds.), *Manual for the ECDEU Assessment Battery* (pp. 12–6). USA: National Institute of Mental Health.

Nezu, A. M., Nezu, C. M., & McMurran, M. (2009). Problem-solving therapy. In W. T. O'Donohue & J. E. Fisher (Eds.), *General principles and empirically supported techniques of cognitive behavior therapy* (pp. 500–505). New York, NY: John Wiley & Sons.

Obler, M., & Terwilliger, R. F. (1970). Pilot study on the effectiveness of systematic desensitization with neurologically impaired children with phobic disorders. *Journal of Counseling and Clinical Psychology, 34*(3), 314–318.

Ollendick, T. T., & Cerny, J. A. (1981). *Clinical behavior therapy with children*. New York, NY: Plenum Press.

Ollendick, T. H. (1983). Reliability and validity of the revised fear survey schedule for children (FSSC-R). *Behaviour Research and Therapy, 21*, 685–692.

Ollendick, T., & King, N. (1998). Empirically supported treatments for children with phobic and anxiety disorders: Current status. *Journal of Clinical Child Psychology, 27*(2), 156–167.

Ollendick, T. H., Öst, L.-G., Reuterskiöld, L., Costa, N., Cederlund, R., Sirbu, C., et al. (2009). One-session treatment of specific phobias in youth: A randomized clinical trial in the United States and Sweden. *Journal of Consulting and Clinical Psychology, 77*, 504–516.

Page, H. A., & Hall, J. F. (1953). Experimental extinction as a function of the prevention of a response. *Journal of Comparative and Physiological Psychology, 46*, 33–34.

Palermo, T. M., Eccleston, C., Lewandowski, A. S., Williams, A., & Morley, S. (2010). Randomized controlled trials of psychological therapies for management of chronic pain in children and adolescents: An updated meta-analytic review. *Pain, 148*(3), 387–397.

Pentz, M. A. W. (1980). Assertion training and trainer effects on unassertive and aggressive adolescents. *Journal of Counseling Psychology, 27*(1), 76–83.

Perepletchikova, F., Axelrod, S. R., Kaufman, J., Rounsaville, B. J., Douglas-Palumberi, H., & Miller, A. L. (2011). Adapting dialectical behaviour therapy for children: Towards a new research agenda for paediatric suicidal and non-suicidal self-injurious behaviours. *Child and Adolescent Mental Health, 16*, 116–121.

Rachman, S. S. (1966). Studies in desensitization: II. Flooding. *Behaviour Research and Therapy, 4*, 1–6.

Research Unit on Pediatric Psychopharmacology Anxiety Study Group. (2002). The Pediatric Anxiety Rating Scale (PARS): Development and psychometric properties. *Journal of the American Academy of Child and Adolescent Psychiatry, 4*, 1061–1069.

Reynolds, W. M., & Coats, K. I. (1986). A comparison of cognitive-behavioral therapy and relaxation training for the treatment of depression in adolescents. *Journal of Consulting and Clinical Psychology, 54*(5), 653–660.

Reynolds, C. R., & Richmond, B. O. (2008). *Revised children's manifest anxiety scale* (2nd ed.). Los Angeles, CA: Western Psychological Services.

Reynolds, S., Wilson, C., Austin, J., & Hooper, L. (2012). Effects of psychotherapy for anxiety in children and adolescents: A meta-analytic review. *Clinical Psychology Review, 32*, 251–262.

Rotheram, M. J., & Armstrong, M. (1980). Assertiveness training with high school students. *Adolescence, 15*(58), 267–276.

Rotheram-Borus, M. J. (1988). Assertiveness training with children. In R. H. Price, E. L. Cowen, R. P. Lorion, & J. Ramos-McKay (Eds.), *Fourteen ounces of prevention: A casebook for practitioners* (pp. 83–97). Washington, DC: American Psychological Association.

Saigh, P., Yule, W., & Inamdar, S. (1996). Imaginal flooding of traumatized children and adolescents. *Journal of School Psychology, 34*(2), 163–183.

Sarkova, M., Bacikova-Sleskova, M., Orosova, O., Madarasova Geckova, A., Katreniakova, Z., Klein, D.,…., Dijk, J. P. (2013). Associations between assertiveness, psychological well-being, and self-esteem in adolescents. *Journal of Applied Social Psychology, 43*(1), 147–154. doi: http://dx.doi.org/10.1111/j.1559-1816.2012.00988.x.

Scahill, L., Riddle, M. A., McSwiggin-Hardin, M., Ort, S. I., King, R. A., Goodman, W. K., et al. (1997). Children's Yale-Brown obsessive compulsive scale: Reliability and validity. *Journal of the American Academy of Child and Adolescent Psychiatry, 36*, 844–852.

Schab, L. M. (2009). *Cool, calm, and confident: A workbook to help kids learn assertiveness skills.* Oakland, CA: New Harbinger Publications.

Shirk, S. R., Kaplinski, H., & Gudmundsen, G. (2009). School-based cognitive-behavioral therapy for adolescent depression: A benchmarking study. *Journal of Emotional and Behavioral Disorders, 17*(2), 106–117.

Silverman, W. K., & Albano, A. M. (1996). *Anxiety disorders interview schedule for DSM-IV: Child and parent versions.* San Antonio, TX: Psychological Corporation.

Silverman, W. K., & Nells, W. B. (1988). The anxiety disorders interview schedule for children. *Journal of the American Academy of Child and Adolescent Psychiatry, 27*, 772–778.

Silverman, W. K., & Rabian, B. (1994). Specific phobia. In T. H. Ollendick, N. J. King, & W. Yule (Eds.), *International handbook of phobic and anxiety disorders in children and adolescents* (pp. 87–109). New York, NY: Plenum Press.

Solomon, R. L., Kamin, L. J., & Wynne, L. C. (1953). Traumatic avoidance learning: the outcomes of several extinction procedures with dogs. *The Journal of Abnormal and Social Psychology, 48*, 291–302.

Spiegler, M. D., & Guevremont, D. C. (2003). *Contemporary behavior therapy* (4th ed.). Belmont, CA: Wadsworth.

Sreenivasan, U., Manocha, S. N., & Jain, V. K. (1979). Treatment of severe dog phobia in childhood by flooding: A case report. *Journal of Child Psychology and Psychiatry, 20*, 255–260.

Stallard, P., Simpson, N., Anderson, S., Carter, T., Osborn, C., & Bush, S. (2005). An evaluation of the FRIENDS programme: A cognitive behaviour therapy intervention to promote emotional resilience. *Archives of Disease in Childhood, 90*, 1016–1019.

Stampfl, T. G. (1961). *Implosive therapy: A learning theory derived psychodynamic therapeutic technique.* Unpublished paper presented in the Department of Psychology, University of Illinois.

Stark, K. D., Reynolds, W. M., & Kaslow, N. J. (1987). A comparison of the relative efficacy of self-control therapy and a behavioral problem-solving therapy for depression in children. *Journal of Abnormal Child Psychology, 15*, 91–113.

St-Jacques, J., Bouchard, S., & Bélanger, C. (2010). Is virtual reality effective to motivate and raise interest in phobic children toward therapy? A clinical trial study of in vivo with in virtuo versus in vivo only treatment exposure. *Journal of Clinical Psychiatry, 71*, 924–931.

Sukhodolsky, D. G., Solomon, R. M., & Perrine, J. (2000). Cognitive behavioral, anger-control intervention for elementary school children: A treatment-outcome study. *Journal of Child and Adolescent Group Therapy, 10*(3), 159–169.

The Pediatric OCD Treatment Study (POTS) Team. (2004). Cognitive-behavior therapy, sertraline, and their combination for children and adolescents with obsessive-compulsive disorder. *JAMA, 292*, 1969–1976.

Thompson, K. L., Bundy, K. A., & Broncheau, C. (1995). Social skills training for young adolescents: Symbolic and behavioral components. *Adolescence, 30*, 723–734.

Thompson, K. L., Bundy, K. A., & Wolfe, W. R. (1996). Social skills training for young adolescents: Cognitive and performance components. *Adolescence, 31*(123), 505–21. Retrieved from http://search.proquest.com/docview/195936956?accountid=14068.

Tiwari, S., Kendall, P. C., Hoff, A. L., Harrison, J. P., & Fizur, P. (2013). Characteristics of exposure sessions as predictors of treatment response in anxious youth. *Journal of Clinical Child and Adolescent Psychology, 42*, 34–43.

Ultee, C. A., Griffioen, D., & Schellekens, J. (1982). The reduction of anxiety in children: 'Systematic desensitization in vitro' and 'systematic desensitization in vivo'. *Behavioral Research and Therapy, 20*, 61–67.

Vande Voort, J., Svecova, J., Brown Jacobsen, A., & Whiteside, S. P. (2010). A retrospective examination of the similarity between clinical practice and manualized treatment for childhood anxiety disorders. *Cognitive and Behavioral Practice, 17*, 322–328.

Walkup, J. T., Albano, A. M., Piacentini, J., Birmaher, B., Compton, S., Sherrill, J.T., ..., Kendall, P.C. (2008). Cognitive behavioral therapy, sertraline, or a combination in childhood anxiety. *The New England Journal of Medicine, 359*, 2753–2766.

Watson, J. P., & Raynor, R. (1920). Conditioned emotional reactions. *Journal of Experimental Psychology, 3*, 1–14.

Weisman, D., Ollendick, T. H., & Horne, A. M. (1978). A comparison of muscle relaxation techniques with children. *Unpublished manuscript*, Indiana State University.

Weisz, J., & Jensen, A. (2001). Child and adolescent psychotherapy in research and practice contexts: Review of the evidence and suggestions for improving the field. *European Child and Adolescent Psychiatry, 10*, 1–13.

Wise, K. L., Bundy, K. A., Bundy, E. A., & Wise, L. A. (1991). Social skills training for young adolescents. *Adolescence, 26*, 233–241.

Wolpe, J. (1958). *Psychotherapy by reciprocal inhibition*. Stanford, CA: Stanford University Press.

Wolpe, J. (1969). *The practice of behavior therapy*. Oxford, England: Pergamon.

Wolpe, J. (1990). *The practice of behavior therapy* (4th ed.). New York, NY: Pergamon Press.

Wood, A., Harrington, R., & Moore, A. (1996). Controlled trial of a brief cognitive-behavioural intervention in adolescent patients with depressive disorders. *Journal of Child Psychology and Psychiatry, 37*(6), 737–746.

Zettle, R. (2003). Acceptance and Commitment Therapy (ACT) vs. systematic desensitization treatment of mathematics anxiety. *The Psychological Record, 53*, 197–215.

Part IV
Implementation Concerns and Future Directions

Chapter 14
Transporting Cognitive Behavior Interventions to the School Setting

Matthew P. Mychailyszyn

Today's children and adolescents face many challenges: increasing educational demands (Shepard & Smith, 1988), rising rates of divorce (Heckel, Clarke, Barry, McCarthy, & Selikowitz, 2009), media exposure to messages of violence and terrorism (Comer & Kendall, 2007), and other psychosocial stressors. These contribute to youth's vulnerability to a wide range of associated mental-health difficulties, and, indeed, youth psychopathology prevalence rates have been found to range from 1 to 51 %, with the most reliable estimates suggesting that between 12 and 20 % of youth struggle with clinical-level symptoms of disorder at any given time (Costello, Egger, & Angold, 2005; Roberts, Attkisson, & Rosenblatt, 1998). Such figures are generally consistent with estimates made by the United States Congress, suggesting that between 5.6 million and 6.8 million (18–22 %) youth are in need of mental-health services (U.S. Public Health Service, 2000).

Of greater concern is research suggesting that the incidence and prevalence rates of youth psychopathology are on the rise. In some cases, there is debate as to whether certain forms of mental illness, such as ADHD and autism spectrum disorders, are truly increasing in presence among the general population of children and adolescents or, alternatively, whether rising prevalence rates simply reflect more recent improvements in the field to reliably identify and diagnose disorders (see Fernell & Gillberg, 2010; Kočovská et al., 2012; Pomerantz, 2005). In other cases, however, investigators are pointing to empirical evidence that support real escalations in the prevalence of psychiatric disorders in youth, such as in the case of the anxiety and depressive disorders (Hammen & Rudolph, 2003). In some cases, this may be unique to the specific social context and cultural conditions of the so-called

M.P. Mychailyszyn, Ph.D. (✉)
Department of Psychology, Towson University, Towson, MD, USA

Division of Psychology and Neuropsychology, Mt. Washington Pediatric Hospital, Baltimore, MD, USA
e-mail: matthew.mychailyszyn@gmail.com

© Springer Science+Business Media New York 2015
R. Flanagan et al. (eds.), *Cognitive and Behavioral Interventions in the Schools*, DOI 10.1007/978-1-4939-1972-7_14

"modern" and "westernized" societies, such as that which exists in the United States and the United Kingdom; specifically it has been suggested that it is the especially competitive and divisive social environments of North America and the United Kingdom that may have led to rising levels of internalizing difficulties for children in countries in these regions more significantly than elsewhere in affluent countries (see Dorling, 2009). To complicate matters further, changes to clinical criteria in the recently published 5th edition of the *Diagnostic and Statistical Manual of Mental Disorders* (DSM-5) stand to impact the diagnostic landscape as prevalence rates will be significantly influenced by modifications to the symptom thresholds, age cutoffs, and overall categorization of a number of mental-health disorders.

Problems with Access to Care

Whatever the *true* reality is in terms of the trends in overall prevalence rates, the very simple fact of the matter is that a substantial portion of our youth are in need of mental-health services. Regrettably, many of those children and adolescents never receive any kind of mental-health support. Though as many as 40 % of those with a psychiatric diagnosis and associated impairment may be accessing services across different sectors, only about one in five is receiving care from a specialty mental-health provider (Burns et al., 1995). Less conservative estimates suggest that between two-thirds and three-quarters of those youth in need of help do not have access to appropriate care and are thus left untreated (United States Congress, Office of Technology Assessment, 1991). This issue is especially troublesome for youth suffering with internalizing disorders, as such problems are often less visible to parents and teachers as compared to externalizing conditions. Indeed it has been documented that the majority of youth struggling with anxiety and depression have never received treatment (Chavira, Stein, Bailey, & Stein, 2004; Logan & King, 2002). Perhaps most disturbing of all is that relatively little ground has been gained, as the estimated percentage of those with unmet needs—across all categories of psychopathology—has remained virtually unchanged over a span of nearly three decades (United States Congress, Office of Technology Assessment, 1986).

Moreover, despite strong support in favor of evidence-based practice (EBP) from the American Psychological Association (APA) and the American Academy of Child and Adolescent Psychiatry (AACAP), fewer still of the individuals receiving services are actually administered the type of empirically supported treatments (ESTs) that research evidence has deemed "efficacious" (U.S. Public Health Service, 2000). Although the emphasized importance of reliance on an evidence base is beginning to lead to a greater focus on ESTs in the training of the newest generations of psychologists (Cukrowicz et al., 2005), a considerable gap remains. McCabe (2004) claims that "practical guidelines for professional psychologists who may be interested in incorporating EBPs into their own work setting are not available" (p. 571). Schoenwald and colleagues (2008) state that "little is known about the nation's infrastructure for children's mental health services…the capacity of that infrastructure to support the implementation of (ESTs), and factors affecting that capacity" (p. 85).

The consequence of such a set of circumstances is a host of long-term negative sequelae for youth who are otherwise unable to access quality mental-health services. For instance, youth with attention-deficit/hyperactivity disorder (ADHD) have been found to suffer academic impairments spanning from preschool through adolescence (Daley & Birchwood, 2010), while investigators have found such outcomes to persist into adulthood where ADHD is associated with lower educational attainment as well as lower levels of employment (Kuriyan et al., 2013). The presence of other "disruptive behavior disorders" (e.g., oppositional defiant disorder and conduct disorder) has been shown to be a significant predictor of continuing behavior problems that tends to correspond with a higher rate of criminal justice system involvement and represents a significant financial burden to the general public (Fergusson, Horwood, & Ridder, 2005; Scott, Knapp, Henderson, & Maughan, 2001; Van Bokhoven, Matthys, van Goozen, & van Engeland, 2006). Although often perceived as less troublesome than those exhibiting externalizing symptomatology, youth with internalizing difficulties are nevertheless often comparably distressed and impaired. Anxiety disorders in childhood and adolescence can lead to impairments in school functioning (Mychailyszyn, Mendez, & Kendall, 2010) and increased vulnerability to the development of comorbid conditions and, if left untreated, may persist into adulthood. Untreated anxiety disorders are particularly associated with the development of substance abuse problems (Kendall, Safford, Flannery-Schroeder, & Webb, 2004; Woodward & Fergusson, 2001). Depression is similarly associated with a range of negative outcomes (Collins & Dozois, 2008), with episodes of earlier onset having a longer duration and significantly predicting later episodes of adult depression (Wicks-Nelson & Israel, 2009). Of significant concern is evidence indicating that youth with even subclinical levels of depressive symptoms experience a wide range of psychosocial impairments (Georgiades, Lewinsohn, Monroe, & Seeley, 2006; Gotlib, Lewinsohn, & Seeley, 1995).

Rationale for Enhancing Mental-Health Services in Schools

What all of the above information impresses upon us is that there is a significant need for change with regard to the manner in which quality mental-health services are delivered to children and adolescents. Further, it is imperative for the healthcare community to explore methods for increasing access to mental-health treatment for at-risk children and adolescents. One commonly suggested solution to this problem is to more comprehensively incorporate mental-health services into school systems. Farmer and colleagues (2003) found that the education sector was the most common point of entry as well as the most frequent provider of such services for children and adolescents across all age groups.

Despite—or perhaps more appropriately, *because of*—its role as the primary access point, the education sector bears considerable responsibility to enhance its ability to be a reliable provider of quality mental healthcare services for youth. Indeed, the need for schools to play a larger role in the establishment and maintenance of emotional and psychological well-being for youth is widely noted (Weist, Evans, & Lever, 2003). In the United States, the Surgeon General's Report on Children's Mental Health in 2000 and the President's New Freedom Commission on Mental Health (2003) have advocated for schools to accept a greater role in promoting mental health care for young people, specifically emphasizing the dynamic interplay between emotional well-being and academic success. These sentiments have been echoed by governments around the world. For instance, in establishing its national action plan for mental health from 2006 to 2011, the Council of Australia Governments (COAG) pledged political and financial support to reforming mental-health services and building partnerships that would allow a more effective institution of school-based prevention and early intervention programs for children and adolescents in need of care.

What are the impediments to progress that hinder achievement of the goal of enhancing school-based mental-health service provision? Such a question is multifaceted and involves research that cuts across various domains of investigational inquiry. The remainder of this chapter will review and discuss the topics pertinent to answering this question, in hopes that such consideration may aid the field's advancement toward the realization of such a critical objective.

The Issue of "Transportability"

Based on the accumulation of outcome studies and conclusions reached by literature reviews (e.g., Collins & Dozois, 2008; Eyberg, Nelson, & Boggs, 2008; Horowitz & Garber, 2006; Ollendick, King, & Chorpita, 2006), cognitive-behavioral therapy (CBT) meets established standards to be considered an evidence-based treatment for internalizing disorders and disruptive behavior disorders in youth. Best practice parameters indicate that CBT should be endorsed as the first-line treatment of choice for youth struggling with these problems (American Psychological Association Task Force on the Promotion and Dissemination of Psychological Procedures, 1995; Chambless & Hollon, 1998; Compton et al., 2004). The importance of adhering to evidence-based treatment recommendations is underscored by conclusions drawn from a review conducted by Evans and Weist (2004) who determined that providing interventions that do not have empirical support is likely to provide little to no benefit to students and schools. Even with such knowledge, however, questions remain regarding the potential for empirically supported interventions to be successful when implemented in schools, where they are typically delivered by a variety of professionals and to diverse populations (Owens & Murphy, 2004). For instance, in educational settings, mental-health services may be delivered by teachers, guidance counselors, school social workers, or school psychologists, among others. And although the findings are somewhat mixed in the literature, at least some evidence points to a reduction in outcome effects when programs are conducted by individuals with less training in the intervention (e.g., Brunwasser, Gillham, & Kim, 2009). It is therefore imperative that school-based personnel responsible for such service delivery—most particularly school psychologists, whose focused mental-health training makes them the most well equipped—continue to extend their skills and training in order to deliver interventions with fidelity and comparable effect.

Answers to these questions revolve primarily around features of "transportability"——the degree to which evidence-based treatments work when implemented in community contexts (Schoenwald & Hoagwood, 2001). Issues revolving around this topic are not new. Nearly 20 years ago, the *Journal of Consulting and Clinical Psychology* devoted a special issue to an examination of "how findings from carefully controlled studies of efficacious psychosocial interventions for children can be transported into naturalistic studies of the effectiveness of services" (Hoagwood, Hibbs, Brent, & Jensen, 1995, p. 683). The notion of transportability has continually been discussed at multiple levels, surfacing in the Surgeon General's Conference on Children's Mental Health which promoted increased reliance on the use of "scientifically proven" mental-health services implemented as "cost-effective, proactive systems of behavior support at the school level" as well as a strengthening of schools' capacity to be "a key link to a comprehensive, seamless system of school- and community-based identification, assessment and treatment services" (U.S. Public Health Service, 2000). Ginsburg and colleagues (2008) accurately point out that one challenge which continues to confront psychology is successful dissemination of empirically supported intervention strategies to community treatment settings—especially settings serving youth from diverse racial and ethnic backgrounds. The difficulty is found in the gap between research and service clinics such that results derived from the lab may be difficult to replicate in the community (Weisz, Donenberg, Han, & Weiss, 1995).

Achieving transportability requires a "bridging of the gap," which has also been referred to as "translating science into practice" (Chorpita, 2003). What this entails is essentially a move from "efficacy" to "effectiveness" (Mufson, Dorta, Olfson, Weissman, & Hoagwood, 2004; Schoenwald & Hoagwood, 2001) or from "research therapy" to "clinic therapy" (Weisz et al., 1995). In each case, the former term reflects scenarios characterized by homogeneously comprised samples and therapists with in-depth training in the use of manual-based treatments. The goal of these studies is to specifically test and evaluate the intervention. Conversely, the latter term describes efforts to evaluate applications of these efficacious treatments in community settings, which often lack resources such as research funding, an available team of clinicians in training, and a variety of treatment-related materials, among other things. Thus, an unfortunate consequence of a shift to community settings is often lower adherence to treatment fidelity and a drop-off in treatment effects compared to randomized controlled trials (e.g., RCTs; Henggeler, Melton, Brondino, Scherer, & Hanley, 1997).

One solution to the problem of transportability may lie in what Schoenwald and Hoagwood (2001) refer to as "street-ready" interventions—ones that can be applied in representative settings and systems. Following empirical validation of efficacy, treatments can be adapted in logical and user-friendly ways for application in broader community settings.

The School Context

It is acknowledged that the dissemination and implementation of empirically supported treatments within school systems would mark a considerable change from the way in which mental-health services are traditionally provided to youth (Evans & Weist, 2004). Challenges exist with regard to schools' acceptance of a greater role in children's mental health (Owens & Murphy, 2004; Pincus & Friedman, 2004; Weisz et al., 1995) and questions about the logistics and feasibility of applying EFT protocols in schools abound. For instance, Schoenwald and Hoagwood (2001) inquire: What is the [best] intervention? Who can implement it, under what circumstances, and to what effect? Owens and Murphy (2004) ask: How effective are these treatments when delivered to diverse populations by mental-health professionals in community settings who struggle with the added burdens of higher caseloads and fewer resources? Such questions reflect a procedural challenge for school-based interventions.

Obstacles to Effective Implementation in Schools

While the link between children's mental health and academic success would seemingly provide a natural avenue for collaborative efforts between professionals in psychology and education (Mufson et al., 2004), developing and sustaining such relationships can be difficult, and significant barriers to effective implementation exist.

A particularly problematic obstacle for school-based mental-health interventions can be getting teachers "on board" (Pincus & Friedman, 2004). Teachers are often asked to play an active part in the delivery of such services, with tasks including identification of at-risk students, completion of questionnaires, and even program implementation in some cases. However, these tasks may require training, reflecting a time commitment that competes with an already demanding academic schedule (Owens & Murphy, 2004). Combined with the possibility that children may need to spend time out of the classroom to participate in the intervention, it is understandable that teachers may not be enthusiastic about also adopting a central role in the delivery of mental-health services.

In terms of barriers to transportability/dissemination of ESTs in educational settings, important findings were obtained in a study conducted by Beidas,

Mychailyszyn, and colleagues, (2012). While some of the challenges identified by school mental-health providers mirrored those often faced in standard clinic-based service provision, others were specific to the particular school context. Organizational and systemic constraints were cited including the limited time to conduct individual sessions, the resources available for each child (e.g., clinicians reported an average of 5 sessions over a period of 3 months as contrasted with typical clinic-based treatment which likely comprising 12 sessions over the same span of time), and the support from some principals and members of the school's administration. Qualitative accounts offered by school mental-health providers underscored how difficult implementation of ESTs can be in an educational setting. For instance, one participant was unable to remove students from the class for an hour each week due to the academic instructional time that would be lost. Feedback from those charged with the duty of providing services in schools underscores the significant nature of the obstacles that are present; it may be that such barriers exist to the extent that perfect adherence to the well-validated procedures of ESTs may not be feasible in an educational setting. What then may be done in order to ensure that youth are being delivered services that are consistent with best practice parameters? Beidas and colleagues (2012) have likely stated it best when they assert, "Collaborating with providers to adapt ESTs to be more amenable to the school context is paramount" (p. 204).

Advantages to the School Setting

Despite the pitfalls, numerous advantages make schools a preferred setting for addressing the mental-health needs of youth. Schools are the most youth-accessible location because this is where they spend the most concentrated amount of time each day (New Freedom Commission on Mental Health, 2003). The school setting provides the opportunity to maximize access, affording an increased ability to reach youth by offering interventions "where they are" (Weist et al., 2003). When schools provide mental-health services, they become centers of care that are located within the community. This change can help to eliminate common obstacles that prevent youth from receiving care (Flaherty, Weist, & Warner, 1996), including transportation needs which must often be coordinated around busy and chaotic parental schedules (Storch & Crisp, 2004).

From an ecological contextual perspective considering the varied role of environmental influences (Bronfenbrenner, 1979), schools are a significant part of a child's microsystem, serving as one of the most proximal influences in a youth's development. Schools are also a primary setting in which youth display impairment (Ginsburg, Becker, Kingery, & Nichols, 2008). As the problematic nature of disruptive behavior disorders is essentially grounded in an interpersonal context, the school environment poses extraordinary challenges for such youth who struggle to balance appropriate interactions in a complex social structure that involves both peers and authority figures. For youth fraught with anxiety and depression, many of the situations that cause disorder-related interference are interwoven within the school experience. Anxious youth may be apprehensive about separating from parents to attend school, concerned about social interactions among a network of peers, and worried about evaluation of academic performance (McLoone, Hudson, & Rapee, 2006). For depressed youth, the school setting may force them to confront on a daily basis the aspects of life they are depressed about (e.g., absence of meaningful peer relationships or academic underachievement). School-based interventions are uniquely poised to enhance generalizability, fostering growth in the very situations that lead to difficulty. As such, school demonstrates the type of "ecological validity" (Owens & Murphy, 2004) allowing treatment benefits to be realized in a context that is both clinically and practically meaningful to the everyday lives of children and adolescents. Schools also offer an ideal setting for treatment evaluation by multiple informants (e.g., students, school-based mental-health practitioners, teachers, parents, administrators, etc.), with ongoing adaptations made based on the lessons learned from implementation.

Another benefit of the educational setting is that for school-based mental-health practitioners, their presence in schools allows them to intervene with youth and process problematic situations on a real-time basis. Of particular importance to school systems located in less economically advantaged areas, school-based clinicians can offer programs that are free and much more accessible as compared to traditional private-practice outpatient or hospital-based services which may not be affordable.

Finally, to the extent that parents see schools as familiar or trustworthy, this may also facilitate treatment. Parents who have good relationships with their children's schools may view mental-health services provided in this setting as more acceptable. The naturalistic setting of schools may have the capacity to reduce the stigma that often accompanies mental-health treatment in the greater community (Storch & Crisp, 2004). Such a benefit may translate into important differences regarding access to care, as research suggests that youth are more likely to utilize school-based services than those that are offered through traditional mental-health clinics (Anglin, Naylor, & Kaplan, 1996; Earls, Robins, Stiffman, & Powell, 1989).

Dissemination and Implementation in Schools: Issues for Consideration

Given the discussion above, a major goal in the mental-health field is to disseminate and implement (DI) ESTs for youth psychosocial difficulties in school settings. Dissemination includes the purposeful distribution of relevant information and materials to school mental-health providers, whereas implementation refers to the adoption and integration of ESTs into practice in the school setting (Lomas, 1993). A critical step that is fundamental for effective DI is to train school mental-health providers in the provision of ESTs. Recent literature reviews demonstrate the importance of incorporating training and ongoing consultation into DI efforts across a variety of settings (Beidas & Kendall, 2010; Rakovshik & McManus, 2010).

From an ecological perspective, an important step in the implementation of ESTs in educational settings is examining whether contextual variables, such as individual therapist and organizational-level variables, predict the implementation of ESTs or the treatment outcomes (Beidas & Kendall, 2010). Findings are mixed in the broader training literature pertaining to evidence of an association between therapist variables and training outcomes. While one study found that therapist variables, such as interpersonal style, influenced therapist adherence and skill (Henry, Schacht, Strupp, Butler, & Binder, 1993), another study found no effect of therapist interpersonal styles, personality variables, or prior experience on adherence and skill (Miller, Yahne, Moyers, Martinez, & Pirritano, 2004). Attitudes toward ESTs as predictors of training outcomes and implementation should also be examined (Aarons, 2005), given findings that therapists who held more positive views toward treatment manuals had higher ratings of adherence (Henggeler, Sheidow, Cunningham, Donohue, & Ford, 2008).

Recent research suggests that organizational factors may influence implementation of ESTs. A number of models consistent with an organizational perspective have been applied to implementation of mental-health services in community settings (Glisson et al., 2010; Weiner, Lewis, & Linnan, 2009). Constructs of particular interest include organizational culture and organizational climate, with the former defined as shared beliefs and expectations of a work environment and the latter defined as shared perceptions about the work environment's impact on worker well-being (Glisson & James, 2002). Notably, organizational climate has been associated with youth outcomes in child welfare systems, such that youth served by agencies with higher rated organizational climates demonstrate better outcomes (Glisson & Green, 2011).

Unfortunately, much of the DI literature to date on organizational predictors of training outcomes and implementation of ESTs has focused on child welfare and community mental-health settings, not educational contexts. Research in schools has lagged, despite the acknowledgment that schools are a ripe environment for dissemination of ESTs (Storch & Crisp, 2004). Qualitative research has identified a number of organizational factors as pertinent to the implementation process for school staff, specifically principal/administrator support, teacher support, financial resources, high-quality training and consultation, alignment of the intervention with school philosophy, ensuring that outcomes are visible to stakeholders, and developing ways to address turnover in staff (Forman, Olin, Hoagwood, Crowe, & Saka, 2009).

One recent preliminary study completed in the school setting found that pretraining therapist attitudes toward evidence-based practice did not influence training outcomes in school mental-health providers, whereas organizational-level constructs such as organizational climate were important for school mental-health provider engagement (Lyon, Charlesworth-Attie, Vander Stoep, & McCauley, 2011). Advancing the work in this area, Beidas, Edmunds, Marcus, and Kendall (2012) conducted a randomized trial evaluating the efficacy of three training modalities and the impact of ongoing consultation after training on the delivery of CBT. An examination of a subsample of school mental-health providers (Beidas, Edmunds et al., 2012) suggests "that there is a positive relationship between school mental health provider attitudes and improvement in adherence to an EST. Providers with higher attitudes regarding the appeal of evidence-based practice, openness to using evidence-based practice, and endorsement that evidence-based practices do not diverge from their current practice also demonstrated improvement in adherence following training in an EST" (p. 203). Despite such encouraging emerging work, more research on individual- and organizational-level predictors of training outcomes and implementation is needed, due to the unique context of schools which is distinct from that of community mental-health clinics.

Adapting CBT Implementation for Application in Schools

A few points must first be considered in a discussion regarding alterations to treatment delivery. Perhaps foremost is the notion that, to a certain degree, adaptation must inherently be a part of—as opposed to being incongruous with—ethical and effective service provision. In a discussion of how to "smooth the trail" for dissemination of EBP with youth, Kendall and Beidas (2007) indicate that "to effectively practice EBP, clinicians must apply empirically supported principles toward treatment. However, there is room for clinical expertise to synthesize scientific findings with individual client characteristics" (p. 13). Treatment manuals are thus not to be seen as *cookbooks* that require rigid and uncompromising following of some type of therapy *recipe*. Rather, when following a manual-based intervention protocol, the successful therapist tailors treatment to the particular presenting issues and needs of each unique child.

Helpful Adaptations for Implementation of ESTs in Schools

In a similar spirit, it is necessary to consider how flexible adaptation of interventions may be implemented within educational settings. As the preceding discussion has underscored, not only is a *cookbook* approach to service provision likely to be clinically contraindicated, but within the school context, it simply may not even be feasible. It is incumbent upon all stakeholders to determine which changes may be made to address specific obstacles, while continuing to preserve treatment integrity. This chapter now turns its attention to offering suggestions for how such a goal may be accomplished, integrating findings from emerging research, and concluding with recommendations for future directions.

One of the barriers most commonly identified by school-based mental-health service providers is difficulty with coordinating regularly scheduled weekly sessions lasting for the 50 min typically constituting a "clinical hour" of standard treatment protocols. One of the first time-related logistical challenges is the need for a student to be retrieved from one location (e.g., classroom) and brought to the school counselor's office or other meeting location. Unlike standard outpatient community or university-based clinics (the latter of which being where most treatment protocols are born) where caregivers are responsible for having their child present at the starting time of the session, this burden likely falls to the mental-health professional—especially in a societal age where schools are necessarily having to minimize the possibility of unsupervised student movement within their walls. Although easily overlooked, even if only requiring 5 min of transit time, this reflects a precious 10 % of session time that therapists in the aforementioned outpatient settings do not have to forego. As confidentiality standards would preclude discussing issues of a clinical nature with the student while walking through the halls, a good suggestion would be to use this time for rapport building, a feature that is integral (though unfortunately sometimes itself overlooked) to working with youth. Spending a few minutes engaged in pleasant and psychologically nonthreatening conversation can help to make the child feel at ease, strengthen the relationship bond, and, in so doing, make it easier to get "down to business" upon arrival at the location for the session.

A more difficult time-related issue is that a 50-min block of time—even if the above-described transit time is already included—may simply be impractical for a number of reasons. Of primary concern is the amount of time the student loses from the educational curriculum. As previously noted, youth with mental-health difficulties are already at greater risk for associated academic underachievement; as such, there is concern about exacerbating the potential for such problems. Within middle or high school settings, a standard 50-min session might be an awkward fit given that the length of a typical course "period" is often shorter. These two issues may overlap insofar as attempting to meet at the same weekly time could lead to a disproportionate amount of instructional time being lost from one particular subject area.

When faced with such a dilemma, the school mental-health clinician is encouraged to adopt a flexible approach to session scheduling. What this will likely entail is shortening the clinical session (e.g., divided in half or cut to correspond with the length of a school period). As CBT protocols typically offer multiple activities to familiarize a client with principles during the psychoeducation phase(s) of treatment, sessions may be shortened (e.g., from 50 min to 40–45 min to fit a class period) by selecting only one of the available activity options; importantly, this recommendation demonstrates an adaptation that reflects continued adherence to a protocol while still maintaining treatment integrity. In circumstances where only even shorter blocks of time are available, it is recommended that the school mental-health provider consider holding biweekly (2 per week) sessions lasting 25–30 min. Using the exposure phase of CBT for anxiety disorders as an example, such a structure could be applied to great effect, as the first weekly session may be used for planning of an exposure task and the second for carrying it out; such a format would also carry the added benefit of having the intervening days to make the appropriate preparations (e.g., coordinating the assistance of teachers or peers) which can often be difficult to optimally accomplish within a standard single session. In relation to the concern about sessions regularly coinciding with the same academic subject area, it is recommended that school-based therapists avoid the temptation of defaulting to relying on the student's lunchtime or physical education, music, or art classes. Aside from the contribution that such areas make to a student's education and development, they also often offer a welcome break from the rigors of perceivably more "academic" classes. Expecting students to regularly miss out on such opportunities runs the risk of breeding resentment and disengagement, with past research finding such an approach to be linked with decreased attendance (Quayle, Dziurawiec, Roberts, Kane, & Ebsworthy, 2001). In coordinating a meeting schedule, school mental-health providers are encouraged to strive for some rotation in meeting times throughout the school day, so as to minimize the cumulative loss of time from any one area. Other alternatives include considering whether meeting outside of normal school hours (e.g., after school) may be appropriate on a single or recurring basis, especially as certain sensitive clinical activities (e.g., very distressing exposure tasks) may not be amenable to having a limited window of time within which they must be completed.

Given the number of youth for whom school-based mental-health providers are responsible, adaptations to the total number of therapy sessions may also be necessary, as a standard 16-week course of treatment may prohibitively limit the total number of students that a school-based therapist can practically serve at any given time. This issue brings up an important point in the discussion of transportability. Cognitive-behavioral therapy (CBT) encompasses a broad collection of techniques joined by a common theoretical underpinning regarding the etiology and associated treatment for psychopathology. While implementing such techniques can be said to be *empirically based* as there is research evidence for the utility of the ingredients of treatment, simply drawing upon CBT strategies is not equivalent to delivering *empirically supported treatment* (EST), which signifies that a particular formalized intervention has been scientifically evaluated and judged to meet specific outcome criteria (for a more in depth review on these terms, the interested reader is referred to Chambless & Hollon, 1998; Kendall & Beidas, 2007; Lonigan & Elbert, 1998). The distinction is raised here to underscore the implication of significant deviations from treatment protocols for what may be said regarding the evidence base that exists in support of various forms of treatment. Thus, coming back to the issue raised at the introduction of this paragraph, it is *not* recommended that school-based clinicians simply decide to omit sessions from treatment packages as they see fit. Rather, should there be the need for brief treatments, it is suggested that interventions that have already been developed in this manner are selected. As an example, an 8-session version of the *Coping Cat* (Beidas, Mychailyszyn, Podell, & Kendall, 2013; Crawley et al., 2013) treatment for youth anxiety has been created with initial outcomes indicating that it is a feasible, acceptable, and beneficial treatment option for anxious youth; given its briefer duration, such a treatment package would likely be easier to deliver in schools.

As researchers seek to discover the adaptations necessary for implementation of treatments in the educational settings, a unique development is the incorporation of computer technology. The advent of computer-assisted CBT offers a promising innovation to facilitate the dissemination and sustainability of ESTs in schools (Mychailyszyn et al., 2011). Given the structured and sequential nature of CBT, these treatments are readily translated into engaging computer programs (Selmi, Klein, Greist, Sorrell, & Erdman, 1990). Computer-assisted CBT has advantages including a user-friendly format for youth and school staff, built-in rewards (e.g., video game time), and video modeling of key treatment components and essential skills. Considering the increasing presence of computers in schools and their potential to deliver content to multiple youth at the same time, computer programs carry the potential to increase the transportability of efficacious treatment in a cost-effective manner (Greist, 1998).

Contrasted with efforts to modify existing treatments, an alternative—and highly beneficial—trajectory would be to focus on creating CBT interventions designed and intended specifically for delivery within schools. Masia-Warner and colleagues have obtained encouraging results from initial trials that support the potential of disseminating and implementing school-based CBT (Masia, Klein, Storch, & Corda, 2001; Masia-Warner et al., 2005; Masia-Warner, Fisher, Shrout, Rathor, & Klein, 2007). The intervention developed by Masia and colleagues was based on several important considerations/components that make it particularly well suited to the school context: the school environment is used as the setting for exposure work so as to encourage generalization to meaningful environments, teachers are relied upon to identify students' specific difficulties and assist in the conducting of classroom exposures, and outgoing/prosocial school peers are involved so as to facilitate social interactions.

Modular treatment is an innovative development that holds significant promise for providers seeking to address the behavioral and emotional needs of youth. Recognizing that comorbidity tends to be the rule rather than the exception among youth with psychological difficulties (Brady & Kendall, 1992), and that their problems and treatment needs often shift throughout the course of treatment, researchers have developed a "modular" approach to delivery of services. One such example is the *Modular Approach to Therapy for Children with Anxiety, Depression, or Conduct Problems* (*MATCH*; Chorpita & Weisz, 2005), in which treatment procedures involving cognitive-behavioral therapy are drawn from EBTs for anxiety, depression, and disruptive conduct are structured as free-standing modules. This intervention reflects a wonderful example of "programmed flexibility" in which various treatment modules comprise a menu of options for clinicians to choose from when working with youth. For instance, in clinical practice, separate modules focusing on relaxation, cognitive restructuring, compliance with caregiver commands, or increasing treatment motivation, among others, may be implemented according to what the therapist believes will most greatly enhance outcomes given a youth's particular presentation and needs (Weisz et al., 2012). Modular treatment may reflect a paradigm shift in how psychological services are offered, as this approach embodies the notion of flexible individualized services, with initial findings suggesting that it outperforms usual care and standard single-disorder

EBTs with samples of diverse youth in community settings that include schools (Weisz et al., 2012).

A final consideration in the discussion of adapting CBT for the school setting has to do with involvement of caregivers. When treatment is provided to youth in a clinic, it is nearly always the parent(s) who take the actions necessary to initiate and procure services (e.g., calling the clinic, completing intake, bringing the child for assessment), and as such, there is access to caregiver information regarding the reason for referral. When students come to the attention of school mental-health providers at the referral of teachers or other school staff, however, integral information about home life issues may be absent. Obtaining of informed consent for treatment from caregivers who are the student's legal guardians must not be overlooked. Further, school-based providers of psychological services are therefore strongly exhorted to ensure that they build an open and ongoing collaborative relationship with caregivers by whatever means possible; though meeting in person is most preferred, flexibility is once more encouraged, as alternative modalities of communication (e.g., phone consultation, e-mail, home-school notebook, etc.) should be explored so as to have access to the most important informant(s) in a youth's life. Without open and ongoing communication and collaboration with a child's parental figures, even application of the most sound and evidence-based treatment approaches may not lead to positive and/or lasting results.

Conclusion

This chapter has sought to explore the many issues pertinent to the transporting of cognitive-behavioral interventions to the school setting. As has been reviewed, this is a multifaceted endeavor fraught with numerous barriers, though a variety of adaptations are possible to address and overcome these obstacles. Hope exists for the successful achievement of this objective as recent research has explored the designing of school-specific interventions, the incorporation of innovative technology, and the development of treatment approaches created with flexible implementation for diverse populations in mind. Such efforts reflect important steps forward. However as always, additional work is necessary in order to continue advancing gains in the school context. In this way, CBT can be made more readily available to youth in a setting where identification, access, and service provision have the potential to be the most available, cost-effective, and relevant!

References

Aarons, G. A. (2005). Measuring provider attitudes toward evidence-based practice: Consideration of organizational context and individual differences. *Child and Adolescent Psychiatric Clinics of North America, 14*, 255–271.

Anglin, T. M., Naylor, K. E., & Kaplan, D. W. (1996). Comprehensive school-based health care: High school students' use of medical, mental health, and substance abuse services. *Pediatrics, 97*, 318–330.

APA Task Force on Promotion and Dissemination of Psychological Procedures. (1995). Training in and dissemination of empirically-validated psychological treatments: Report and recommendations. *The Clinical Psychologist, 48*, 3–24.

Beidas, R. S., Edmunds, J. M., Marcus, S. C., & Kendall, P. C. (2012). Training and consultation to promote implementation of an empirically supported treatment: A randomized trial. *Psychiatric Services, 63*, 660–665.

Beidas, R. S., & Kendall, P. C. (2010). Training therapists in evidence-based practice: A critical review of studies from a systems-contextual perspective. *Clinical Psychology: Science and Practice, 17*, 1–30.

Beidas, R. S., Mychailyszyn, M. P., Edmunds, J. E., Khanna, M. S., Downey, M. M., & Kendall, P. (2012). Training school mental health providers to deliver cognitive-behavioral therapy. *School Mental Health, 4*, 197–206.

Beidas, R. S., Mychailyszyn, M. P., Podell, J. L., & Kendall, P. C. (2013). Brief cognitive behavioral therapy for anxious youth: The inner workings. *Cognitive and Behavioral Practice, 20*, 134–146.

Brady, E. U., & Kendall, P. C. (1992). Comorbidity of anxiety and depression in children and adolescents. *Psychological Bulletin, 111*, 244–255.

Bronfenbrenner, U. (1979). *The ecology of human development*. Cambridge, MA: Harvard University Press.

Brunwasser, S. M., Gillham, J. E., & Kim, E. S. (2009). A meta-analytic review of the Penn Resiliency Program's effect on depressive symptoms. *Journal of Consulting and Clinical Psychology, 77*, 1042–1054.

Burns, B. J., Costello, E. J., Angold, A., Tweed, D., Stangl, D., Farmer, E. M. Z., et al. (1995). DataWatch: Children's mental health service use across service sectors. *Health Affairs, 14*, 147–159.

Chambless, D. L., & Hollon, S. D. (1998). Defining empirically supported therapies. *Journal of Consulting and Clinical Psychology, 66*, 7–18.

Chavira, D. A., Stein, M. B., Bailey, K., & Stein, M. T. (2004). Child anxiety in primary care: Prevalent but untreated. *Depression and Anxiety, 20*, 155–164.

Chorpita, B. F. (2003). The frontier of evidence-based practice. In A. E. Kazdin & J. R. Weisz (Eds.), *Evidence-based psychotherapies for children and adolescents* (pp. 42–59). New York, NY: Guildford.

Chorpita, B. F., & Weisz, J. R. (2005). *Modular approach to therapy for children with anxiety, depression, or conduct problems*. Honolulu, HI/Boston, MA: University of Hawaii at Manoa/ Judge Baker Children's Center, Harvard Medical School.

Collins, K. A., & Dozois, D. J. A. (2008). What are the active ingredients in preventative interventions for depression? *Clinical Psychology: Science and Practice, 15*, 313–330.

Comer, J. S., & Kendall, P. C. (2007). Terrorism: The psychological impact on youth. *Clinical Psychology: Science and Practice, 14*, 178–212.

Compton, S. N., March, J. S., Brent, D., Albano, A. M., Weersing, V. R., & Curry, J. (2004). Cognitive-behavioral psychotherapy for anxiety and depressive disorders in children and adolescents: An evidence-based medicine review. *Journal of the American Academy of Child and Adolescent Psychiatry, 43*, 930–959.

Costello, J. E., Egger, H. L., & Angold, A. (2005). 10-year research update review: The epidemiology of child and adolescent psychiatric disorders: I. Methods and public health burden. *Journal of the American Academy of Child and Adolescent Psychiatry, 44*, 972–986.

Council of Australian Governments (COAG). *National action plan for mental health 2006-2011*. Retrieved March 2013, from http://www.coag.gov.au/sites/default/files/NAP%20on%20 Mental%20Health%20-%20Fourth%20Progress%20Report.pdf

Crawley, S., Kendall, P. C., Benjamin, C., Brodman, D., Wei, C., Beidas, R., et al. (2013). Brief Cognitive-Behavioral Therapy (BCBT) for anxious youth: Feasibility and initial outcomes. *Cognitive and Behavioral Practice, 20*, 123–133.

Cukrowicz, K. C., White, B. A., Reitzel, L. R., Burns, A. B., Driscoll, K. A., Kemper, T. S., et al. (2005). Improved treatment outcome associated with the shift to empirically supported treatments in a graduate training clinic. *Professional Psychology: Research and Practice, 36*, 330–337.

Daley, D., & Birchwood, J. (2010). ADHD and academic performance: Why does ADHD impact on academic performance and what can be done to support ADHD children in the classroom? *Child: Care, Health and Development, 36*, 455–464.

Dorling, D. (2009). The age of anxiety: Living in fear for our children's mental health. *Journal of Public Mental Health, 8*, 4–10.

Earls, R., Robins, L. N., Stiffman, A. R., & Powell, J. (1989). Comprehensive healthcare for high-risk adolescents: An evaluation study. *American Journal of Public Health, 79*, 999–1005.

Evans, S. W., & Weist, M. D. (2004). Implementing empirically supported treatment in the schools: What are we asking? *Clinical Child and Family Psychology Review, 7*, 263–267.

Eyberg, S. M., Nelson, M. M., & Boggs, S. R. (2008). Evidence-based psychosocial treatments for children and adolescents with disruptive behavior. *Journal of Clinical Child & Adolescent Psychology, 37*, 215–237.

Farmer, E. M. Z., Burns, B. J., Phillips, S. D., Angold, A., & Costello, E. J. (2003). Pathways into and through mental health services for children and adolescents. *Psychiatric Services, 54*, 60–66.

Fergusson, D. M., Horwood, L. J., & Ridder, E. M. (2005). Show me the child at seven: The consequences of conduct problems in childhood for psychosocial functioning in adulthood. *Journal of Child Psychology and Psychiatry, 46*, 837–849.

Fernell, E., & Gillberg, C. (2010). ASD diagnoses in Stockholm preschoolers. *Research in Developmental Disabilities, 31*, 680–685.

Flaherty, L. T., Weist, M. D., & Warner, B. S. (1996). School-based mental health services in the United States: History, current models and needs. *Community Mental Health Journal, 32*, 341–352.

Forman, S., Olin, S., Hoagwood, K., Crowe, M., & Saka, N. (2009). Evidence-based intervention in schools: Developers' views of implementation barriers and facilitators. *School Mental Health, 1*, 26–36.

Georgiades, K., Lewinsohn, P. M., Monroe, S. M., & Seeley, J. R. (2006). Major depressive disorder in adolescence: The role of subthreshold symptoms. *Journal of the American Academy of Child & Adolescent Psychiatry, 45*, 936–944.

Ginsburg, G. S., Becker, K. D., Kingery, J. N., & Nichols, T. (2008). Transporting CBT for childhood anxiety disorders into inner-city school-based mental health clinics. *Cognitive and Behavioral Practice, 15*, 148–158.

Glisson, C., & Green, P. (2011). Organizational climate, services, and outcomes in child welfare systems. *Child Abuse and Neglect, 35*, 582–591.

Glisson, C., & James, L. R. (2002). The cross-level effects of culture and climate in human service teams. *Journal of Organizational Behavior, 23*, 767–794.

Glisson, C., Schoenwald, S. K., Hemmelgarn, A., Green, P., Dukes, D., Armstrong, K. S., et al. (2010). Randomized trial of MST and ARC in a two-level evidence-based treatment implementation strategy. *Journal of Consulting and Clinical Psychology, 78*, 537–550.

Gotlib, I. H., Lewinsohn, P. M., & Seeley, J. R. (1995). Symptoms versus a diagnosis of depression: Differences in psychosocial functioning. *Journal of Consulting and Clinical Psychology, 63*, 90–100.

Greist, J. H. (1998). Treatment for all: The computer as a patient assistant. *Psychiatric Services, 49*, 887–889.

Hammen, C., & Rudolph, R. D. (2003). Childhood mood disorders. In E. J. Mash & R. A. Barkley (Eds.), *Child psychopathology* (2nd ed., pp. 233–278). New York, NY: Guilford Press.

Heckel, L., Clarke, A., Barry, R., McCarthy, R., & Selikowitz, M. (2009). The relationship between divorce and the psychological well-being of children with ADHD: Differences in age, gender, and subtype. *Emotional & Behavioural Difficulties, 14*, 49–68.

Henggeler, S. W., Melton, G. B., Brondino, M. J., Scherer, D. G., & Hanley, J. H. (1997). Multisystemic therapy with violent and chronic juvenile offenders and their families: The role of treatment fidelity in successful dissemination. *Journal of Consulting and Clinical Psychology, 65*, 821–833.

Henggeler, S. W., Sheidow, A. J., Cunningham, P. B., Donohue, B. C., & Ford, J. D. (2008). Promoting the implementation of an evidence-based intervention for adolescent marijuana abuse in community settings: Testing the use of intensive quality assurance. *Journal of Clinical Child and Adolescent Psychology, 37*, 682–689.

Henry, W. P., Schacht, T. E., Strupp, H. H., Butler, S. F., & Binder, J. L. (1993). Effects of training in time-limited dynamic psychotherapy: Mediators of therapists' responses to training. *Journal of Consulting and Clinical Psychology, 61*, 441–447.

Hoagwood, K., Hibbs, E., Brent, D., & Jensen, P. (1995). Introduction to the special section: Efficacy and effectiveness in studies of child and adolescent psychotherapy. *Journal of Consulting and Clinical Psychology, 63*, 683–687.

Horowitz, J. L., & Garber, J. G. (2006). The prevention of depressive symptoms in children and adolescents: A meta-analytic review. *Journal of Consulting and Clinical Psychology, 74*, 401–415.

Kendall, P. C., & Beidas, R. S. (2007). Smoothing the trail for dissemination of evidence-based practices for youth: Flexibility within fidelity. *Professional Psychology: Research and Practice, 38*, 13–20.

Kendall, P. C., Safford, S., Flannery-Schroeder, E., & Webb, A. (2004). Child anxiety treatment: Outcomes in adolescence and impact on substance abuse and depression at 7.4 year follow-up. *Journal of Consulting and Clinical Psychology, 72*, 276–287.

Kočovská, E., Biskupstø, R., Gillberg, I. C., Ellefsen, A., Kampmann, H., Stórá, T., et al. (2012). The rising prevalence of autism: A prospective longitudinal study in the Faroe Islands. *Journal of Autism and Developmental Disorders, 42*, 1959–1966.

Kuriyan, A. B., Pelham, W. E., Jr., Molina, B. S. G., Waschbusch, D. A., Gnagy, E. M., Sibley, M. H., et al. (2013). Young adult educational and vocational outcomes of children diagnosed with ADHD. *Journal of Abnormal Child Psychology, 41*, 27–41.

Logan, D. E., & King, C. A. (2002). Parental identification of depression and mental health service use among depressed adolescents. *Journal of the American Academy of Child and Adolescent Psychiatry, 41*, 296–304.

Lomas, J. (1993). Diffusion, dissemination, and implementation: Who should do what? *Annals of the New York Academy of Science, 703*, 226–235.

C. Lonigan, & J. Elbert (Eds.). (1998). Special issue on empirically supported psychosocial interventions for children [special issue]. *Journal of Clinical Child Psychology, 27*(2), 138–145.

Lyon, A., Charlesworth-Attie, S., Vander Stoep, A., & McCauley, E. (2011). Modular psychotherapy for youth with internalizing problems: Implementation with therapists in school-based health centers. *School Psychology Review, 40*, 569–581.

Masia, C. L., Klein, R. G., Storch, E. A., & Corda, B. (2001). School-based behavioral treatment for social anxiety disorder in adolescents: Results of a pilot study. *Journal of the American Academy of Child and Adolescent Psychiatry, 40*, 780–786.

Masia-Warner, C., Klein, R. G., Dent, H. C., Fisher, P. H., Alvir, J., Albano, A. M., et al. (2005). School-based intervention for adolescents with social anxiety disorder: Results of a controlled study. *Journal of Abnormal Child Psychology, 33*, 707–722.

Masia-Warner, C. M., Fisher, P. H., Shrout, P. E., Rathor, S., & Klein, R. G. (2007). Treating adolescents with social anxiety disorder in school: An attention control trial. *Journal of Child Psychology and Psychiatry, 48*, 676–686.

McCabe, O. L. (2004). Cross the quality chasm in behavioral health care: The role of evidence-based practice. *Professional Psychology: Research and Practice, 35*, 571–579.

McLoone, J., Hudson, J. L., & Rapee, R. M. (2006). Treating anxiety disorders in a school setting. *Education and Treatment of Children, 29*, 219–242.

Miller, W. R., Yahne, C. E., Moyers, T. B., Martinez, J., & Pirritano, M. (2004). A randomized trial of methods to help clinicians learn motivational interviewing. *Journal of Consulting and Clinical Psychology, 72*, 1050–1062.

Mufson, L. H., Dorta, K. P., Olfson, M., Weissman, M. M., & Hoagwood, K. (2004). Effectiveness research: Transporting interpersonal psychotherapy for depressed adolescents (IPT-A) from the lab to school-based health clinics. *Clinical Child and Family Psychology Review, 7*, 251–261.

Mychailyszyn, M. P., Beidas, R. S., Benjamin, C. L., Edmunds, J. L., Podell, J. L., Cohen, J. S., et al. (2011). Assessing and treating child anxiety in schools. *Psychology in the Schools, 48*, 223–232.

Mychailyszyn, M. P., Mendez, J. L., & Kendall, P. C. (2010). Anxiety disorders and school functioning in youth: Comparisons by diagnosis and comorbidity. *School Psychology Review, 39*, 106–121.

New Freedom Commission on Mental Health. (2003). *Achieving the promise: Transforming mental health care in America*. Final Report. DHHS Pub. No. SMA-03-3832. Rockville, MD.

Ollendick, T. H., King, N. J., & Chorpita, B. F. (2006). Empirically supported treatments for children and adolescents. In P. C. Kendall (Ed.), *Child and adolescent therapy: Cognitive-behavioral procedures* (3rd ed., pp. 492–520). New York, NY: Guildford Press.

Owens, J. S., & Murphy, C. E. (2004). Effectiveness research in the context of school-based mental health. *Clinical Child and Family Psychology Review, 7*, 195–209.

Pincus, D. B., & Friedman, A. G. (2004). Improving children's coping with everyday stress: Transporting treatment interventions to the school setting. *Clinical Child and Family Psychology Review, 7*, 223–240.

Pomerantz, J. M. (2005). ADHD: More prevalent or better recognized? *Drug Benefit Trends, 17*, 220–221.

Quayle, D., Dziurawiec, S., Roberts, C., Kane, R., & Ebsworthy, G. (2001). The effect of an optimism and lifeskills program on depressive symptoms in preadolescence. *Behaviour Change, 18*, 194–203.

Rakovshik, S. G., & McManus, F. (2010). Establishing evidence-based training in cognitive behavioral therapy: A review of current empirical findings and theoretical guidance. *Clinical Psychology Review, 30*, 496–516.

Roberts, R. E., Attkisson, C. C., & Rosenblatt, A. (1998). Prevalence of psychopathology among children and adolescents. *American Journal of Psychiatry, 155*, 715–725.

Schoenwald, S. K., Chapman, J. E., Kelleher, K., Hoagwood, K. E., Landsverk, J., Stevens, J., et al. (2008). A survey of the infrastructure for children's mental health services: Implications for the implementation of empirically supported treatments (ESTs). *Administration and Policy in Mental Health and Mental Health Services Research, 35*, 84–97.

Schoenwald, S. K., & Hoagwood, K. (2001). Effectiveness, transportability, and dissemination of interventions: What matters when? *Psychiatric Services, 52*, 1190–1197.

Scott, S., Knapp, M., Henderson, J., & Maughan, B. (2001). Financial cost of social exclusion: Follow up study of anti-social children into adulthood. *British Medical Journal, 323*, 191–194.

Selmi, P. M., Klein, M. H., Greist, J. H., Sorrell, S. P., & Erdman, H. P. (1990). Computer-administered cognitive-behavioral therapy for depression. *American Journal of Psychiatry, 147*, 51–56.

Shepard, L. A., & Smith, M. L. (1988). Escalating academic demand in kindergarten: Counterproductive policies. *The Elementary School Journal, 89*, 135–145.

Storch, E. A., & Crisp, H. L. (2004). Taking it to the schools——Transporting empirically supported treatments for childhood psychopathology to the school setting. *Clinical Child and Family Psychology Review, 7*, 191–193.

U.S. Public Health Service. (2000). *Report on the surgeon general's conference on children's mental health: A national action agenda*. Washington, DC: U.S. Government Printing Office.

United States Congress, Office of Technology Assessment. (1986). *Children's mental health: Problems and services. (OTA-H-33)*. Washington, DC: US Government Printing Office.

United States Congress, Office of Technology Assessment. (1991). *Adolescent health (OTA-H-33)*. Washington, DC: US Government Printing Office.

Van Bokhoven, I., Matthys, W., van Goozen, S. H. M., & van Engeland, H. (2005). Prediction of adolescent outcome in children with disruptive behaviour disorders: A study of neurological, psychological, and family factors. *European Child and Adolescent Psychiatry, 14*, 153–163.

Weiner, B. J., Lewis, M. A., & Linnan, L. A. (2009). Using organization theory to understand the determinants of effective implementation of worksite health promotion programs. *Health Education and Research, 24*, 292–305.

Weist, M. D., Evans, S. W., & Lever, N. A. (2003). Introduction: Advancing mental health practice and research in schools. In M. D. Weist, S. W. Evans, & N. A. Lever (Eds.), *Handbook of school mental health: Advancing practice and research* (pp. 1–7). New York, NY: Kluwer Academic/Plenum Publishers.

Weisz, J. R., Chorpita, B. F., Palinkas, L. A., Schoenwald, S. K., Mirand, J., Bearman, S. K., et al. (2012). Testing standard and modular designs for psychotherapy treating depression, anxiety, and conduct problems in youth: A randomized effectiveness trial. *Archives of General Psychiatry, 69*, 274–282.

Weisz, J. R., Donenberg, G. R., Han, S. S., & Weiss, B. (1995). Bridging the gap between laboratory and clinic in child and adolescent psychotherapy. *Journal of Consulting and Clinical Psychology, 63*, 688–701.

Wicks-Nelson, R., & Israel, A. (2009). *Abnormal child and adolescent psychology* (7th ed.). Upper Saddle River, NJ: Pearson Education.

Woodward, L. J., & Fergusson, D. M. (2001). Life course outcomes of young people with anxiety disorders in adolescence. *Journal of the American Academy of Child and Adolescent Psychiatry, 40*, 1086–1093.

Chapter 15
Professional Issues in Cognitive and Behavioral Practice for School Psychologists

Rosemary Flanagan

Much has been written about the practice of child CBT in private practice and other clinical settings, yet important distinctions become apparent when looking toward the implementation of these techniques in school settings. For example, the school psychologist must incorporate into treatment planning systemic factors such as the involvement of multiple personnel (e.g., classroom and special area teachers), scheduling restrictions, and the specific details of service delivery (e.g., who will provide the treatment and in what capacity). Further, consideration must be given to deciding which individuals will provide the service (e.g., a service planned by a school psychologist might be implemented by an appropriately trained classroom teacher). It is also important to balance the relationships among the individuals involved in the child's progress (see Mychailyszyn, Chap. 14, this volume, for a discussion). Balancing relationships involves meeting children's needs while working within the constraints of the instructional program and working collaboratively with teachers and the other school personnel involved in delivering the intervention. This all takes place while working to ensure that treatment integrity is maintained. This chapter will examine professional issues that the psychologist must be mindful of when implementing these practices in schools, including the need for appropriate supervision, gaining entry and bringing a program of cognitive and behavioral therapies/interventions into schools, and special issues in the implementation of school-based CBT group therapy, a commonly utilized treatment modality.

R. Flanagan, Ph.D., A.B.P.P. (✉)
Graduate School of Psychology, Touro College, New York, NY, USA
e-mail: rflanaganabpp@gmail.com

© Springer Science+Business Media New York 2015
R. Flanagan et al. (eds.), *Cognitive and Behavioral Interventions in the Schools*, DOI 10.1007/978-1-4939-1972-7_15

Supervision

Ethical and professional practice standards require that psychologists limit practice to areas within their areas of competence (American Psychological Association, 2002). This means that one must have had appropriate instruction in and supervised practice in carrying out the particular interventions they use. These standards apply to both trainees and fully credentialed professional psychologists. Thus, if one is expanding his or her practice repertoire to new areas, it is imperative to obtain appropriate supervision while working toward clinical competency. Clinical competency is important from the vantage points of multiple members of the school community, including the client (in this case a student), parents, school administrators, the practicing psychologist, and the supervising psychologist, although it can mean different things to different members of the school community. For example, the child client might appreciate the practitioner being able to persuade significant adults to offer more privileges, or the school administrators might value seeing a child for disciplinary reasons less often. The practitioner, in contrast, may value the attainment and effective application of an increasingly sophisticated set of practice skills.

When considering the role of supervision in schools, it is important to recognize that there are varied levels and forms of supervision within these settings (Flanagan & Miller, 2010; Harvey & Struzziero, 2008). In general, school-based supervision falls into two main categories: clinical supervision and administrative supervision.

Definitions of Clinical Supervision in Professional Psychology

Clinical supervision in psychology is an individual developmental situation in which the supervisor helps develop competence in the supervisee (Loganbill, Hardy, & Delworth, 1982). McIntosh and Phelps (2000) reviewed definitions of supervision in school psychology and offered a definition that expands this idea: "Supervision is an interpersonal interaction between two or more individuals for the purpose of sharing knowledge, assessing professional competencies, and providing objective feedback with the terminal goals of developing new competencies, facilitating effective delivery of psychological services, and maintaining professional competencies" (p. 33). Hawkins and Shohet (2006) further describe clinical supervision as a relationship involving mutual professional growth. Each supervision situation can be a new learning experience for both the supervisor and the supervisee because each case is unique and can be considered from multiple perspectives. This provides an opportunity for the supervisor and supervisee to learn from one another. Additional learning for seasoned supervisors may come from the supervisee sharing contemporary information from the didactic part of his or her training.

Fouad et al. (2009) proposed a model of foundational competencies in professional psychology, one of which is supervision. The essential elements are supervisor skills and characteristics that include: (1) understanding the complexity of the supervisory role, including ethical, legal, and contextual issues; (2) knowledge of procedures and practices of supervision; (3) engaging in professional reflection about one's clinical relationships with supervisees, as well as supervisee's relationships with clients; (4) understanding of other individuals and groups and intersecting dimensions of diversity in the context of supervision practice and the ability to reflect on the role of one's self in therapy and in supervision; and (5) having a command of and application of relevant ethical, legal, and professional standards and guidelines. This model might also be considered a template for ongoing professional growth.

The Supervisory Process

Stoltenberg and Delworth (1987) offer a model of supervision that deconstructs the process of supervision to illustrate how the supervisee's development parallels the process of becoming a therapist. The model is applicable to all areas of professional psychology, including school and clinical child psychology. Competence in the supervisee is conceptualized according to three dimensions: developmental level, psychological structures (self/other awareness, autonomy, and motivation) and practice domains; these levels may not be uniform.

The first dimension characterizes the trainee who is learning specific interventions and skills. Exercises in this phase of supervision might include: learning how to present "cognitive restructuring" to children of different developmental stages, setting up a token economy, or writing behavioral contracts for children and adolescents. The second dimension characterizes a supervisee who can empathize with and understand the client's perspective. Supervision activities might include learning to be nonjudgmental toward clients while simultaneously being authoritative in conceptualizing problems and proposing interventions. For example, a supervisee would learn how to genuinely accept the child's reasons for refusing to attend school, yet be able to insist on the child's attendance despite the anxiety that this insistence may incur in the child. It might also include learning to be accepting of and nonjudgmental toward the parent who "gives in" to such a child while having the clinical sensitivity needed to support and empower the parent in following through with the intervention. The third dimension, comprised of practice domains, involves integrated functioning, characterized by the ability to be self-aware, while showing the client empathy and understanding. An individual functioning in this dimension can work with the client's perspective as well as his or her own strengths and weaknesses and can utilize practice domains as needed. Thus, a psychologist who recently experienced a death of a family member might be called upon to help a child in a similar circumstance. The skill set needed to address this task is potentially daunting in that the individual has to learn to place his or her emotions, attitudes, values, and biases aside, so that he or she can focus on the client. Practice domains include: intervention skill competence, assessment approaches and techniques, individual/cultural differences, interpersonal assessment, theoretical orientation, problem conceptualization, goal selection and treatment planning, and professional ethics (Stoltenberg & Delworth, 1987). A practitioner showing integrated functioning is providing what is needed at the moment because he or she is in tune with what is transpiring in the situation on multiple levels. In cognitive and behavioral practice, this may sometimes involve knowing when to put the "agenda" for the session aside and to attend to the client's immediate needs.

Clinical supervision needs will vary according to the point at which an individual psychologist is in his or her career trajectory. Some examples might include a psychology faculty member and a graduate student in a classroom setting, a school psychologist in school-based practice whose work is supervised, or a psychologist employee of a clinic or hospital who is supervising a practicum student, extern, or intern. Supervisory situations also include a practitioner accruing postdoctoral hours prior to taking the licensing exam. Although the terminology might not seem to fit, supervision can also be between fully qualified colleagues who are conferring on challenging clinical problems.

Because supervisors are expected to competently provide the services they supervise, clinical supervision includes discussing the following elements of the case: background history, assessment of the problem, case conceptualization and formulation, treatment planning, theoretical and scientific underpinnings, specific strategies and techniques, and the evaluation of client progress.

Implementation issues are also a critical topic for discussion in the supervision of school-based cognitive and behavioral practice. Aspects of implementation that require particular attention in supervision include: (1) the need to limit interruptions to the child's educational program while planning an intervention; (2) coordination of care, as most interventions involve dealing with multiple adults in addition to the child client(s); (3) the feasibility maintaining treatment integrity while conducting a particular intervention, treatment, technique in the school setting; (4) anticipating difficulties in conducting the intervention, treatment, technique, or strategy in the school setting; and (5) adapting the intervention, treatment, technique, or strategy while keeping its scientific underpinnings intact, allowing for the regular evaluation of progress. This last notion is particularly important because it involves knowing which elements of a treatment are essential to its success.

Supervision in Cognitive and Behavioral Practice

Supervisors teach technique and correct misconceptions (Haynes, Corey, & Moutlon, 2003) about cognitive and behavioral practice, particularly in regard to tasks and responsibilities within the session. Parallel to CBT sessions with clients, supervision sessions are focused and structured, with both the supervisee and the supervisor responsible for the session content (Liese & Beck, 1997). Likewise, the steps in a supervision session include following up from the prior session, using some of the same techniques pedagogically in supervision that are used in therapy, such as role play and role reversal. A unique feature of CBT-based supervision is that supervisors typically ask for feedback from the supervisee (see Liese & Beck, 1997, for a discussion). These elements bear similarity to the supervision of practice domains in the developmental model (Stoltenberg & Delworth, 1987).

Haynes et al. (2003) reviewed and critiqued a number of supervision methods in order to identify different approaches to the supervisory process. Verbal exchange and case consultation are often used, although these are limited by what the supervisee reveals. More effective supervision methods include co-therapy and observational methods, as they provide a firsthand view of the supervisee's skills. Videotapes are preferred over audiotapes for these observations, as they also give access to an analysis of the supervisee's body language. Role playing and role reversal (e.g., supervisor takes the role of the client) are particularly effective techniques because they provide opportunities to practice skills. Modeling of techniques is a particularly effective supervisory approach. For example, assigning homework to supervisees—such as assigning readings and assessing if the readings are carried out—allows the supervisee to see how the supervisor negotiates the technique of giving homework. Moreover, assigning homework to the supervisee provides additional opportunities to build skills.

An additional important element is how the supervisee's view of his or her skills impacts his or her ability as a therapist. Cognitive and behavioral practitioners are mistaken if they think skill proficiency is all there is to interventions and therapy. Skill as a cognitive and behavioral therapist goes beyond the techniques and includes developing competencies in the creation of a therapeutic alliance. This can include the ability to recognize what the client's needs are at a particular moment, as a therapeutic situation is first and foremost an interpersonal interaction. It is important to learn that it is sometimes appropriate to relegate the techniques and strategies to a secondary role because the client (child, teacher, principal, or parent) needs support and understanding at the moment. Just as learning the techniques is a process for clients, it is one for supervisees!

Another important task of supervision as it might relate to school settings will be for the supervisee to learn that the multiple members of the school community or consumers of school psychological services (child, teacher, principal, or parent) are not always ready to do the work that is needed to make an intervention work. This is one reason why clear psychoeducation that explains the overall plan for an intervention and its rationale is essential. Moreover, fledgling (as well as experienced) therapists might neither anticipate nor understand such barriers to intervention. This is therefore an important lesson for supervision—particularly as it relates to helping the therapist to maintain the therapeutic alliance so that therapy can go forward. These descriptions of the elements of the supervision process bear similarity to the therapist developmental levels and the growth of therapist psychological structures in the model of supervision proposed by Stoltenberg and Delworth (1987).

The quality of supervision is important. Good supervisors are flexible, able to see multiple perspectives, working with diversity, broadly knowledgeable about the field, able to manage negative emotions, committed to being a continual learner, sensitive to the work context, able to handle power in a non-oppressive manner, and have personal characteristics such as patience, humility, and humor (Hawkins & Shohet, 2006). Competent clinical supervisors are able to perform the services that are supervised (Knapp & VandeCreek, 2006). Most important, as indicated earlier, is that the particulars of the supervisory situation vary according to whether the work is being done in a school or other clinical setting. Understanding the ways in which the credentialing for school-based psychologists differs from other professional psychologists provides an important context for the supervisory process in the school setting.

Supervision in School Settings

The administrative structure of school settings creates a unique supervision situation within professional psychology as it requires both setting-specific administrative supervision (which is legally and ethically appropriate in schools) and clinical supervision.

Administrative supervision includes accountability for compliance with state and federal guidelines, internal procedures in the school, timeliness, and meeting deadlines. Administrative supervisors in schools generally do not have practice credentials in professional psychology. Schools have multiple levels of supervision, with complexity, multiplicity, and uniqueness within each level (Harvey & Struzziero, 2000, 2008). In schools, the lead administrative supervisor is the superintendent, who has in turn other persons accountable to him or her who have administrative responsibility to act as his or her agent in many matters, such as pupil personnel directors, special education administrators, and building principals. All of these individuals are first qualified as classroom teachers; although it is possible for a school psychologist to serve in one of these roles, it is relatively uncommon. A school system may have a lead (school) psychologist; this varies by locale and is more common in large urban school districts.

Because supervision of a school psychologist by a either a certified school psychologist or a licensed psychologist is neither required by law nor regulation in schools, it is not always available (Harvey & Struzziero, 2000). Thus, alternative arrangements may be needed for the school psychologist in need of clinical supervision. Arrangements can include formal clinical supervision provided by a licensed psychologist who is employed in the setting. If this is not available, supervision can be arranged for on a contractual basis. Lastly, one can call on colleagues to discuss cases, providing these individuals have appropriate training and supervised experience for the case consultations they are providing.

Although school administrative supervisors are generally not trained to provide supervision on clinical matters (because they are typically not psychologists), they are responsible for quality assurance and service integrity (Harvey & Struzziero, 2000; Hawkins & Shohet, 2006). This suggests the need for trust and respect across school psychologist/administrator dyads; if this trust is not present, there may be concerns with confidentiality that could potentially undermine clinical supervision and ultimately compromise treatment integrity. For example, a school psychologist employee can be considered insubordinate if he or she refuses to discuss details of a case with a school administrator. Confidentiality in schools clearly applies to external third parties; but within the school building, it is on a need-to-know basis (see Jacob, Decker, & Hartshorne, 2011, for a discussion). So, for example, only individuals with a legitimate educational interest would be informed about a child's academic or social-emotional problem. School personnel in clerical roles would not need this information, nor would teachers who are not the child's current teacher. While many school psychologists have the trust and respect of their school-based superiors, there is the possibility of this reality negatively impacting service delivery. A case in point is an administrative supervisor asking the school psychologist if he or she knows which individuals from their caseload attended a student-run meeting to promote an understanding and acceptance of sexual diversity.

Finally, supervision for those in school settings should include the enhancement of multicultural competencies . While clearly important in all settings, it is essential in school settings because of the diversity in the school-aged population. Given that there is compulsory education in the United States, those working in school settings are theoretically faced with serving individuals from any racial/ethnic background, religion and health-related or education-based disability (for a discussion of diversity in school psychology see Flanagan & Miller, 2010). Culturally competent supervisors have the dual task of applying multicultural competencies to their direct interactions with supervisees and to their indirect interaction with clients via the supervisee. Cultural competence is defined as an awareness of one's own biases and values, having an understanding of the worldview of supervisees and clients, and a commitment to develop culturally appropriate interventions (Haynes et al., 2003). Resources are available to assist with this task (e.g., Costantino & Malgady, 2005; Frisby & Reynolds, 2005; Malgady, 2010).

Credentialing and Service Provision in School Psychology

In order to serve as a school psychologist employed in a public school, a credential issued by the respective State Department of Education is required. The vast majority of school psychologists are credentialed at the subdoctoral level (Curtis, Grier, & Hunley, 2004), with at least 60 credits post-baccalaureate that includes a master's degree (or equivalent) and a full-time university approved supervised internship (Flanagan & Miller, 2010). It is not uncommon for such programs to require more than the state minimums for coursework because the practice and knowledge base in school psychology continues to expand. This entry-level credential is the only necessary credential for school-based practice.

Individuals holding doctoral degrees can also be credentialed as school psychologists. Providing that the school psychology-specific requirements for the state are met, they can earn the same entry-level credential as an individual practicing at the subdoctoral level. Similarly, providing that state-specific requirements are met, a doctoral-level school psychologist may also be credentialed as a psychologist who can practice independently. Thus, there are two sets of credentialing standards regulated by two governmental offices, a state department of education and a (professional) psychology licensing board. There is often additional pay for possessing the doctoral degree in school settings, but it is typically nominal given the personal and financial commitment needed to obtain the doctorate.

Doctoral-level psychologists might also serve schools as independent contractors by meeting specific needs or carrying out particular tasks; these duties will differ from the district-employed school psychologist, who is typically a member of a collective bargaining unit. In these cases, payment is typically from a budget line set aside for external consultants. It is worth noting that in 1983, New York's Education Commissioner, Gordon Ambach, rendered a decision indicating that contracting for school psychologists to provide routine school psychological services is not acceptable if this results in a contracted position replacing a salaried one (see Matter of Freidman, 19 Ed. Dept.Rep.522).

Thus, it follows that contracted psychologists would offer a service that is either different from, or above and beyond, that which the in-house school psychologist is trained to provide. Psychologists can also work in schools as staff members of a school-based mental health clinic; such a clinic would be operating under the purview of its own license, rather than a part of a public school district. Individuals serving in either capacity are required to have the credential issued by the respective State Board for Psychology that permits independent practice as a psychologist. For these scenarios, supervision is provided in a similar manner to other areas of professional psychology.

Gaining Entry into School Systems/Classrooms

Although psychologists have the knowledge and skills that can help youngsters with academic and social-emotional concerns, they may struggle to get their programs accepted or to convince other members of the school community of the value of the service they are offering members of the school community. When entry into the "system" is problematic, the task may be facilitated by supervision. If one is not an employee of the school system, a strategy is needed to gain entry, which is a precondition to members of the school community buying into a project. If one is an employee of the school system (i.e., the in-house school psychologist), there is still the task of getting members of the school community to buy into a novel method of service delivery. That said, there are common elements applicable to getting one's intervention (or research) project off the ground, whether or not one is an employee of the school system. Central to gaining entry is being able to demonstrate a strong commitment to professional and ethical standards. Many of the detailed procedures and policies in schools are put into place to avoid problems in these domain areas.

Practitioners and researchers wishing to provide a school-based intervention should consider several items. First, one may be more successful gaining entry if the problem or concern to be addressed is something that the school is already invested in. It is important to solve the problems they want solved (Vane, 1985). Thus, targets for intervention fall into two broad categories: (1) concerns/problems connected to media events and/or federal/state regulations that potentially impact the majority of youngsters and (2) behavioral and mental health problems of individual youngsters that either consume considerable amounts of the administrator's work day or that make it difficult for a teacher to maintain an instructional environment conducive to learning. Buy-in will be increased by keeping these parameters in mind. Cognitive and behavioral interventions can be effectively applied to individuals or larger groups, irrespective of the presence of an educational disability or a diagnosable (i.e., DSM-5; American Psychiatric Association, 2013) disorder. Similar to therapeutic situations, a working relationship with the administrators (and teachers) needs to be established. This will be more similar to a consultation alliance (Conoley, Conoley, & Reese, 2009) than a therapeutic alliance.

So how does one start? In the absence of previously established connections to school personnel, it is best to start through consultation with the superintendent. For researchers who are offering an intervention as part of a study, it is highly desirable to have an already approved proposal from the researcher's affiliated Institutional Review Board (IRB) and to share this with the superintendent. In the case of a practitioner who is not conducting research, the practitioner must be credentialed for independent practice and must be ready to discuss the financial arrangements such as whether the compensation will come from insurance monies or local funds. Importantly, procedures in the proposal must show sensitivity to the constraints of the school day. If a project is overly disruptive to the instructional program, it will most likely be rejected, no matter how well conceived it is. The practitioner or researcher should take direction from the superintendent's office as to the next steps which set the stage for the buy-in at the school building level. Whether the superintendent' office shares the proposal with the principals, or the researcher (practitioner) contacts the principals directly, it is essential to determine if there is interest in the project. A telephone call to the principal's administrative assistant is the next step. Concisely explain the project and ask if a copy of the proposal would be helpful, provide it in mode they prefer (i.e., email, hard copy) and provide contact information. Be willing to meet with the school personnel promptly. Present the project concisely and underscore its value. Respond to their questions and indicate the voluntary nature of the project. Some individuals will respond immediately, others may wish to consider it—it is their choice! It is wise not to be overly rigid; it makes it far more likely that the working relationship will then be cooperative and collaborative. Flexibility in scheduling is important. It is wise to compromise on details that are not expected to negatively impact research design or treatment integrity. The overall entry strategy will be highly similar for a building-based school psychologist who wants to attempt a new intervention. Parent consent and child assent must be obtained prior to beginning the project.

Research on implementation and sustainability (i.e., the extent to which members of the school community continue to implement the intervention after the person delivering the intervention is gone) issues (Forman, Olin, Hoagwood, Crowe, & Saka, 2009) provides information that not only facilitates the research progress by leading to greater treatment integrity but may lead to greater buy-in by members of the school community. Well-conceived and worthwhile projects are destined for failure without stakeholder buy-in. From the vantage point of members of the school community, keys to successful implementation are the development of principal and other administrator support; the development of teacher support, financial resources to sustain practice; the provision of high-quality training to ensure fidelity of practice; working to ensure that the intervention dovetails with what is important to the school's goals, programs, and policies; ensuring that the program outcomes are apparent to members of the school community; and having a plan to deal with employee turnover and training new employees. A survey of school psychologists indicates (Forman, Fagley, Chu, & Walkup, 2012) that treatment acceptability, the efficacy of a particular intervention, and organizational support are important considerations for implementation of evidence-based interventions. This suggests that both the implementing school psychologists and the members of the school community have similar views as to what is necessary for a successful partnership. This may in turn facilitate sustainability (i.e., ongoing use of the intervention) when the psychologist's task is completed.

The task of gaining entry also involves offering an intervention that the members of the school community (teachers, parents, administrators, and children) feel has the potential to significantly improve some aspect of school life. It is therefore important to consider current problems or concerns when attempting to gain initial entry; in other words, solve the problems *they* want solved (Vane, 1985). These problems will most typically be broad-based educational or social issues that impact large numbers of children, such as high-stakes testing. While it is possible that an intervention to address a highly specific problem or one for a particular group of students might also be well received, it is often better advised to save that proposal for when the psychologist has already shown the value of cognitive and behavioral interventions. Some examples include helping teachers become more effective in managing their classrooms and/or dealing with challenging child behaviors. The psychologist can advocate for these interventions by citing research that more effective learning environments and behavioral management by teachers translate into positive outcomes such as the principal having fewer problems to address after recess, children completing their work more effectively, children having more and better peer relations, and so forth.

Group Therapy

Groups are a popular treatment modality in schools; they are cost- and time-effective and provide opportunities for primary prevention (Krieg, Simpson, Stanley, & Snider, 2002). Change in groups is governed by four mechanisms: (1) cohesiveness among participants; (2) the universal nature of the issues commonly addressed in groups; (3) the emphasis on learning something about oneself while learning to practice desirable behaviors (Perusse, Goodenough, & Lee, 2009) such as empathy, intimacy, and involvement within the group setting; and (4) learning to apply the skills learned (Gladding, 2008; Greenberg, 2003) in the group to situations outside of it (Krieg et al., 2002). While ideal groups are comprised of a heterogeneous mix of youth whose strengths and weaknesses are balanced, this is not always the case in schools because some groups are comprised of youngsters from the same classroom, or youngsters who appear to need attention because they exhibit behaviors disruptive to the instructional program. Thus, the group may tend toward homogeneity rather than heterogeneity.

Topics for groups vary with most being categorized as addressing developmental milestones and rites of passage, the climate and culture of the school (including residential settings) as well as developing/strengthening coping and problem-solving skills. Work that focuses on affective and behavioral skills often addresses issues that impact smaller numbers of students such as divorce, or larger numbers of students such as the Sandy Hook school shooting in 2012. Given that there is a wide range of topics and problems that school-based groups might address, the knowledge and training base for a school psychologist to conduct a group competently and effectively is potentially broad. A recent meta-analysis of school counseling outcome studies indicate that overall, groups are effective (see Whiston, Tai, Rahardja, & Eder, 2011, for a discussion).

Because cognitive and behavioral interventions have skill components that are built via practice, group therapy is a modality that can be particularly effective. While often utilized in response to problems that arise and that impact large numbers of children, it can be used in a proactive or preventive way for smaller numbers of youngsters. For example, scenarios can be crafted to simulate common childhood situations that might be addressed through self-talk comprised of self-generated coping statements. Another possibility might be to practice assertive responding or to work as a group to generate and review possible solutions for problems common to group members. Within schools and residential treatment settings however, there are a number of important considerations that impact treatment that would not arise in clinical practice settings. By discussing the commonalities and differences in group treatment by setting, these important points are readily made. Group leaders in all settings will typically deal with developing trust as well as an array of negative emotions that are expressed during the sessions as a function of the nature and extent of self-disclosure.

In clinical settings, groups are typically organized by gender, age group, or presenting problem; sessions typically take place outside of the school day. Youngsters do not know one another prior to commencing the group; it is also possible that some have been in individual treatment. It is common for therapists in clinic settings to refer children who are in individual treatment to ongoing skill-based or problem-focused groups in the clinic, or make referrals to a group to ease the transition from individual therapy, while making it possible to "monitor" the youngster following termination from individual treatment. Thus, it is possible that members will often come and go; thus, the group composition may often change. Confidentiality and privacy issues are more complex than in individual treatment, but can typically be managed by requiring participants to abide by the notion of what is discussed in the group remains in the group. Parents and guardians should be advised of this requirement and the reasons behind it; the group leader should make it clear that he or she will address the concerns raised by parents or guardians of the participating youngsters. Such limits should work well because the group can be limited to individuals who are otherwise unknown to one another; this is not the case in schools.

In schools, group treatment is often seen as an efficient way of reaching youngsters (Krieg et al., 2002; Perusse et al., 2009). There are a number of differences between clinic-based groups and school-based groups. First, the sessions typically take place during the school day. One unfortunate correlate of this is that some youngsters (many of which can least afford to miss instruction) will miss some time in the classroom. Next, the duration of a session may vary from a clinic-run group which is typically 90 min; the duration of group sessions in schools tends to be the class period, typically 40–45 min. Moreover, school-based groups typically would not continue after the school year ends. Thus, provisions may be needed for youngsters with ongoing treatment requirements. These considerations suggest the need to set limits in terms of who is in the group and what kinds of problems are addressed.

It may be wise to address skill-related problems in school-based groups, as opposed to problems that are more affectively based. Group membership may be determined by grade, class, gender, and scheduling or by needs/presenting problem. Youngsters usually know one another; thus, prior history/interactions and knowledge of one's disposition, strengths, and weaknesses are already known to group members; this means there may be important social history before the group commences! If the group is taking place in a special education setting, these potential concerns are compounded because the youngsters share even more history, as they are often in the same classroom for much of the school day, and tend to progress through the grades as a unit that does not redistribute from year to year. If the group is taking place at a residential school/treatment setting, there is the possibility of additional complexities because there is even greater familiarity, as the group members are together for schooling and housing. The increased familiarity and the strong possibility that the reason the group is taking place because of problems occurring in the school make it critical to have clear ground rules and expectations for one's behavior in the group and outside the group. Clearly, similar issues arise for youngsters in residential treatment settings.

All of these variables make privacy issues paramount. While confidentially within the school setting applies when the group leader is communicating with *external* (emphasis added) third parties, this does not apply to communication with parents, guardians, school administrators, and teachers. It must be explained to these adults that legitimate legal access aside, information sharing should be on a need to know basis (Jacob et al., 2011) and, in the case of parents, guardians, and teachers, will be limited to information about their particular individual children. Thus, only if a third party outside of the school setting (meaning not an educator or administrator) received information from a psychologist without a properly completed release form would there be a breach of confidentiality. For example, Johnny's mother cannot be told what Mary reveals in the group even if it impacts Johnny. These concerns can complicate school psychological practice considerably.

Additional problems may arise related to the youngsters who are participants. But this is not the only problem! The youngsters who are participants in the group have no such legal requirement to abide by professional standards for confidentiality. Theoretically, they are free to discuss what took place in the group with anyone they choose. Yet, this is clearly inappropriate and could be counterproductive, ultimately undermining or sabotaging the group experience. Thus, it is extremely important to have each youngster "buy-in" to clear boundaries and limits by carefully explaining the limits of confidentiality and privacy (Crespi, 2009) as well as the potential consequences for failure to "buy-in." The simplest (and probably safest) course of action is to create a climate with the expectation that what takes place in this room remains in this room. Youngsters may initially balk at such a boundary, yet will follow the rationale and accept the boundary because they will not want peers outside the group (or some adults in the setting) to know what they said about them in the group. Youngsters speaking with the group leader privately about concerns related to how the group is going should be permitted. The group leader can then determine whether the concern is one best left private or is one that should be discussed with the group, providing the youngster who raised the concern is in agreement.

Group leaders can take additional actions that may reduce the likelihood of sensitive personal information being revealed by group members to third parties. Groups organized around specific skill development, such as managing low frustration tolerance, can be conducted by using predetermined scenarios that group members are commonly faced with, such as school rules. Prior to the start of a group, leaders might include group members in developing ways to relate to a member who breached confidentiality; appropriate consequences developed by peers will often be more aversive than consequences determined by adults. Incorporating psychoeducational strategies to further the goal of "learning to think twice before speaking" might also be beneficial. Should there be a member-initiated breach, well-reasoned school-based disciplinary consequences that use the unfortunate incident as an opportunity to teach appropriate behavior might be invoked, and apologies required. It is the group leader's job to privately address affective concerns of the youngster (and family) who was compromised.

Conclusions

Complex professional activities were discussed in this chapter: supervision, gaining entry to schools, and managing groups in schools. Similar to other professional activities, each activity is best left to a professional who has the requisite training and experience. These activities share commonalities in that (1) a broad professional knowledge base is required for effective practice, (2) the training and experience requirements are substantial, (3) ethical issues and concerns must be considered and addressed, and (4) each activity requires one to work with, and within, a context to realize change.

Cognitive and behavioral practitioners are well positioned to be successful with these tasks, as they draw on skills common to effective cognitive and behavioral practice with individuals. These include rapport building, goal setting, work to effect change, and the ongoing evaluation of the efficacy of professional activities. Similar to the growth of intervention skills, the professional learning process is ongoing.

References

American Psychiatric Association. (2013). *Diagnostic and statistical manual of mental disorders* (5th ed.). Washington, DC: Author.

American Psychological Association. (2002). *Ethical principles of psychologists and code of conduct.* Washington, DC: Author. Retrieved from http://www.apa.org/ethics/code/index.aspx.

Conoley, C., Conoley, J., & Reese, R. (2009). Changing a field of change. *Journal of Educational and Psychological Consultation, 19*, 236–247. doi:10.1080/10474410903106836.

Costantino, G., & Malgady, R. (2005). TEMAS narrative treatment: An evidence-based culturally competent therapy modality. In E. D. Hibbs & P. S. Jensen (Eds.), *Psychosocial treatments for child and adolescent disorders: Empirically based strategies for clinical practice* (2nd ed., pp. 717–742). Washington, DC: American Psychological Association.

Crespi, T. D. (2009). Group counseling in the schools: Legal, ethical and treatment issues in school practice. *Psychology in the Schools, 46*, 273–280. doi:10.1002/pits.20373.

Curtis, M. J., Grier, E. C., & Hunley, S. A. (2004). The changing face of school psychology: Trends in data and projections for the future. *School Psychology Review, 33*(435–444), 49–66. Retrieved from http://web.ebscohost.com/ehost/pdfviewer/pdfviewer?sid=4ad4a678-05b3-4a80-9fed-314d34544e65%40sessionmgr114&vid=8&hid=23.

Flanagan, R., & Miller, J. A. (2010). *Specialty competencies in school psychology.* New York, NY: Oxford University Press.

Forman, S. G., Fagley, N. S., Chu, B. C., & Walkup, J. T. (2012). Factors influencing school psychologists' "willingness to implement" Evidence-based interventions. *School Mental Health, 4*, 207–218. doi:10.1007/s12310-012-9083-z.

Forman, S. G., Olin, S. S., Hoagwood, K. E., Crowe, M., & Saka, N. (2009). Evidence-based interventions in schools: Developers' views of implementation barriers and facilitators. *School Mental Health, 1*, 26–36. doi:10.1007/s12310-008-9002-5.

Fouad, N. A., Grus, C. L., Hatcher, R. L., Kaslow, N. J., Hutchings, P. S., Madson, M. B., et al. (2009). Competency benchmarks: A model for understanding and measuring competence in professional psychology across training levels. *Training and Education in Professional Psychology, 3*, S5–S26. doi:10.1037/a0015832.

Frisby, C., & Reynolds, C. R. (2005). *Comprehensive handbook of multicultural school psychology.* New York, NY: Wiley.

Gladding, S. T. (2008). *Group work: A counseling specialty* (5th ed.). Columbus, OH: Merrill Prentice Hall.

Greenberg, K. R. (2003). *Group counseling in K-12 schools: A handbook for school counselors.* Boston, MA: Allyn & Bacon.

Harvey, V. S., & Struzziero, J. (2000). *Effective supervision in school psychology.* Bethesda, MD: National Association of School Psychologists.

Harvey, V. S., & Struzziero, J. (2008). *Professional Development and Supervision of School Psychologists: From Intern to Expert* (2nd ed.). Bethesda, MD: NASP/Corwin Press.

Hawkins, P., & Shohet, R. (2006). *Supervision in the helping professions* (3rd ed.). Berkshire, UK: Open University Press.

Haynes, R., Corey, G., & Moutlon, P. (2003). *Clinical supervision in the helping professions: A practical guide*. Pacific Grove, CA: Brookes-Cole.

Jacob, S., Decker, D. M., & Hartshorne, T. M. (2011). *Ethics and law for school psychologists* (6th ed.). Hoboken, NJ: Wiley.

Knapp, S. J., & VandeCreek, L. D. (2006). *Practical ethics for psychologists*. Washington, DC: American Psychological Association.

Krieg, F. J., Simpson, C., Stanley, R. E., & Snider, D. A. (2002). Best practices in making school groups work. In A. Thomas & J. Grimes (Eds.), *Best practices in school psychology* (4th ed., pp. 1195–1216). Bethesda, MD: National Association of School Psychologists.

Liese, B. S., & Beck, J. S. (1997). Cognitive therapy supervision. In C. E. Watkins (Ed.), *Handbook of psychotherapy supervision* (pp. 114–133). New York, NY: John Wiley & Sons.

Loganbill, C., Hardy, E., & Delworth, U. (1982). Supervision: A conceptual model. *The Counseling Psychologist, 10*, 3–42. doi:10.1177/0011000082101002.

Malgady, R. G. (2010). Treating Hispanic children and adolescents using narrative therapy. In J. R. Weisz & A. Kazdin (Eds.), *Evidence-based psychotherapies for children and adolescents* (2nd ed., pp. 391–400). New York, NY: Guilford.

McIntosh, D. E., & Phelps, L. (2000). Supervision in school psychology: Where will the future take us? *Psychology in the Schools, 37*, 33–38. doi:10.1002/(SICI)1520-6807(200001)37:1<33::AID-PITS4>3.0.CO;2-F.

Perusse, R., Goodenough, G. E., & Lee, V. V. (2009). Group counseling in the schools. *Psychology in the Schools, 46*, 225–231. doi:10.1002/pits.20369.

Stoltenberg, C. D., & Delworth, U. (1987). *Supervising counselors and therapists*. San Francisco, CA: Jossey-Bass.

Vane, J. R. (1985). School psychology: To be or not to be. *Journal of School Psychology, 23*, 101–112.

Whiston, S. C., Tai, W. L., Rahardja, D., & Eder, K. (2011). School counseling outcome: A meta-analytic examination of interventions. *Journal of Counseling and Development, 89*, 37–55. doi:10.1002/j.1556-6678.2011.tb00059.x.

Chapter 16
Technology-Based Cognitive-Behavioral Therapy in School Settings

Yvette N. Tazeau and Dominick A. Fortugno

Introduction

Technology has dramatically altered how we interact with one another. From telephone to email to instant messaging, long-distance communication has undergone a phenomenal evolution in only a few decades. Nearly 200 years passed between the establishment of the US Postal Service system and the first uses of email. In the past 40 years since the introduction of email, electronic communication has grown to dominate our written exchanges. As our methods of communicating are changing, mental health and counseling professionals are adapting their tools for providing service. The different modes of communication and interaction have given rise to new mediums of didactic learning and new techniques for the counseling relationship. Telephones, short message services (SMS) (i.e., text or instant messaging), computers, Web sites, email, video conferencing, telehealth, and now smartphones have all been used to simulate direct face-to-face contact with clients for the provision of services to a larger audience. Research over the past few decades has explored the efficacy of these methods for treating psychological and physical ailments and has uncovered important variables moderating success in their use.

This chapter briefly describes the history of early computer-assisted therapy efforts. First, the chapter includes a description of technology-based techniques used with cognitive-behavioral therapy (CBT) and research on their treatment effectiveness. Second, we focus on the use of digital technology in delivering CBT with the K-12 student population. Third, we discuss the benefits and challenges inherent

Y.N. Tazeau, Ph.D. (✉)
Independent Practice, P.O. Box 20684, San Jose, CA 95160, USA
e-mail: ytazeau@ix.netcom.com

D.A. Fortugno, Ph.D.
School of Health Sciences, Touro College, 1700 Union Blvd., Bay Shore, NY 11706, USA
e-mail: dominick.fortugno@gmail.com

© Springer Science+Business Media New York 2015
R. Flanagan et al. (eds.), *Cognitive and Behavioral Interventions
in the Schools*, DOI 10.1007/978-1-4939-1972-7_16

in using these techniques, including guidelines to maximize their potential and cautions for their use and situations to avoid. Finally, we take a look at technological advances for the future and how they might shape CBT in the years to come.

Early History: Intersection of First Computers and CBT

Although a comprehensive review of the Digital Age (Ceruzzi, 2012) is beyond the scope of this chapter, there are key advances that shaped and inform today's current technology practice of CBT. In the 1960s, computers were used in industry to automate business processes such as scheduling and information management. Relevant to psychology, Weizenbaum (1966) developed ELIZA, a natural language program based loosely on Rogerian psychotherapy. Later that same year, Colby, Watt, and Gilbert (1966) established a similar program that, like Weizenbaum's, attempted to mimic the open-ended questions posed to clients in a therapeutic setting. Although these cases represented a quantum leap in using computers to augment traditional therapy, they had limited flexibility and were unable to provide interactive dialogue, contributing to a concern that computer technology could be dehumanizing to patients. Nonetheless, also during this time, Colby (1968) conducted one of the first studies using computer-assisted therapy for children with autism. Examining ten case studies, he found that children responded well to the computers, which used various visual and auditory "games" to promote language use. Colby attributed the success to the system's consistency, suggesting the nonhuman interface was more engaging and less confrontational for these children.

In the early 1970s, the mental health industry was at a time that Lanyon (1971) called a "pretechnological" phase, one characterized by "an emphasis on individually provided services, a minimal number of tools, lack of standardization, and the apprenticeship system" (p. 1073). Electronic technologies as applied to mental health and counseling did not predominate at the time. Lanyon noted a deep undercurrent of resistance that he attributed to the notion that mental health providers and clients preferred the craftsman status awarded to an individual practitioner who relied solely on their knowledge base, rather than the role of a technician utilizing equipment. However, he offered an impassioned argument for the potential efficiency technology offered, including standardizing diagnostic criteria, automating assessments and patient care, and augmenting counseling and behavior modification. Other researchers echoed these potential benefits suggesting that computers play a role in not only analysis but also treatment procedures (Hogan, 1971).

Computer-assisted models for therapy continued to focus on automated responses throughout the early 1970s. In the mid-1970s, a number of important technological innovations were taking place that would revolutionize computers' power and availability. Microprocessors and floppy drives appeared, which set the stage for the first commercial and "personal" computers. Seemingly overnight, computer mainframes that had filled rooms and cost hundreds of thousands of dollars were replaced by affordable desktop devices with internal memory and many times the processing power. As computers became more accessible, their utility and potential as a therapeutic tool increased. Although psychologists appeared to have accepted that computer algorithms simply lacked the empathy to establish a therapeutic relationship (Spero, 1978), studies emerged that examined other aspects of treatment. Sidoruk (1976) incorporated an interactive graphics computer program system for standardizing both the diagnostic and treatment aspects of schizophrenia. Angle, Ellinwood, Hay, Johnsen, and Hay (1977) used an interactive computer to collect participant self-report data. Yet another study was based on a customized, automated computer-based simulation to examine marriage decisions and values (Smith & Debenham, 1979).

In the 1980s, researchers continued exploring the use of computers for behavioral aspects of additional disorders (Neumann, 1986), as well as began examining the efficacy of using computer-based techniques for aspects of greater treatment interactivity. Overall, early findings indicated computer-assisted models of therapy, and assessment showed promise, despite being based primarily on case studies and small samples (Zarr, 1984). Studies considered the effectiveness of computer-assisted CBT for conditions such as depression (Selmi, Klein, Greist, Johnson, & Harris, 1982). Foree-Gävert and Gävert's (1980) study of obesity included a computer-feedback mechanism for planning and analyzing participants' diets. Another obesity study included an ambulatory computer-assisted component, i.e., a portable microcomputer system, and the participants who used the method lost more weight than the group of participants who used the traditional paper-and-pencil method of accountability (Burnett, Taylor, & Agras, 1985). Microcomputers, as applied to clinical testing, were examined in Bartram and Bayliss' (1984) study of automating occupational assessments. In a study of obsessive-compulsive disorder (Baer, Minichiello, Jenike, & Holland, 1988), a portable computer program was introduced for treatment, along with the use of a laptop computer, and greater compliance was demonstrated with the portable device. A study of stress introduced the use of a computer for the induction of relaxation (Baer & Surman, 1985). Regarding anxiety, some studies of phobias (Ghosh & Marks, 1987; Ghosh, Marks, & Carr, 1988) concluded that psychiatric treatment, a self-help book, and computer programmed instruction all provided substantial improvement, i.e., the researchers found no significant differences between the treatment modalities.

Studies in the 1990s were more sophisticated in their treatment of computer-assisted components as variables and as tools. Taylor, Agras, Losch, Plante, and Burnett (1991) used a pocket computer in a weight loss program and included groups that used the computer alone or in conjunction with a diet plan. The authors noted that the participants were attitudinally positively disposed toward the use of the pocket computers for treatment. Newman, Kenardy, Herman, and Taylor (1996) used a handheld computer program in a case study of panic disorder treatment with CBT. Newman and Consoli's (1997) review of computer technology and CBT for anxiety disorders highlighted useful features of the technology for the treatment and went one step further in suggesting a role for computerized treatment as a sole CBT treatment intervention. Such a recommendation no doubt reflected the growing comfort with computer-assisted treatments and the developing literature base showing similar results in computer- and counselor-based treatments. Also, self-directed projects and other "homework" assignments conducted on computers appeared to enhance treatment efficacy in a manner similar to having written assignments reviewed by a counselor. CD-ROM applications would also become available, providing for self-paced, interactive multimedia forms of treatment intervention (Khanna & Kendall, 2010; Whitfield, Hinshelwood, Pashely, Campsie, & Williams, 2006). In summary, however, computer assistance at this time was limited to mimicking techniques typically performed by counselors. The arrival of the Internet would soon accelerate change yet again.

Rise of the Internet

The Internet was envisioned as futuristic libraries with advanced information access and storage capacities (Licklider, 1960). Licklider's idea was "a network of such centers, connected to one another by wide-band communication lines and to individual users by leased-wire services" (p. 7). These ideas formed the foundation for early network computing. Years later, Web pages and browsers would become the World Wide Web. When Dow, Kearns, and Thornton (1996) published their review of how the Internet has developed and its effects on psychology practice, they estimated 11.7 million active Web pages existed on just over 100,000 servers. The authors grouped Internet activities in two general groups, email and Web pages, and described several of CBT aspects on which the Internet was likely to have a profound effect, including marketing, assessment, progress monitoring, records access, and service delivery. They noted a number of specific ways in which the Internet would allow CBT practitioners to enhance their practice and expand their influence. For example, they suggested that counselors could take a more active role in educating the public on matters such as behavioral risk factors and therapeutic techniques. Bibliotherapy and practice techniques could be enhanced through the use of Web pages with dynamic multimedia content. Email and instant messages could provide real-time communication, and new breakthroughs in voice and even video chat would allow counselors to interact directly with their clients in ways that could not be accomplished via telephone. Consultation and research would be profoundly altered by the Internet. The authors also pointed out potential negative consequences, including security concerns and the explosion of misinformation, dishonesty, and plagiarism. While many of their observations proved prophetic, Dow and his colleagues provided a limited scope of how the Internet would be used specifically in CBT. In some ways, this was to be expected given the Internet's subsequent unanticipated growth. It would have been difficult for the authors to imagine the Internet's growth, much less predict the effects on one single area of psychology practice. Yet, the authors very accurately predicted that the Internet would have profound effects on psychological practice, including CBT, in terms of disseminating information to the public, enhancing communication, and even providing a medium for direct service delivery.

CBT and the Internet

By 2003, studies exploring the use of Internet-based therapies seemed to be exploding in the research literature. The journal *Cognitive Behavior Therapy* devoted an entire special issue to the topic, collecting a series of studies that explored the efficacy, benefits, and challenges of using Internet-based CBT treatments for a variety of ailments, including posttraumatic stress (Lange, Van De Ven, & Schrieken, 2003), panic disorder (Richards, Klein, & Carlbring, 2003), eating disorders and obesity (Zabinski, Celio, Wilfley, & Taylor, 2003), and stress management (Zetterqvist, Maanmies, Ström, & Andersson, 2003). Other articles published around the same time conducted similar explorations, i.e., randomized trials of CBT, (Carlbring, Ekselius, & Andersson, 2003; Christensen, Griffiths, & Jorm, 2004), ushering in what would be more widespread research on the use of CBT treatments conducted over the Internet.

What these early researchers found, and what others have found since, is that the Internet provides a medium for enhancing CBT delivery as long as a distinction is made between different treatment formats and that there is an understanding of the drawbacks and unintended consequences of using the Internet to promote therapy. Several reviews and meta-analyses have found broad support for the efficacy of computer-based and Internet-based therapeutic techniques (Barak, Hen, Boniel-Nissim, & Shapira, 2008; Wantland, Portillo, Holzemer, Slaughter, & McGhee, 2004; Webb, Joseph, Yardley, & Michie, 2010) and for the effectiveness of Internet-based CBT in particular (Cuijpers, van Straten, & Andersson, 2008; Spek et al., 2007). A comprehensive review by Andersson, Carlbring, Berger, Almlöv, and Cuijpers (2009) found that Internet treatments based on CBT met established criteria as "empirically supported" when used to treat moderate depression, panic disorder, anxiety, posttraumatic stress, and even headaches. Moreover, effect sizes for these treatments tend to be equivalent to those of face-to-face CBT. Secondary research studies such as these have also begun to explore variables that may moderate treatment, and researchers have outlined suggestions for design and implementation. For example, Spek et al. (2007) found clear evidence that therapist support is vital for the effectiveness of Internet-based treatments for depression.

Just as contributors noted in a review of technologies that support evidence-based behavioral health practices (Cucciare & Weingardt, 2010), Internet-based CBT offers a number of obvious advantages over traditional face-to-face therapy, including flexibility, access, and anonymity. Treatments using email and Web-based "homework" assignments usually do not require a set hour for a response. Instead, therapy exercises and interactions can be completed at the client's preferred pace. Early researchers (Dow et al., 1996) predicted that these indirect media might also reduce social barriers to self-disclosure and information sharing by providing a less intensive form of interaction. Even video conferencing, e.g., telehealth, which requires live support from the therapist, saves valuable time traveling between sites and allows the client to engage from a familiar, comfortable location if they choose. This increased flexibility could be especially important for individuals suffering from disorders that limit their mobility or otherwise hamper their ability to seek therapy outside of their home. For example, Herbst et al. (2012) found a telemental health intervention effective and economical for treatment of obsessive-compulsive disorder. Internet treatments can disseminate information on a continuous basis over great distances and may be especially appealing to individuals who are already familiar and comfortable with social media, video, and electronic communication.

While the Internet as a medium for CBT offers useful advantages, its open, indirect, impersonal nature also lends itself to certain drawbacks and opportunities for misuse. Technical issues such as computer support and Internet access are common challenges, particularly for clients in low socioeconomic areas. Also, while email and instant messaging offer opportunities for convenient communication, individuals can have experiences of misinterpreting an email or instant message because of the lack of visual cues and inability to note facial expressions. These issues can be compounded substantially for some clients and may undermine the therapist's best efforts to establish trust. Issues of confidentiality and broader privacy have loomed largely over the general, public debate on Internet security during the past several years. Finally, while the Internet has become a useful source of information on disorders and treatments, mental health professionals contend with the "downside" of widespread dissemination, including pop-culture and amateur quizzes that blur the line between nonprofessional and clinical assessment (Buchanan, 2003) and even the intentional promotion of dangerous behaviors like pro-anorexia nervosa Web sites (Gotthelf, 2001).

Mobile Devices: The Emergence of Apps

The year 2013 marked the first time that most adults in the United States owned a smartphone, i.e., 56 % of Americans (Smith, 2013). Other handheld mobile device use, such as that associated with tablets, also increased. Also in 2013, tablet shipments exceeded that of computer notebooks (NPD DisplayResearch, 2013). With such levels of mobile device usage, it is not surprising that technology companies such as Apple (Apple Press, 2013) reported 40 billion app downloads in 2012 on its AppStore, an application source that had launched only a few years earlier, in 2008.

Internet access continues to shift away from desktop and laptop computers to handheld mobile devices, with one in three cell phone owners using smartphones as a way to access health information (Fox & Duggan, 2012). Whether it is for smartphones or tablets, these wireless mobile communication devices provide health information in the form of apps, known broadly as mobile health, mHealth (U.S. Department of Health and Human Services, 2013). Indeed, the new mobile app technology formats are opportunities to extend the reach of counseling and health care to clients and clinicians/counselors alike (Tazeau, 2012). What this latest technology frontier means for CBT is that there is another form of treatment intervention in the form of mobile software applications, "apps." App developers appear to have made the most of these notable trends and have created CBT apps for these newest technology formats. One review of mobile mental health apps indicated that the tools have the potential for reducing symptoms in various conditions including depression, anxiety, stress, and possibly substance abuse (Donker et al., 2013).

Users of mobile technology are not limited to adults. Three out of four teens ages 12–17 access the Internet with mobile devices (Madden, Lenhart, Duggan, Cortesi, & Gasser, 2013), and 38 % of young children under the age of 2 are reported to use mobile devices for watching videos and playing games (Common Sense Media, 2013). It is not surprising then that the field of education has been one of the earlier adopters of mobile technologies (Barber, 2012). School settings are a natural environment for the use of mHealth apps for students, particularly given the incidence and prevalence rates of mental illness in childhood. For example, a study that surveyed mental health in youth for six years, beginning in 2005, indicated that in a given year, 13–20 % of US children experience a mental disorder such as attention-deficit/hyperactivity disorder, behavioral or conduct problems, anxiety, depression, autism spectrum disorders, and Tourette syndrome (Centers for Disease Control and Prevention, 2013). Costello, He, Sampson, Kessler, and Merikangas (2013) noted that only 45 % of adolescents who have disorders of mental health received treatment, and the treatment received was primarily from pediatricians, school counselors, or probation officers. The authors noted that regarding services, teens with phobias and any anxiety disorder were least likely to receive help. Such information suggests that there are opportunities for using mobile app technology in school counseling settings to augment pediatric mental health care.

CBT Mobile Health Technology and School Counseling

Computer-based (e.g., CD-ROM) and Internet-based CBT treatments, such as those previously discussed, can be therapist assisted or self-guided. Some of these same treatments have been adapted for the mobile app-based format. For example, Watts et al. (2013) found that CBT delivered by way of mobile phone was as effective as computer-based delivery. Many mobile apps for CBT appear to be self-guided interventions of self-monitoring, including thought records, mood tracking, relaxation exercises, and other treatment components of CBT. The increasing number of mHealth apps available notwithstanding, there are few studies on the efficacy of mobile health apps in general, for mental health and for CBT interventions specifically, and fewer for their use in school environments. One review of mobile apps for adolescents revealed that most such apps were made with the idea of enhancing the treatment aspects of participation and adherence (Seko, Kidd, & Wiljer, 2013). Enock and McNally's (2013) review of mobile apps and Web-based interventions reported that in adult populations, the technologies did provide a reduction in symptoms for anxiety but noted that studies did not account for student populations. This limited research on mobile mental health apps would suggest that users proceed with a certain degree of healthy skepticism as to any untested claims of treatment efficacy of specific apps. Indeed, app creation has outpaced its research validation

(Riley et al., 2011). Still, it is mostly the United States that lags in this research, as Australia and the United Kingdom lead the way. Australia is responsible for approximately one-half of the world's e-mental health programs, and it has exceeded all other countries in related research publications (Jorm, Morgan, & Malhi, 2013).

Despite the relative lack of US-based efficacy studies of mobile mental health apps, practitioner common sense and reliance on evidence-based practice guidelines for traditional CBT can help guide users by recognizing that a mobile app that is based on CBT as a scientific practice can serve as a useful adjunctive tool/device to their interventions. Just as CBT utilizes a thought record that can be completed by the user on a piece of paper, so can it be done in electronic format. Similarly, just as relaxation exercises can be done in vivo in a session, they can also be audio recorded for repeated or later use. These tools are the same in content, what varies is the delivery format. An appropriate and useful question that research can address is whether or not, if as a homework device, a given format is preferred or utilized more than another.

Luxton, McCann, Bush, Mishking, and Reger (2011) point out that mobile health apps have many useful applications for behavioral health care, including their usefulness in symptom assessment, psychoeducational resources, tracking of resources, and managing of treatment progress. Aguilera and Muench (2012) indicate that CBT practitioners tend to include technology-based innovations in the practice of CBT. Thus, blending software with human intervention can have the potential to impact a student's learning of CBT in ways that are flexible and tailored in a personalized manner. For example, bibliotherapy has been a traditional tool in the use of psychotherapy. With the advent of digital books, these same books can reside on a mobile device that can afford greater accessibility to a student who already uses a tablet for other school-related learning tasks. Other aspects of mobile technology can suggest opportunities for greater client engagement in the therapeutic process. Particularly for children, the use of a gaming format, i.e., gamification, may create a greater level of interest and sustained attention based on this type of interactivity. Some CBT apps geared toward youth are including this aspect in mobile formats. For teens, the aspect of social networking is appealing, and some apps can include this approach to user engagement. For example, if school counselors are limited in their interactions with students, the apps can help extend and bridge the counselor-student connection.

However, apps that allow social networking, transmitting data, text messaging, location status, and sending photos pose challenges to the issue of treatment confidentiality when the youth is working with a school counselor. Notably, in 2013, the US Federal Trade Commission (FTC) updated the Children's Online Privacy Protection Act (COPPA). COPPA provides for parental control over the information Web sites collect from and about children. The updated COPPA rule is a privacy policy that outlines guidelines regarding Web sites and online services directed to children. The rule imposes limits on various aspects of mobile device capabilities, including photographs, videos, audio recordings, geolocation data, and the like. The updated rule also requires makers of apps to confirm, i.e., verify parental consent. For example, parents must allow access for the sharing of their child's personal information. Parents are also the arbiters for the notification of any information disclosures to third parties. In general, app makers are limited in the information they can collect about a child via the child's use of the app.

Determining the appropriateness of an app for a child is a challenging task. One set of guidelines (American Health Information Management, 2013) suggests that consumers consider three aspects in the selection of a mobile health app—Advice, Privacy, and Personal (APP)—and that thoughtful consideration should include knowing about the security aspects of the app and what personal health information will be shared through the app.

Just as COPPA rules help app developers create apps for youth that follow privacy protection guidelines, there are additional heuristics that can help the school counselor identify a most useful app for a particular student. In reviewing an app, a school counselor will want to determine if the app is appropriate for the student based on the chronological and developmental age of the student. Another important aspect to consider is the app's operability, i.e., how user-friendly it is based on the app's graphical interface and features. The school counselor will want to consider if the CBT app provides strengths and/or advantages over the other, more conventional CBT adjunctive tools such as therapeutic board games, traditional worksheets, bibliotherapy, and workbook-based protocols. In selecting an app for use, the counselor may also want to consider the apps' suitability for use with other staff or teachers who may be part of the student's intervention team. Providing staff with additional time to become acquainted with the new technology before implementing its use can enhance the ease with which the technology is integrated and accepted by the student.

One of four US elementary and high school students is Hispanic (US Census Bureau, 2012). Mobile apps can provide an additional advantage for the treatment of mental health issues within the Hispanic population and in other communities of color. Lopez, Gonzalez-Barrera, and Patten (2013) report that Latinos are the greatest online users and owners of cell phones. The greater availability of mental health interventions delivered through these mediums therefore has the potential to shape healthcare availability and to promote greater health equity.

The Future of Technology and Mental Health in Schools

Traditional CBT that is delivered in a classroom environment has been demonstrated to be efficacious in helping adolescents experiencing depression (Stallard et al., 2012). While there will continue to be a place for this type of traditional delivery format of CBT, technology provides opportunities for CBT to be delivered in novel and less traditional ways. For example, the American Psychological Association (2013) partnered with Microsoft Corporation to deliver classroom presentations by way of its Microsoft's Skype software, a voice, video calling, and instant messaging electronic communication system. Responding to the White House National Conference on Mental Health (2013), 100 psychologists help deliver a series of classroom lessons in one hour presentation format via Skype. Students are able to dialogue with the presenters on mental health issues including anxiety, depression, anger, and resilience. The year-long program of Skype-delivered lessons is a unique way in which to connect with students across vast distances and to provide specialized resources to the nearly 70,000 teachers world-wide who are reported to be Skype users.

Another technology that will likely make its way to the classroom is known as "wearable tech." These are computer-based measurement devices that can be worn by individuals and that provide for continuous monitoring thereby allowing for immediate feedback. Often referred to as the technology category of "personalized medicine," the wearable tech tools can assess almost any measurable variable and convert it into a form of notification to the user. For example, physiological states that can infer mood can provide cues for self-correction or cognitive disputing of the monitored data. Facial expressions, perspiration levels, muscle tension, gait, etc. are all potential sources of data that could potentially assist in predicting physiological symptoms related to anxiety, depression, and other mental health concerns.

Summary

This chapter outlined CBT's use as expressed through digital technology, including the general evolution of digital technology from the first computers, then the Internet, and now mobile technology. A description was provided regarding how researchers and practitioners have adapted these innovations to enhance and expand mental health and counseling service delivery. Discussed were the advantages and challenges that these new inventions pose for mental health practice. The chapter explored the research on specific treatments and contexts, including applications for school counseling. Finally, introduced were groundbreaking new technologies still in development and the ways in which they might impact CBT implementation in the future. The Internet and its easy accessibility through mobile devices provide both exciting opportunities and significant challenges for increased delivery of mental health interventions. As the use of the electronic technologies becomes more widespread among youth (Shipp, 2010), school counselors and therapists can anticipate research on the treatment and cost-effectiveness of these technologies in assisting interventions with school-age populations.

References

Aguilera, A., & Muench, F. (2012). There's an App for that: Information technology applications for cognitive behavioral practitioners. *The Behavior Therapist, 35*(4), 65–73.
American Health Information Management Association (2013, July) Mobile health apps 101: A primer for consumers. *Just think APP.* Retrieved from http://myphr.com/HealthLiteracy/MX7644_myPHRbrochure.pdf

American Psychological Association. (2013). APA teams with Microsoft to bring mental health into the classroom. *Monitor on Psychology, 44*(11), 12.

Andersson, G., Carlbring, P., Berger, T., Almlöv, J., & Cuijpers, P. (2009). What makes Internet therapy work? *Cognitive Behavior Therapy, 38*(S1), 55–60.

Angle, H. V., Ellinwood, E. H., Hay, W. M., Johnsen, T., & Hay, L. R. (1977). Computer-aided interviewing in comprehensive behavioral assessment. *Behavior Therapy, 8*(4), 747–754.

Apple Press Info (2013, January). *App store tops 40 billion downloads with almost half in 2012.* Retrieved from http://www.apple.com/pr/library/2013/01/07App-Store-Tops-40-Billion-Downloads-with-Almost-Half-in-2012.html

Baer, L., Minichiello, W. E., Jenike, M. A., & Holland, A. (1988). Use of a portable computer program to assist behavioral treatment in a case of obsessive compulsive disorder. *Journal of Behavior Therapy and Experimental Psychiatry, 19*(3), 237–240.

Baer, L., & Surman, O. S. (1985). Microcomputer-assisted relaxation. *Perceptual and Motor Skills, 61*(2), 499–502.

Barak, A., Hen, L., Boniel-Nissim, M., & Shapira, N. A. (2008). A comprehensive review and a meta-analysis of the effectiveness of Internet-based psychotherapeutic interventions. *Journal of Technology in Human Services, 26*(2–4), 109–160.

Barber, D. A. (2012, January). 5 K-12 Ed tech trends for 2012. *The Journal.* Retrieved from http://thejournal.com/Articles/2012/01/10/5-K-12-Ed-Tech-for-2012.aspx?p=1

Bartram, D., & Bayliss, R. (1984). Automated testing: Past, present and future. *Journal of Occupational Psychology, 57*(3), 221–237.

Buchanan, T. (2003). Internet-based questionnaire assessment: Appropriate use in clinical contexts. *Cognitive Behaviour Therapy, 32*(3), 100–109.

Burnett, K. F., Taylor, C. B., & Agras, W. S. (1985). Ambulatory computer-assisted therapy for obesity: A new frontier for behavior therapy. *Journal of Consulting and Clinical Psychology, 53*(5), 698–703.

Carlbring, P., Ekselius, L., & Andersson, G. (2003). Treatment of panic disorder via the Internet: A randomized trial of CBT vs. applied relaxation. *Journal of Behavior Therapy and Experimental Psychiatry, 34*(2), 129–140.

Centers for Disease Control and Prevention (2013, May). Mental health surveillance among children—United States, 2005-2011. *MMWR Supplements, 62*(02), 1–35. Retrieved from http//www.cdc.gove/mmwr/preview/mmwrhtml/su6202a1.htm?s_cid=su6202a1?w

Ceruzzi, P. E. (2012). *Computing: A concise history.* Cambridge, MA: MIT Press.

Christensen, H., Griffiths, K. M., & Jorm, A. F. (2004). Delivering interventions for depression by using the internet: Randomised controlled trial. *BMJ, 328*(7434), 265.

Colby, K. M. (1968). Computer-aided language development in nonspeaking children. *Archives of General Psychiatry, 19*(6), 641–651.

Colby, K. M., Watt, J. B., & Gilbert, J. P. (1966). A computer method of psychotherapy: Preliminary communication. *The Journal of Nervous and Mental Disease, 142*(2), 148–152.

Common Sense Media. (2013, October). *Zero to eight: Children's media use in America, a common sense media research study.* Retrieved from http://www.commonsensemedia.org/research/zero-to-eight-childrens-media-use-in-america-2013

Costello, E. J., He, J., Sampson, N. A., Kessler, R. C., & Merikangas, K. R. (2013). Services for adolescents with psychiatric disorders: 12-Month data from the national comorbidity survey-adolescent. *Psychiatric Services.* doi:10.1176/appi/ps.201100518.

Cucciare, M. A., & Weingardt, K. R. (Eds.). (2010). *Using technology to support evidence-based behavioral health practices: A clinician's guide.* New York, NY: Routledge.

Cuijpers, P., van Straten, A., & Andersson, G. (2008). Internet-administered cognitive behavior therapy for health problems: A systematic review. *Journal of Behavioral Medicine, 31*(2), 169–177.

Donker, T., Petrie, K., Proudfoot, J., Clarke, J., Birch, M., & Christensen, H. (2013). Smartphones for smarter delivery of mental health programs: A systematic review. *Journal of Medical Internet Research, 5*(11), e247. doi:10.2196/jmir.2791.

Dow, M. G., Kearns, W., & Thornton, D. H. (1996). The Internet II: Future effects on cognitive behavioral practice. *Cognitive and Behavioral Practice, 3*(1), 137–157.

Enock, P. M., & McNally, R. J. (2013). How mobile apps and other web-based interventions can transform psychological treatment and the treatment development cycle. *The Behavior Therapist, 36*(3), 56–66.

Foree-Gävert, S., & Gävert, L. (1980). Obesity: Behavior therapy with computer-feedback versus traditional starvation treatment. *Cognitive Behaviour Therapy, 9*(1), 1–14.

Fox, S., & Duggan, M. (2012, November). Mobile health 2012. *Pew Internet: Pew Internet & American Life Project.* Retrieved from http://www.pewinternet.org/Reports/2012/Mobile-Health.aspx

Ghosh, A., & Marks, I. M. (1987). Self-treatment of agoraphobia by exposure. *Behavior Therapy, 18*(1), 3–16.

Ghosh, A., Marks, I. M., & Carr, A. C. (1988). Therapist contact and outcome of self-exposure treatment for phobias. A controlled study. *The British Journal of Psychiatry, 152*(2), 234–238.

Gotthelf, M. (2001, August). The new anorexia outrage. *Self,* 82–84.

Herbst, N., Voderholzer, U., Stelzer, N., Knaevelsrud, C., Hertenstein, E., Schlegl, S., Nissen, C., & Kulz, A. K. (2012). The potential of telemental health applications for obsessive-compulsive disorder. *Clinical Psychology Review, 32,* 454–466.

Hogan, R. A. (1971). Research thoughts toward a computerized therapy. *Behavior Therapy, 2*(1), 107–109.

Jorm, A. F., Morgan, A. J., & Malhi, G. S. (2013). The future of e-mental health. *Australian & New Zealand Journal of Psychiatry, 47*(2), 104. Retrieved from http://anp.sagepub.com/content/47/2/104.

Khanna, M. S., & Kendall, P. C. (2010). Computer-assisted cognitive behavioral therapy for child anxiety: Results of a randomized clinical trial. *Journal of Consulting and Clinical Psychology, 78,* 737–745.

Lange, A., Van De Ven, J. P., & Schrieken, B. (2003). Interapy: Treatment of post-traumatic stress via the Internet. *Cognitive Behaviour Therapy, 32*(3), 110–124.

Lanyon, R. I. (1971). Mental health technology. *American Psychologist, 26*(12), 1071–1076.

Licklider, J. C. R. (1960). Man-computer symbiosis. *IRE Transactions on Human Factors in Electronics, 1,* 4–11.

Lopez, M. H., Gonzalez-Barrera, A., & Patten, E. (2013, March). *Closing the digital divide: Latinos and technology adoption.* Pew Research, Hispanic Center. Retrieved from http://www.pewhispanic.org/2013/03/07/closing-the-digital-divide-latinos-and-technology-adoption/

Luxton, D. D., McCann, R. A., Bush, N. E., Mishking, M. C., & Reger, G. M. (2011). mHealth for mental health: Integrating smartphone technology in behavioral healthcare. *Professional Psychology: Research and Practice, 42*(6), 505–512.

Madden, M., Lenhart, A., Duggan, M., & Cortesi, S., Gasser, U. (2013, March). Teens and technology 2013. *Pew Internet: Pew Internet & American Life Project.* Retrieved from http://www.pewinternet.org/Reports/2013/Teens-and-Tech/Main-Findings.aspx?view=all

Neumann, D. (1986). A psychotherapeutic computer application: Modification of technological competence. *Behavior Research Methods, Instruments, & Computers, 18*(2), 135–140.

Newman, M. G., & Consoli, A. (1997). Computers in assessment and cognitive behavioral treatment of clinical disorders: Anxiety as a case in point. *Behavior Therapy, 28*(2), 211–235.

Newman, M. G., Kenardy, J., Herman, S., & Taylor, C. B. (1996). The use of hand-held computers as an adjunct to cognitive-behavior therapy. *Computers in Human Behavior, 12*(1), 135–143.

NPD DisplayResearch. (2013, January). *Tablet PC market forecast to surpass notebooks in 2013.* Retrieved from http://www.displaysearch.com/cps/rde/xchg/displaysearch/hs.xsl/130107_tablet_pc_market_forecast_to_surpass_notebooks_in_2013.asp

Richards, J., Klein, B., & Carlbring, P. (2003). Internet-based treatment for panic disorder. *Cognitive Behaviour Therapy, 32*(3), 125–135.

Riley, W. T., Rivera, D. E., Atienza, A. A., Nilsen, W., Allison, S. M., & Mermelstein, R. (2011). Health behavior models in the age of mobile interventions: Are our theories up to the task? *Translational Behavioral Medicine, 1*(1), 53–71.

Seko, Y, Kidd, S., & Wiljer, D. (2013, October). *Apps for those who help themselves: Mobile self-guided interventions for adolescent mental health*. Selected Papers of Internet Research, North America, 3. Retrieved from http://spir.aoir.org/index.php/spir/article/view/833

Selmi, P. M., Klein, M. H., Greist, J. H., Johnson, J. H., & Harris, W. G. (1982). An investigation of computer-assisted cognitive-behavior therapy in the treatment of depression. *Behavior Research Methods & Instrumentation, 14*(2), 181–185.

Shipp, A. E. (2010). Review of 'Born digital: Understanding the first generation of digital natives'. *Professional School Counseling, 13*(5), 270–271.

Sidoruk, W. (1976). Application of interactive graphics technology to the problem of standardizing diagnosis and therapy of schizophrenic patients. *Schizophrenia Bulletin, 2*(4), 595–607.

Smith, A. (2013, June) Smartphone ownership 2013. *Pew Internet: Pew Internet & American Life Project*. Retrieved from http://www.pewinternet.org/Reports/2013/Smartphone-Ownership-2013.aspx

Smith, G. W., & Debenham, J. D. (1979). Computer automated marriage analysis. *American Journal of Family Therapy, 7*(1), 16–31.

Spek, V., Cuijpers, P. I. M., Nyklícek, I., Riper, H., Keyzer, J., & Pop, V. (2007). Internet-based cognitive behaviour therapy for symptoms of depression and anxiety: A meta-analysis. *Psychological Medicine, 37*(3), 319–328.

Spero, M. H. (1978). Thoughts on computerized psychotherapy. *Psychiatry, 41*(3), 279–288.

Stallard, P., Sayal, K., Phillips, R., Taylor, J. A., Speares, M., Anderson, R., et al. (2012). Classroom based cognitive behavioural therapy in reducing symptoms of depression in high risk adolescents: Pragmatic cluster randomized controlled trial. *BMJ, 345*, e6058. doi:10.1136/bmj.e6058.

Taylor, C. B., Agras, W. S., Losch, M., Plante, T. G., & Burnett, K. (1991). Improving the effectiveness of computer-assisted weight loss. *Behavior Therapy, 22*(2), 229–236.

Tazeau, Y. N. (2012). Making the most of mobile technology in private practice. *The California Psychologist*, May/June, 11–14.

The White House Blog. (2013, June). *The national conference on mental health*. Retrieved from http://www.whitehouse.gov/blog/2013/06/03/national-conference-mental-health

U.S. Census Bureau. (2012, October). *Enrollment status of the population 3 years old and over, by Hispanic Origin*. Retrieved from http://www.census.gov/hhes/school/data/cps/2012/tables.html

U.S. Department of Health and Human Services, Health Resources and Services Administration, Health Information Technology and Quality Improvement. (2013). *What is mHealth?* Retrieved 1 June 2013, from http://www.hrsa.gov/healthit/mhealth.html

U.S. Federal Trade Commission. (2013). *Children's online privacy protection act (COPPA)*. Retrieved from www.coppa.org

Wantland, D. J., Portillo, C. J., Holzemer, W. L., Slaughter, R., & McGhee, E. M. (2004). The effectiveness of Web-based vs. non-Web-based interventions: A meta-analysis of behavioral change outcomes. *Journal of Medical Internet Research, 6*(4), 40.

Watts, S., Mackenzie, A., Thomas, C., Griskaitis, A., Mewton, L., Williams, A., et al. (2013). CBT for depression: A pilot RCT comparing mobile phone vs. computer. *BMC Psychiatry, 13*, 49. doi:10.1186/1471-244X-13-49.

Webb, T. L., Joseph, J., Yardley, L., & Michie, S. (2010). Using the Internet to promote health behavior change: A systematic review and meta-analysis of the impact of theoretical basis, use of behavior change techniques, and mode of delivery on efficacy. *Journal of Medical Internet Research, 12*(1), e4.

Weizenbaum, J. (1966). ELIZA—A computer program for the study of natural language communication between man and machine. *Communications of the ACM, 9*(1), 36–45.

Whitfield, G., Hinshelwood, R., Pashely, A., Campsie, L., & Williams, C. (2006). The impact of a novel computerized CBT CD rom (overcoming depression) offered to patients referred to clinical psychology. *Behavioural and Cognitive Psychotherapy, 34*(1), 1–11.

Zabinski, M. F., Celio, A. A., Wilfley, D. E., & Taylor, C. B. (2003). Prevention of eating disorders and obesity via the Internet. *Cognitive Behaviour Therapy, 32*(3), 137–150.

Zarr, M. L. (1984). Computer-mediated psychotherapy: Toward patient-selection guidelines. *American Journal of Psychotherapy, 38*(1), 47–62.

Zetterqvist, K., Maanmies, J., Ström, L., & Andersson, G. (2003). Randomized controlled trial of Internet-based stress management. *Cognitive Behaviour Therapy, 32*(3), 151–160.

Index